Health & Medical Horizons

1989

MACMILLAN EDUCATIONAL COMPANY

A Division of Macmillan, Inc.

NEW YORK

COLLIER MACMILLAN PUBLISHERS

LONDON

Health & Medical Horizons 1989 is not intended as a substitute for the medical advice of physicians. Readers should regularly consult a physician in matters relating to their health and particularly regarding symptoms that may require diagnosis or medical attention.

For Your Health

How can you help yourself and your family stay healthy? What are the latest advances in preventing and treating disease? This book will give you the most current answers to these important questions—in expert articles written in language that is easy to understand.

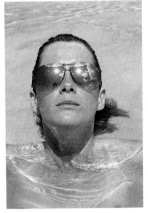

Page 4

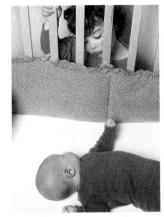

Page 16

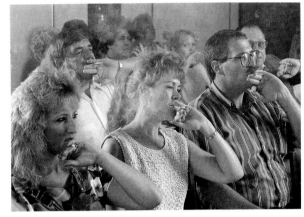

Page 104

FEATURE ARTICLES

SAFETY IN THE SUN _____ 4
Sensible precautions for those who love to have fun in the sun.

SIBLING RIVALRY _____ 16
Jealousy . . . arguments . . . tussles over toys! What parents can do to minimize the inevitable conflicts between their children.

DESIGNS FOR THE DISABLED _____ 24
From specially designed bathroom fixtures to seeing-eye robots, a wide range of devices are available to help the handicapped lead full and independent lives.

A NEW LOOK AT MEAT _____ 34
If red meat is carefully selected and prepared, and served in moderate portions, it need not be banished from the dinner table.

ASPIRIN _____ 46
Long a standby for aches and fever, aspirin may also prevent heart attacks and strokes, and perhaps even help the immune system ward off disease.

CHOOSING LONG-TERM CARE _____ 58
The services available for the special care that many older people need: from at-home assistance to nursing homes.

LYME DISEASE _____ 70
Fifteen years ago, no one had heard of this debilitating, tick-borne disease; today it is spreading through large areas of the United States.

DANCING FOR FUN AND FITNESS _____ 80
Dancing can be a healthful experience—good for both body and mind. And if that's not enough, it can also be great fun.

ALL ABOUT ALLERGIES _____ 94
Affecting up to 50 million Americans, allergies are nothing to sneeze at.

WELLNESS IN THE WORKPLACE _____ 104
Companies are helping their employees to keep fit, eat right, stop smoking, and generally stay well.

HOW TO PREVENT CHILDHOOD OBESITY _____ 118
Practical steps can be taken to keep children from becoming overweight.

MANIA AND DEPRESSION _____ 130
Effective treatments are now available to help the millions of people who suffer from depression or manic-depression.

HAVING A FIRST CHILD AFTER 35 _____ 144
Some women over 35 may face special problems during pregnancy, but thanks to dramatic improvements in prenatal care, the chances of delivering a healthy baby are good.

WHAT KILLED NAPOLEON? _____ 156
Was Mozart poisoned by a rival composer? Did Henry VIII really have syphilis? Medical detective work is shedding light on the afflictions of many historical figures.

PREMATURE BABIES _____ 166
There has been a virtual revolution in the care of premature infants. Today babies born 3-4 months early stand a good chance of survival, although some will have lifelong disabilities.

Contents Continues

SPOTLIGHT ON HEALTH

A series of concise reports on practical health topics.

Facts About Oat Bran — 176

How Drugs Are Approved — 178

Anemia — 181

Dealing With a Colicky Baby — 184

Visiting Someone in the Hospital — 186

Yeast Infections — 189

Child Abuse — 191

Fluoridation: A Success Story — 194

Update on "Shock" Therapy — 197

Children With AIDS — 199

Hemorrhoids — 202

Obstetrics and Malpractice — 204

The Right to Die — 207

Rheumatic Fever — 210

What Are Dental Implants? — 213

Dyslexia: A Reading Disorder — 215

Stocking Your Medicine Cabinet — 218

Sjogren's Syndrome — 221

Toilet Training — 224

Detecting Cancer Early — 226

Chicken Pox — 230

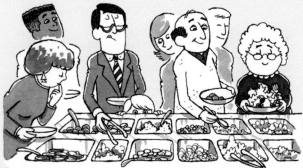

Safety at the Salad Bar — 232

Impotence: A Treatable Problem — 234

The Retinoids: Wonder Drugs? — 236

AGING AND THE AGED   240

Undergoing Surgery • New Findings on Alzheimer's Disease • Exercise and Aging

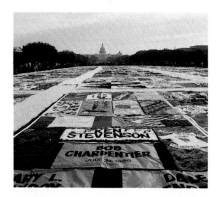

AIDS   242

New Knowledge About the Virus • New Drugs and Treatment Strategies • Concern Over Discrimination • Quilt Commemorates AIDS Victims

BIOETHICS   246

Funding Cutoff for Fetal Tissue Research • Right-to-Die Plea Rejected • Who Owns Human Tissue? • Minors and Abortion

BONES, MUSCLES, AND JOINTS   249

Improved Treatment for Trauma Patients • Advances in Imaging Techniques

BRAIN AND NERVOUS SYSTEM   251

Preventing and Treating Stroke • Cocaine, Speed, and the Nervous System • Update on Parkinson's Disease

CANCER   255

Progress Against Cancer • Prevention and Early Detection • Treating Early Breast Cancer • Biological Weapons Against Cancer

DIABETES   260

Transplant Drug Offers Hope • Marker for Type I Diabetes • Preventing Kidney Damage • Doctor-Patient "Therapeutic Alliance"

DIGESTIVE SYSTEM   262

Heredity and Colorectal Cancer • Salmonella-Infected Grade A Eggs • Dangers of Eating Raw Fish

Health and Medical News

DRUG ABUSE   265

Addicts and AIDS • New Treatments for Cocaine Addiction • New Strategies for Prevention and Law Enforcement

EARS, NOSE, AND THROAT   268

Technology Aids Those With Hearing Loss • Treating Head and Neck Cancers

ENVIRONMENT AND HEALTH   269

The Long Hot Summer • Increased Concern Over the Greenhouse Effect • Health Hazards From Nuclear Weapons Plants • Lead and Children's Health

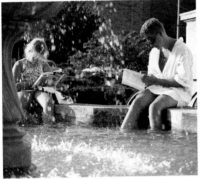

EYES   275

Freezing Technique Reduces Eye Damage in Newborns • Drug Treatment for Squint and Eyelid Spasms • Progress on "Living Contact Lenses"

FAMILY PLANNING   277

New Options Available • Ongoing Controversy Over Abortion Pill • Injectable and Implantable Contraceptives

GENETICS AND GENETIC ENGINEERING   280

Genes That Prevent Cancer • Hormone Affects Women's Skills • Advances in Genetic Testing • Understanding Garbled DNA

GOVERNMENT POLICIES AND PROGRAMS   283

United States
Improvements in Medicare • AIDS Bill Passed • Surgeon General Speaks Out
Canada
Abortion Debate • Tougher Antitobacco Laws • Policy on AIDS Drugs • New Efforts to Rein in Ontario Healthcare Costs

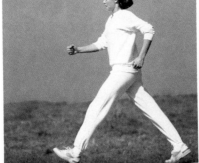

HEART AND CIRCULATORY SYSTEM   289

Type A's After a Heart Attack • Hypertension: Which Drug First? • Benefits of Walking

LIVER   294

Hepatitis Virus Discovered • Advance in Liver Transplants • Treating Gallstones

MEDICAL TECHNOLOGY   295

New Type of Pacemaker • Laser Probe for Blocked Blood Vessels

MEDICATIONS AND DRUGS   298

New Infection Fighters • Preventing Pneumonia in AIDS Patients

MENTAL HEALTH   303

Genetic Marker for Schizophrenia • How Mental State Affects the Immune System

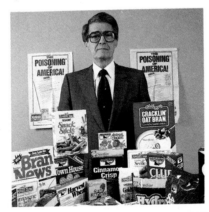

NUTRITION AND DIET   306

Campaign Against Palm and Coconut Oils • Very-Low-Calorie Diets • Yo-Yo Dieting • Apples and Cancer

OBSTETRICS AND GYNECOLOGY   310

The Pill and Breast Cancer: Is There a Link? • The Expanding Role of Ultrasound • Looking Through the Laparoscope

PEDIATRICS   312

Reducing Deafness From Meningitis • Cause of Roseola Identified? • Preventing Asthma Attacks • Breast-Feeding and Childhood Cancer

PUBLIC HEALTH   315

New Evidence Linking Ultraviolet Light and Cataracts • Move to Regulate Computer VDTs • U.S. Radon Advisory

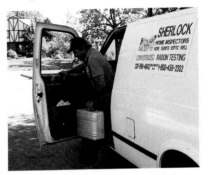

SEXUALLY TRANSMITTED DISEASES   319

Rebirth of the Condom • Chancroid Comeback • Treatment for Recurrent Herpes • Rising Incidence of Syphilis

SKIN   320

Vitamin D for Psoriasis • New Weapons in the Battle Against Wrinkles

SMOKING   322

Warning About Nicotine Addiction • New Smoking Regulations • Tobacco Company Found Liable

TEETH AND GUMS   325

Oral Health in Children • Periodontal Disease Treatments • AIDS Inhibitor in Saliva • Composite Fillings for Back Teeth

WORLD HEALTH NEWS   327

AIDS Around the World • Diseases of Affluence • Cholera Outbreak in India • Animals Spreading Rare Illnesses

CONTRIBUTORS   330
INDEX   332

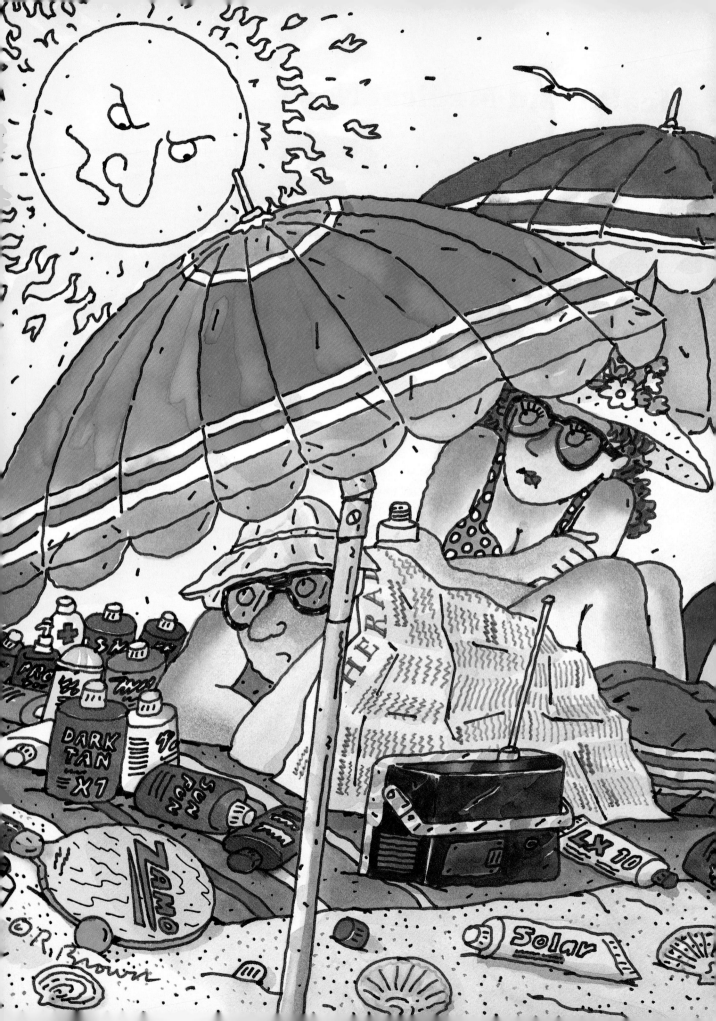

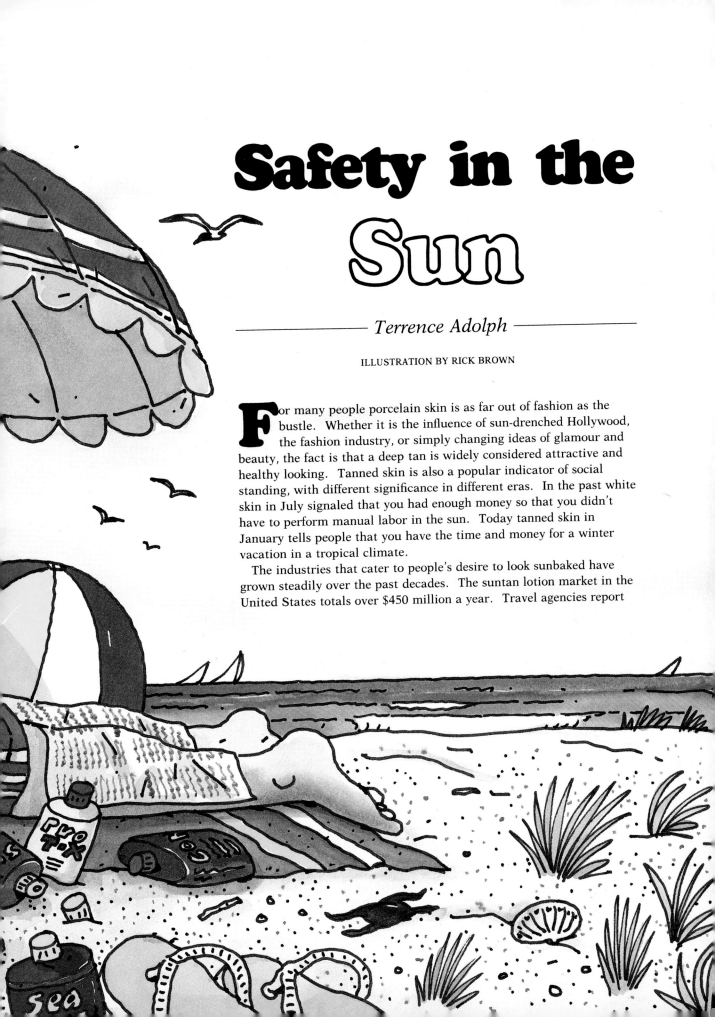

Safety in the Sun

Terrence Adolph

ILLUSTRATION BY RICK BROWN

For many people porcelain skin is as far out of fashion as the bustle. Whether it is the influence of sun-drenched Hollywood, the fashion industry, or simply changing ideas of glamour and beauty, the fact is that a deep tan is widely considered attractive and healthy looking. Tanned skin is also a popular indicator of social standing, with different significance in different eras. In the past white skin in July signaled that you had enough money so that you didn't have to perform manual labor in the sun. Today tanned skin in January tells people that you have the time and money for a winter vacation in a tropical climate.

The industries that cater to people's desire to look sunbaked have grown steadily over the past decades. The suntan lotion market in the United States totals over $450 million a year. Travel agencies report that bookings for midwinter vacations to sun spots have steadily increased. When people can't get away to someplace warm, they now artificially tan with tanning machines, some 275,000 of which can be found across the United States in health clubs and in more than 18,000 tanning salons.

Fun in the sun and a bronzed body can have psychological and even physical benefits, but too much sun exposure can be dangerous. Consumer polls indicate that while people are generally knowledgeable about the dangers, they are not particularly cautious when spending time in the sun. A recent University of Florida survey found that more than 90 percent of those questioned knew that exposure to the sun can cause skin cancer and premature aging, and more than 80 percent understood the necessity of using a sunscreen and the meaning of the SPF (Sun Protection Factor) numbers sunscreens carry. But most of those same people admitted that they still thought that a "tan is healthy," and half of them did not use a sunscreen regularly.

While the sun can provide physical and psychological benefits, too much sun can be dangerous.

Effects of Too Much Sun

A tan is, simply put, the skin's way of indicating that it has been damaged. Tans are caused by the sun's ultraviolet rays. When it comes in contact with the skin, ultraviolet light dilates blood vessels to produce the redness and burning sensation of a sunburn. It also causes the body to produce more melanin—the colored pigment in the skin—so that the skin turns darker. Melanin helps protect the skin by absorbing and scattering further doses of ultraviolet rays. But it cannot absorb all the rays, and further exposure can still damage the skin.

There are different types of ultraviolet rays. Ultraviolet alpha rays (UVA) have longer wavelengths and are more predominant in morning and late afternoon. They are less likely to cause sunburn than ultraviolet beta rays (UVB), which are shorter and are most intense in the middle of the day. Both types can be dangerous, though.

Repeated exposure to ultraviolet light causes physical changes in the skin that are collectively referred to as photoaging. Many of the grosser ravages of the skin do not result from any natural aging process. It is a fact that skin protected from the sun over time generally looks much younger than constantly exposed skin. The visible signs of chronic sun damage take 15 to 20 years to appear. Whereas normal skin gets thinner as it ages, photoaged skin actually gets thicker. It becomes wrinkled, leathery, and tough—and susceptible to unsightly brown spots and warty growths that may become cancerous.

Exposure to the sun's ultraviolet rays may also cause immune system damage, which may make constant sunners more likely to develop skin cancer. Since at any one time about 10 percent of a person's blood is near the surface of the skin, ultraviolet radiation affects it, causing a reduction in the number of blood cells that fight invading organisms and an increase in the number of cells that actually suppress the immune system's response.

Terrence Adolph is a staff editor.

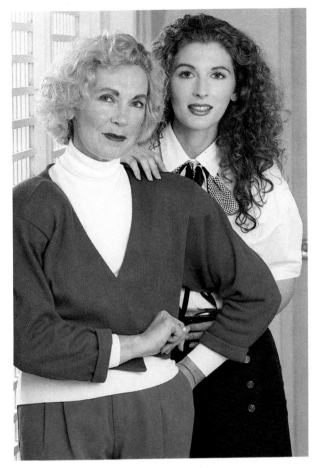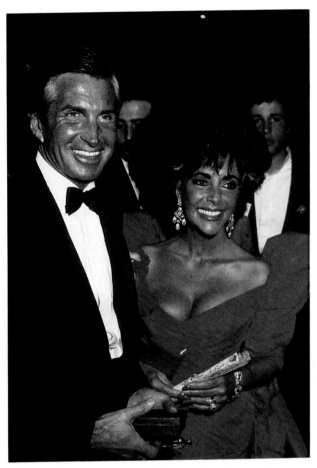

Many medical experts think that repeated and prolonged exposure to ultraviolet light can also cause vision problems, including cataracts (clouding of the lens of the eye) and eye cancer. A 1988 study involving Chesapeake Bay watermen found that those who had greater exposure to ultraviolet light were indeed at increased risk of developing cataracts. Aside from such potential long-term damage, ultraviolet light can burn the eye's cornea, the protective outer layer of the eye, causing discomfort and in some cases severe pain.

Some people may also suffer photosensitive reactions to sunlight—consisting of a rash, redness, or swelling—either from an inherent susceptibility or from a drug or cosmetic. Such reactions to the sun are commonly caused by perfumes and deodorant soaps and such drugs as tranquilizers, oral contraceptives, and the antibiotic tetracycline.

According to the director of a Vancouver modeling agency (at left with one of her models), pale skin is in, but the bronzed look of actors George Hamilton and Elizabeth Taylor (right) is still considered fashionable by many.

Skin Cancer

Probably the most serious result of overexposure to the sun is skin cancer. Since 1930 there has been a 900 percent increase in the annual number of reported cases in the United States. Currently, over 500,000 people in the United States and 40,000 people in Canada get skin cancer each year. About 95 percent of these are less serious cancers that are curable, especially if diagnosed early. Repeated exposure to the sun's ultraviolet rays is a contributing factor in many skin cancers. Indeed, 90 percent of all skin cancers occur on parts of the body that have been exposed to the sun.

Among the reasons experts cite for increases in cases of skin cancer are that Americans have more leisure time than in the past and tend to wear skimpier clothing in warm weather. Large numbers of people have flocked to the Sunbelt states, where skin cancer rates are much higher than in northern states. And the atmosphere's ozone layer, which partially blocks the sun's ultraviolet rays, has been depleted in recent decades.

Skin cancer has in recent years received a good deal of publicity because of the famous people who have had it. Former President Ronald Reagan and his wife, Nancy, President George Bush, Senator Edward Kennedy, and TV newsman Ted Koppel have all had skin cancers removed from their faces, the place where the cancer most frequently occurs.

The most common form of skin cancer is called basal cell carcinoma.

With more melanin (pigment) in their skin, blacks have more but not complete protection from the sun.

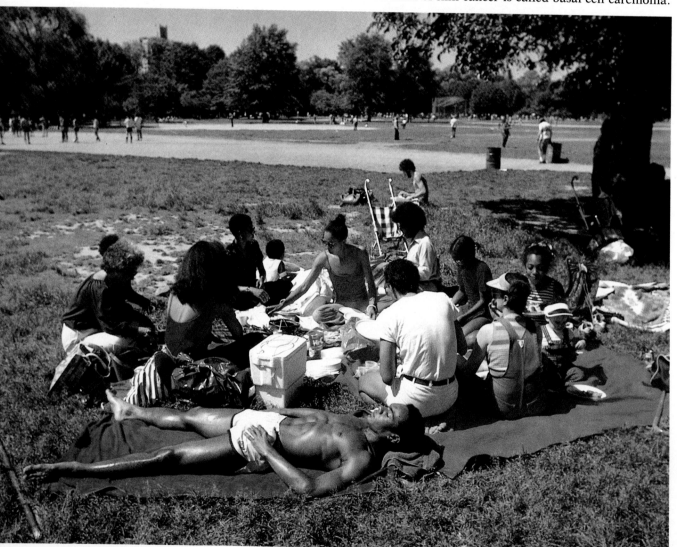

This cancer usually occurs on the head, neck, and upper extremities (hands and arms) and appears as pearly nodules with a depressed central crater. A growth is usually from one-sixteenth to one-half inch in diameter and may occasionally crust over and bleed. The cancer seldom spreads to other tissues of the body and so is the least serious type of skin cancer—and also the easiest to cure. Growths can be removed surgically (the most common treatment), burned away with an electric needle, treated with X rays, or frozen off. Studies indicate, however, that 36 percent of people who get one basal cell carcinoma get a second within five years. Removal of the cancer can be disfiguring or leave unattractive scars.

A second type of highly curable skin cancer is squamous cell carcinoma. These cancers usually appear as raised, pink or reddish, opaque nodules or patches that frequently ulcerate in the center. They are sometimes rough and scaly, more irregular in shape than basal cell carcinomas, and more likely to bleed. This type of skin cancer is also more apt to spread to other parts of the body—and therefore more dangerous if not detected early. Removal of a growth is the same as for basal cell carcinoma.

In recent decades the incidence of a much more serious kind of skin cancer, malignant melanoma, has also greatly increased. This type of cancer—which arises from the cells that produce melanin—looks brown or black or, if larger, multicolored. It is patchy, has irregular borders, may crust or bleed, and can cause disfiguring growths. Over 27,000 Americans get the disease each year, and 6,000 die from it annually. (Some 2,200 people die from other types of skin cancer each year.) Early detection is essential for curing malignant melanoma, since this type of cancer almost always spreads. Melanoma can be surgically removed if detected early, but once it has spread to other organs only a few cases respond to treatment.

Avoiding the Damage

Not all the news about the sun's effects is bad. Sunlight is necessary for the body's production of vitamin D, which is essential for forming bones and teeth. Only a few minutes of sunlight a day produces enough vitamin D for the body's proper functioning. Sunlight can also lift people's moods, alleviate depression, and even improve such conditions as psoriasis, acne, asthma, and arthritis.

Nor are all people equally susceptible to the effects of ultraviolet light. The more pigment, or melanin, skin contains, the more natural protection a person has. Black skin lets only one-fourth to one-fifth of the sun's ultraviolet rays penetrate. For this reason many older black people have more youthful skin than their white counterparts and blacks as a whole have a much lower incidence of skin cancer—though their skin can still be damaged by the sun and does need protection. White people—especially those with light hair, fair complexions, and light eyes, who never tan or do so only barely—have the most to worry about in the sun. Living at a high altitude or near the equator also increases the chances that the sun's rays will be more harmful.

People should be aware that *any* time spent in the sun, not just those

---

Warning Signs of Malignant Melanoma

Early detection is essential in curing malignant melanoma, the most serious type of skin cancer. Follow the ABCD rule to distinguish harmless moles from melanoma:

- **A**symmetry: Harmless moles are usually round and symmetrical; early melanomas are usually irregularly shaped.

- **B**orders: Harmless moles generally have smooth edges; the outside edges of melanomas are usually notched or uneven.

- **C**olor: Benign moles are usually one uniform color (brown); melanomas are variegated, ranging from brown to black, and may have blue, red, or white areas within them.

- **D**iameter: Benign moles are usually relatively small; melanomas tend to be wider than a pencil eraser.

Other warning signs to look for include:

- sudden appearances of new moles or skin spots or the sudden enlargement of an existing mole;

- persistent pain, itching, or tenderness near a mole;

- a crusting, bleeding, ulcerating, or scaling area of skin;

- pigment that spreads out from the edges of a mole to the surrounding skin.

If you note any of these changes on your skin, see a doctor as soon as possible.

hours lying on the beach or by a lake, contributes to the cumulative lifetime damage to the skin from the sun. A light cloud cover may block some of the sun's heat but allows 80 percent of the ultraviolet rays through; snow and ice reflect 90 percent of the sun's rays. Some dermatologists suggest that most people do not spend enough total time at beaches or ski resorts to earn the skin cancer and premature wrinkling that come from overexposure. It's the time spent in the garden, on the golf course or tennis court, or running that adds up over a lifetime to cumulative sun damage. And most of that time people are unaware that they need any special protection.

Sunscreens

For people who enjoy outdoor activities but want to protect their skin, perhaps the best precaution is to use a sunscreen. Sunscreens are products that absorb or reflect the sun's ultraviolet rays. They do not stop tanning or burning, but they can slow the process considerably. A U.S. Food and Drug Administration panel in 1982 found that 21 chemicals on the market are safe and effective in blocking ultraviolet rays. The most commonly used are PABA (para-aminobenzoic acid), which absorbs the burning ultraviolet beta rays, and benzophenones, which protect against ultraviolet alpha rays. Zinc oxide, the white paste you see on lifeguards' noses, reflects ultraviolet rays.

SPFs. In 1978 the FDA proposed that sunscreen manufacturers adopt the Sun Protection Factor system, which the industry took up with eagerness. Sunscreens are labeled with a number that indicates how much protection they offer. Many health experts suggest that people should always use a sunscreen with a minimum SPF of 15, which means that a person using the product will take 15 hours to get the same degree of redness that that person would get in one hour with no protection. Manufacturers consider an SPF of between 2 and 4 to offer "minimal" protection, between 4 and 6 to offer "moderate" protection, between 8 and 15 to offer "maximum" protection, and over 15 to offer "ultra" protection. There are products on the market with SPFs in the high 30s, and cosmetic companies find that the higher numbers are their best sellers.

Proper application. Most people do not know how to use a sunscreen properly. They use too little and apply it too infrequently. They buy a bottle and expect it to last a full season, which it may, though at least partly because people often forget to use it at all.

Sunscreens should be applied at least 15 to 30 minutes before you go out into the sun, so that the chemicals in them can bind to your skin. If you remember to apply them only after you've been in the sun for an hour, your skin has already been damaged. At the beach, sunscreens should be used liberally—as much as nine dollops the size of a quarter at any one time. You cannot really apply too much of a sunscreen; too little, however, can lead to skin damage. It is better to err on the side of safety.

Reapply the sunscreen frequently, at least every 60 to 90 minutes. People tend to sweat a lot lying in the sun and sweat even more if they do any physical activity. Sweating, toweling off, or swimming will

Sunscreens can help protect people who enjoy outdoor activities.

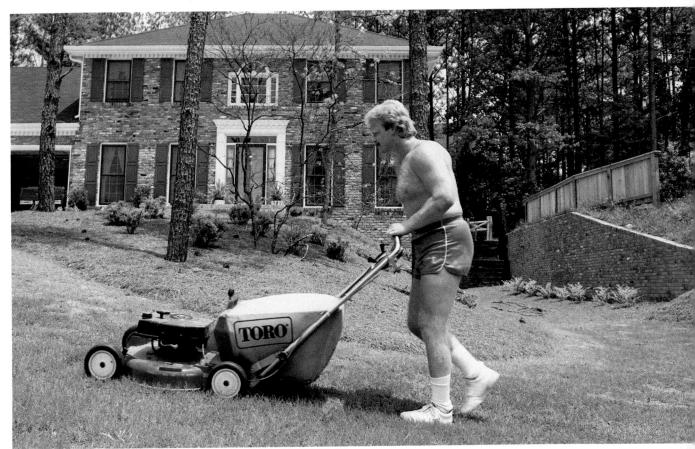

wash off sunscreen already applied. Even so-called waterproof sunscreens should be frequently reapplied. To be called waterproof, a sunscreen must offer undiluted protection after 80 minutes in the water. Some sunscreens are labeled with two SPFs—a higher, nonwaterproof number and a lower, waterproof one.

Many sunscreens also have moisturizing ingredients, such as cocoa butter and lanolin, which provide an added boon to ardent sunbathers by counteracting the sun's drying effect on the skin.

Precautions against sun exposure should be taken during everyday activities like mowing the lawn.

Other Tips

Between 10 in the morning and 2 in the afternoon (or between 11 A.M. and 3 P.M. daylight saving time), the sun's rays are at their strongest—and most immediately damaging. If possible, plan your activities for early morning or late afternoon. Also, work on acquiring your tan gradually, starting with relatively brief sun exposure (as little as 15 minutes at first) and slowly increasing that exposure day by day. Remember that water on the skin acts like a magnifying glass, increasing the harmful effects of the sun's rays. Be cautious about time spent in pools, and avoid spraying yourself with water to increase your tan.

Sand and concrete can reflect up to 40 percent of the sun's ultraviolet rays, so sitting under an umbrella or in the shade will not keep you completely protected from the sun. Products are available specially designed to protect those parts of your body not generally covered by a sunscreen—lips, eyes, and ears. Since many people's noses burn most easily—even with sunscreen—you may want to use a special product there, too, such as zinc oxide, which manufacturers are now producing in a variety of bright colors. Products for your hair can keep it from becoming dry and, if it is colored, from having that color altered.

Sunglasses are also important for sun activities, since ultraviolet light can pass through closed eyelids, and even short-term exposure can damage the eye's cornea. Just because sunglasses are dark doesn't mean they will screen out ultraviolet light. However, manufacturers' labels often now tell how much ultraviolet light their glasses filter out, and some filter close to 100 percent.

Many people pay no particular attention to children out in the sun, but children need perhaps even more protection than adults. By the time most people reach the age of 20, they have received about 80 percent of their total lifetime exposure to the sun. Some medical

Parents should be sure that children wear protective clothing and use sunscreens at the beach.

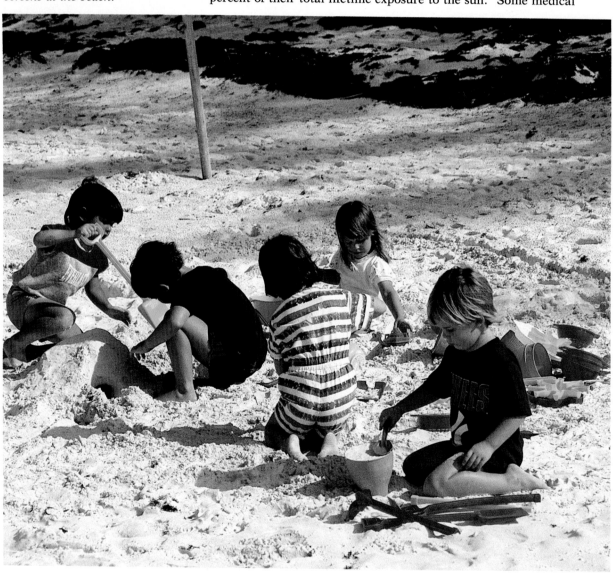

experts estimate that one severe sunburn during childhood or adolescence can double (some even say triple) the risk of developing malignant melanoma later in life. Parents should start using suncreens with maximum protection on their children when they are six months old, keeping infants under that age out of the sun altogether. They should try to moderate children's sun exposure and make them wear protective clothing when possible.

If You Burn

Take a cool bath or shower after sunning, and use a moisturizer on your skin to keep it from becoming dry (which leads, of course, to premature wrinkling). If your skin has burned, take aspirin and soak in a cool bath or apply cold towels to your skin. This may ease some of the soreness and help alleviate the dilated blood vessels in the skin that cause the redness and pain. An over-the-counter topical ointment like calamine lotion or an anesthetic spray or lotion may also help. Most sunburns are first-degree burns and can be treated at home. If you develop fever, chills, nausea, or widespread blistering or infections, see a doctor.

Sunstroke

The most serious immediate problem that too much sun can cause is sunstroke, also known as heatstroke. This is a medical emergency, and immediate medical attention must be sought for the victim.

Most sunstroke occurs in hot, humid weather, and its victims are usually the elderly or physically debilitated. Victims feel hot to the touch, and their skin is red and dry. Essentially, the body's natural cooling mechanism has stopped functioning, and body temperatures rise dangerously high—104°F or higher. The person usually does not sweat, although sunstroke from exercise in the hot sun (known as exertional sunstroke), which occurs mostly in athletes, may leave victims sweating. Sunstroke victims usually have rapid heartbeats, are confused, agitated, lethargic, or stuporous, and sometimes lose consciousness. They should be taken to a hospital emergency room as soon as possible.

While waiting for an ambulance to arrive, there are some things you can do for the victim. Take the person indoors into air-conditioning if possible, or at least to a shady spot. Cool the person down with sheets soaked in cold water; a fan will help lower body temperature. If you have a thermometer, check the patient's temperature every ten minutes, and stop cooling procedures when it drops to 102°F. Further attempts to reduce temperature can actually induce hypothermia—unusually low body temperature.

On extremely hot, humid days, take special precautions to avoid sunstroke, especially if you are in one of the categories of people likely to suffer from it. Wear light clothes, drink plenty of fluids, and avoid overexposure to the sun. Take a cool bath or shower once or twice a day, and rest in air-conditioned places. Avoid strenuous physical activity.

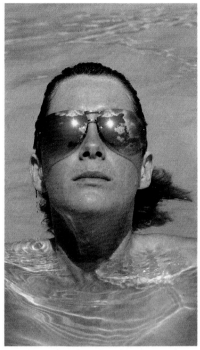

Sunglasses that screen out ultraviolet light help protect the eye's cornea.

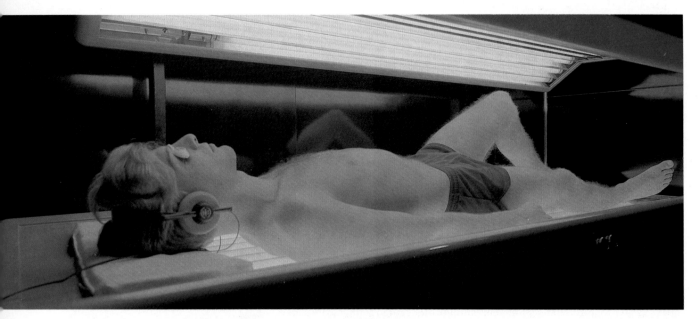

Tanning beds pose the same health risks as unprotected sunning and call for similar precautions.

Tanning Machines

For those who feel socially unpresentable in the long winter months when they cannot tan outside, the tanning machine industry has provided an alternative, albeit a potentially hazardous one. Practically every city across the United States and Canada has at least one tanning salon with those shell-like Plexiglas beds that people lie in for half an hour—paying up to $30 or more for the privilege.

The first tanning machines and sunlamps used ultraviolet beta rays, which are the ones that cause the most immediate burns. Currently, most machines and lamps use ultraviolet alpha rays, which many people erroneously presume is safer. Actually, though the physical damage from UVA rays may not be as immediately apparent in the form of burned skin, tanning machines that use these rays can cause the same long-term damage that regular sunning does—including premature aging of the skin, cataracts, and skin cancer.

In addition to these long-term problems, there are other risks. In 1987 the U.S. Consumer Product Safety Commission received reports of 1,781 emergency hospital visits in the United States that were the result of immediate injuries caused by tanning booths. Few states regulate the industry. The U.S. Food and Drug Administration requires that manufacturers label tanning machines with safe exposure schedules, a warning to users to wear safety goggles, and a warning of the harmful effects of ultraviolet rays. But once the machines are bought by tanning salons or health clubs, the FDA has no easy means of policing their use. The agency usually responds only to specific complaints from consumers. In 1986 the FDA did issue 350 warnings to salons not complying with labeling regulations.

If you are taking any drug that causes you to be photosensitive, consult your doctor before using a tanning machine. Always wear safety goggles, since ultraviolet rays can penetrate closed eyelids. There have been reports of people who did not wear goggles suffering severe and extremely painful cornea burns and temporary or even permanent blindness. Only time will reveal whether a single incident of such damage will eventually lead to cataracts or eye cancer.

Products for Enhancing Skin Color

Many products on the market purportedly offer the consumer either a glowing tan without sun exposure or an enhanced tan with sun exposure. Most of them don't work very well. Tanning pills are often made with canthaxanthin, a chemical that is used as a food coloring. In tanning pills it imparts a temporary yellowish-orange cast to the skin, which doesn't look much like a real tan. The chemical has not been approved by the FDA in the high concentrations found in tanning pills, and the pills are sold illegally. They may cause liver damage and temporary vision problems. Their long-term safety is not known.

Another class of products are known as tan accelerators, which are intended to provide the maximum tan with the minimum of sun exposure. They are generally applied to the skin for three consecutive days before sun exposure and promise to spur the body's production of melanin, so that it takes a shorter time to achieve a tan. Cosmetic companies claim to have an 80 percent success rate with the products, although a recent study by dermatologists at the Cleveland Clinic Foundation found that the accelerators do not increase skin pigmentation or enhance tanning.

A controversial product whose French manufacturers will likely seek FDA approval for marketing in the United States is Bergasol, a lotion currently available in Europe. It promises a fast tan for all types of skin, again by increasing melanin production. But the product contains the chemical psoralen, which is derived from citrus oils and is used to treat psoriasis; psoralen causes skin cancer in high doses.

Finally, there are on the market a number of self-tanning products, which are also applied to the skin. These are basically skin dyes. They often contain a chemical known as dihydroxyacetone, which reacts with protein in the upper layers of skin, giving it a yellow-brown color. Full color is achieved in about three hours, and the color is sloughed off in a few days with the outer layers of skin. These products are generally harmless, according to the FDA. Sometimes, though, they stain the skin unevenly, especially if skin is not smooth, and they do not provide the skin with any protection from the sun as a natural tan would. □

Consumers should be wary of products that offer a tan without the sun.

SUGGESTIONS FOR FURTHER READING

For Every Child Under the Sun: A Guide to Sensible Sun Protection. New York, Skin Cancer Foundation, 1987. Available from the Skin Cancer Foundation, Box 561, Dept. K, New York, NY 10156 (include a self-addressed, stamped legal-size envelope).

LILLYQUIST, MICHAEL J. *Sunlight and Health: The Positive and Negative Effects of the Sun on You.* New York, Dodd, Mead, 1985.

THOMPSON, RICHARD C. "Out of the Bronzed Age." *FDA Consumer,* June 1987, pp. 21-23.

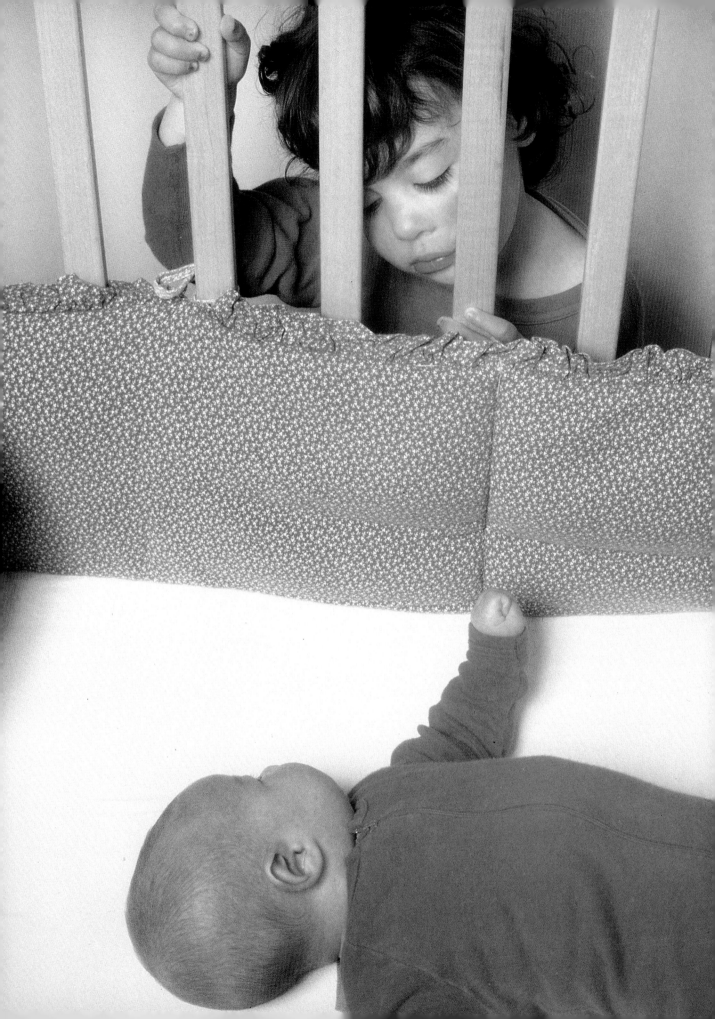

Sibling Rivalry

Judy Dunn, Ph.D.

"It's the fighting that gets me down. They know just how to needle each other, and it's bicker, bicker, bicker. Then one of them lashes out, and they're really at each other. It's worse when Robbie gets home from school—I suppose they're both tired—but every day we have the same kind of scene. It drives me wild, really."

Mother of Charlie and Robbie,
three and six years old.

"It's not fair. He gets his way all the time—and I get the blame. Mom always listens to him, not me. I hate him!"

Annie, nine years old,
talking about her younger brother.

To any parent with more than one child, these quotations sound only too familiar. It is very common indeed for young brothers and sisters to fight and argue and to be endlessly competitive. Many siblings are jealous of one another not just as preschoolers but throughout childhood and beyond. Such jealousy is a theme running through mythology, history, and literature from Cain and Abel onward, and it has been viewed by Sigmund Freud and writers both before and after him as having lifelong effects on personality.

While psychologists and child-rearing experts may argue about the

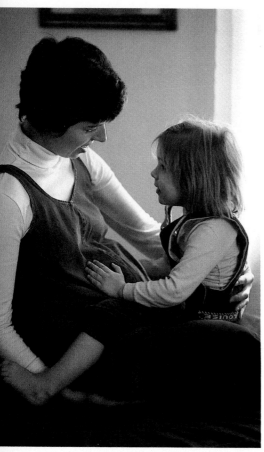

A mother prepares her firstborn child for the arrival of a sibling.

long-term effects of sibling rivalry on children, it definitely has an immediate impact on parents. One study of 700 families with school-aged children found that the parents' most common cause of concern about their children was the jealousy, quarreling, and other conflict among them. Parents have only a limited knowledge of how much fighting and arguing goes on among children in other families, and they often believe that their own children get along exceptionally badly. How common is it for children to be very jealous of their siblings? Does such jealousy really have long-lasting effects? And what, if anything, can parents do about it?

The Oldest Child

For firstborn children jealousy begins very soon after the arrival of a baby brother or sister. Several large-scale studies have found that nearly all firstborn children show signs of emotional upset just after a new baby is born, though the ways they show this disturbance vary. Some children misbehave and become demanding, being particularly difficult with their mothers. Others withdraw and become miserable; they sit for hours sucking their thumb or clutching a favorite toy or other "comfort object" and are often unable to play happily and independently.

The older child's jealousy is evident at this early stage not so much in aggression directed at the new baby—that usually comes later—but in the child's reaction to the parents' or grandparents' attention to the baby. Children often insistently, desperately, demand attention and are clearly disturbed by the change in daily life. Commonly, children regress to more babylike ways, demanding to be treated like the favored newborn. Children who have been toilet trained may revert to wetting or soiling themselves, and sleep problems may occur.

While the great majority of firstborn children show some of these reactions, there are considerable differences among children in the intensity of their reactions and in how long they last. The three questions that most concern parents are: How long do the behavior problems beginning at the birth of a sibling last? Which children are most likely to be jealous? And how can they best be helped?

The answer to the first question is an encouraging one. Although jealousy continues and there are often frequent conflicts between the siblings, the disturbances in sleep, the crying and clinging, and the misbehavior of the older child usually disappear within six months or so. Unfortunately, however, those few children who react to the sibling's birth by becoming very withdrawn tend to develop a poor relationship with that sibling over the years that follow. They need special love, attention, and support from their parents. On the other hand, the children who show their jealousy by being naughty and demanding often develop excellent relationships with their secondborn brothers and sisters. It may be some comfort to parents battling with a

---

Judy Dunn is professor of human development at Pennsylvania State University and the author of several books on child development.

contrary, difficult preschooler that this troublesome behavior seems to be a good way for children to "work off" jealousy.

Factors Affecting Jealousy

What, then, determines which children are most vulnerable to jealousy of a new sibling? Studies show that older children's behavioral disturbances are not simply related to their age—a matter that parents often worry about in planning their families. Although children under five are more likely to be upset than older children, a child's specific age seems to be much less important than the child's personality. Children who tend to be emotional, irritable, moody, and difficult to manage and who find changes in their routines bothersome are the most likely to be upset and to show the most intense jealousy after the baby is born. Unfortunately, a child's temperament is not something that parents can easily control or change.

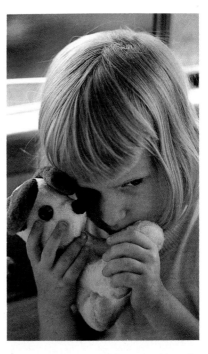

The firstborn child's relationship with his or her parents before the birth of the baby also influences the degree of jealousy. Children who have a close relationship with their fathers tend to be less jealous and upset after the baby's arrival and to be less difficult with their mothers.

After a second child is brought home, first children may respond by withdrawing (such as the child above) or by regressing to more babylike ways of behaving. The girl below clings to her mother and drinks from a bottle—just like her new brother.

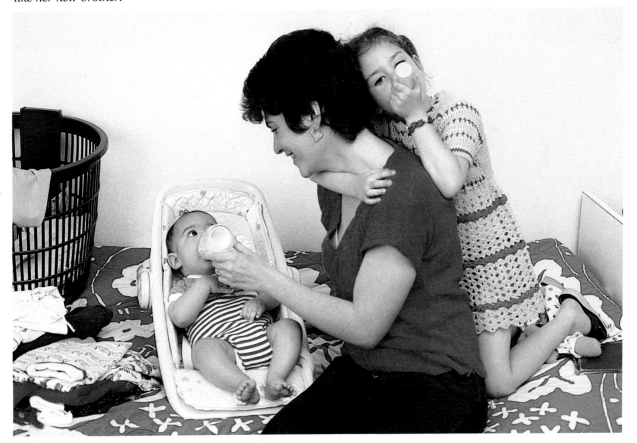

19

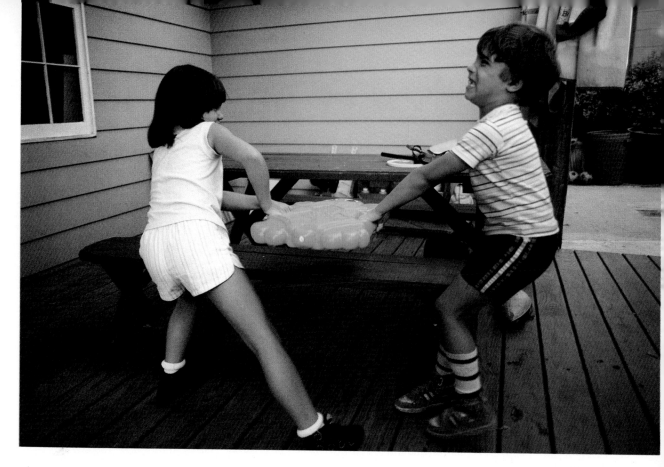

Parents can assure themselves that it is not at all unusual for their children to argue and fight frequently.

On the other hand, one study reports that firstborn girls who have a close and intense relationship with their mothers often become particularly jealous after the birth of a sibling. Another important variable is how tired and stressed the mother is following the baby's birth. The older child is more likely to be withdrawn and jealous if the mother is exhausted and depressed. (It is possible, however, that the child's behavior contributes to the mother's depression as well as vice versa.) Rather than blaming themselves for jealousy, parents should be making sure they—and especially the mother—get as much support as possible during a time that is difficult for everyone.

Helping the Jealous Child

Parents must accept rivalry as a fact of sibling life, but how can they ease the pain and stress for a jealous child? Research indicates that preparing a firstborn child for the shock of a new arrival does surprisingly little to avert jealousy. Most parents talk to their firstborn children about the impending birth, and most young children have had some contact with babies. But while it is a good idea to answer children's questions about the expected arrival and to include them in the preparations, research shows that however clearly children seem to understand what the addition to the family will involve, they may well be overwhelmed by an emotional reaction to the actual event. Visiting the mother in the hospital is often a mixed blessing, too. Many young children find it a tiring and stressful experience. In fact, there is little connection between children's first reaction to the baby and their behavior over the next few weeks.

But there are some clear practical lessons parents can learn from recent studies. First, it is important to try to minimize the changes in the older child's life, which are frequently marked. It is especially important for parents to avoid drastically reducing the attention and time given to the first child after the baby arrives. These changes contribute to jealousy. Also, the times that are most upsetting for the firstborn child are the moments when the mother is caring for the new baby—feeding, bathing, and cuddling. To avoid trouble, mothers should have distractions ready for the older child before they get involved with the new baby.

Advice books on child rearing disagree on whether parents should talk to their older children about the baby and encourage them to help in caring for the baby, or whether the two children should be separated as much as possible. The evidence from research is clear on this point: it is much better to explain to the older child that the baby is a person with needs and feelings and to let the older one take part in caring for the baby. In families in which this happens, the siblings develop much closer and friendlier relationships as the months and years go by.

In contrast to the advice that is often given to parents, research shows that breast-feeding does not appear to be any more upsetting for the older child to witness than bottle-feeding. Mothers need not feel that by choosing to breast-feed they are increasing the stress for the older child.

Later Competition and Conflict

The jealousy of firstborn children at the arrival of a sibling is only the beginning of a continuing story. And jealousy is by no means limited to the firstborn. Competition and squabbles continue throughout childhood, and every child in the family is likely to show some jealousy at some stage, though firstborn children tend to feel the most injured and jealous. Often within a family one pair of siblings is particularly competitive, or one child is mainly responsible for the fights. In these cases, since the other children in the family get along well, the parents' child rearing is not chiefly responsible for the rivalry. Pronouncements are often made about the significance of the age gap between siblings— and of the siblings' gender. It is true that children of the same sex tend to be less rivalrous, in early childhood at least, and siblings close in age tend to be more hostile. But the results of research are inconsistent, and once again the strongest findings are that the siblings' individual personalities matter more than age or sex.

Rivalry between children takes many forms, including competitive remarks and insults, efforts to command parental attention, attempts to disrupt interactions between sibling and parent, and expressions of pleasure when a sibling suffers difficulties. But the most difficult behavior for parents to deal with is direct verbal and physical conflict between the children over possessions, food, play—the list is endless.

Such conflict is extremely common. One large-scale study of seven-year-olds found that 64 percent of children were said by their parents to fight physically with their brothers and sisters, although fewer than half were reported to fight with children outside the family. An interesting

Siblings who one minute may be battling fiercely may at another be peaceably playing together.

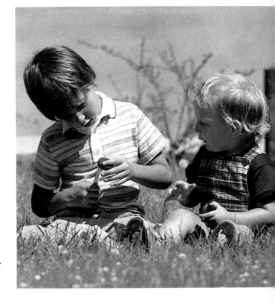

21

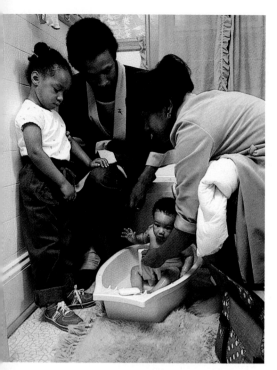

Parents can help ease an older child's jealousy by involving that child in caring for the new baby.

difference between boys and girls was found here: twice as many boys as girls were involved in fights outside the family, but within the family girls were just as likely as boys to come to blows.

It is not hard to understand why conflict is so common. First, the children are, after all, competing for a fixed amount of parental time and attention on a daily basis. No wonder there's emotional urgency to the conflict. Second, brothers and sisters don't choose one another; they are forced to live together in very close, intimate circumstances. Often they have very different personalities, and they know all too well how to rub each other the wrong way.

Two further points about this conflict stand out. First, brothers and sisters who argue a lot often also play together happily, support each other in trouble, and show a good deal of affection and concern for each other. They feel both affection and competition; although the dislike and anger expressed so uninhibitedly may be all too real at any one moment, it is part of a relationship that can also be very friendly. Young children strongly express their feelings about their siblings. Yet the same pair who scream "I hate you!" at each other may be happily playing together a few minutes later.

The second point is that while quarrels are common, there are also startling differences between families in the violence and frequency of conflict. How can these differences be explained? And is there anything parents can do to lessen the conflict?

Parents' Roles in Sibling Conflict

Parents can learn some important lessons from recent research on sibling rivalry. One consistent finding is that rivalry and conflict are more common in families in which the parents tend to treat the children very differently. While it is clearly important to be sensitive to the different needs and interests of individual children, it is also important to remember that children are extremely sensitive to differentiation within the family and inequities in treatment. From a remarkably early age children closely monitor how their parents behave with their siblings, both older and younger, and they respond very directly to differences in affection, attention, and control.

Children are also extremely sensitive to comparisons between themselves and their siblings ("Why can't you make an effort like your brother?" or "Sally could do that at your age, what's the matter with you?"). They are equally sensitive to labels ("He's the shy one of the family" or "She's the bright one" or "Johnny's the worrier, not like his brother"). Even though it's difficult for parents to avoid making comparisons and these comments may be made half-jokingly, they are usually taken very much to heart by children. They cast a long shadow, often reinforcing children's anxieties about themselves and their inadequacies and exacerbating the rivalry between children.

Parents vary widely in their opinions about whether they should let their children sort things out among themselves or whether they should intervene in conflicts. Some parents think they should act as arbitrators and try to get each child to see the other's point of view. Others emphasize that the children will have to cope with conflict outside the home and that they have to learn to stand on their own without parental help.

The usual advice of experts on child rearing is that parents should stay out of sibling quarrels. The argument is that since conflict reflects rivalry for parental attention, the jealousy will only be made worse by parental intervention. However, this advice is mostly a matter of opinion and is not well established by research. Research does offer advice about effective *ways* to intervene if that is the option chosen. Parents should be firm, draw each child's attention to the distress he or she has caused another person, explain the rules, and make quite clear that physical aggression is unacceptable. (Parents should also be careful not to use it themselves.)

On the Bright Side

Only rarely does rivalry and aggression between siblings reach extreme proportions, and in these cases parents should seek help from a family counselor. But some rivalry between young siblings simply has to be accepted as unavoidable and natural. While the endless arguments are trying for parents, they do not usually reflect a failure on their part. In fact, there is a positive side to sibling rivalry. Children can learn useful lessons from disputes with their siblings, lessons about themselves and about other people. There is some evidence, for instance, that children who have frequent arguments with their siblings develop a better understanding of other persons' feelings and motives than children who have less experience in sibling disputes. The emotional urgency of the rivalry that pushes children to quarrel with their siblings also, it seems, pushes them to understand how family relationships work.

While rivalry often continues into adulthood, the majority of siblings develop a special closeness.

Rivalry continues in adulthood, and family crises such as disputes over inheritances often bring back the sharpest jealousies of childhood. But studies of brothers and sisters in adulthood show that for a high proportion of siblings, even for those who fought frequently in childhood, the relationship between them is an important source of comfort and support in later life. Most striking of all, research on the elderly shows that as many as 80 percent of siblings report that they feel close to one another. When asked about the source of this closeness, they attribute their good relationship to shared early childhood and family experiences. The rivalry that was so intense fades in importance, yet the intimacies built up between young siblings—in which rivalry plays a key part—last a lifetime. □

SUGGESTIONS FOR FURTHER READING

BRAZELTON, T. BERRY. *Toddlers and Parents.* New York, Dell, 1986.

DUNN, JUDY. *Sisters and Brothers.* Cambridge, Mass., Harvard University Press, 1985.

DUNN, JUDY, AND CAROL KENDRICK. *Siblings: Love, Envy, and Understanding.* Cambridge, Mass., Harvard University Press, 1982.

REIT, SEYMOUR V. *Sibling Rivalry.* New York, Ballantine Books, 1985.

Designs for the Disabled

More than 35 million people in the United States alone have some sort of permanent physical disability as a result of an accident, illness, or age. Yet until recently many of the devices to aid the handicapped were clumsy or inadequate. In contrast, new designs for the disabled are well-crafted, unobtrusive, and effective. There is a growing awareness that making life easier for the handicapped involves more than designating special parking spaces and installing occasional wheelchair ramps outside public buildings (although these developments are important). It involves helping individuals to make the most of their abilities so that they can be independent and lead full and satisfying lives.

Above, a collapsible knife that allows the user to cut with minimal effort, by either a sawing or a rocking motion with the knife. At right, a vertical platform wheelchair lift enables the wheelchair user to get in and out of the house without navigating stairs.

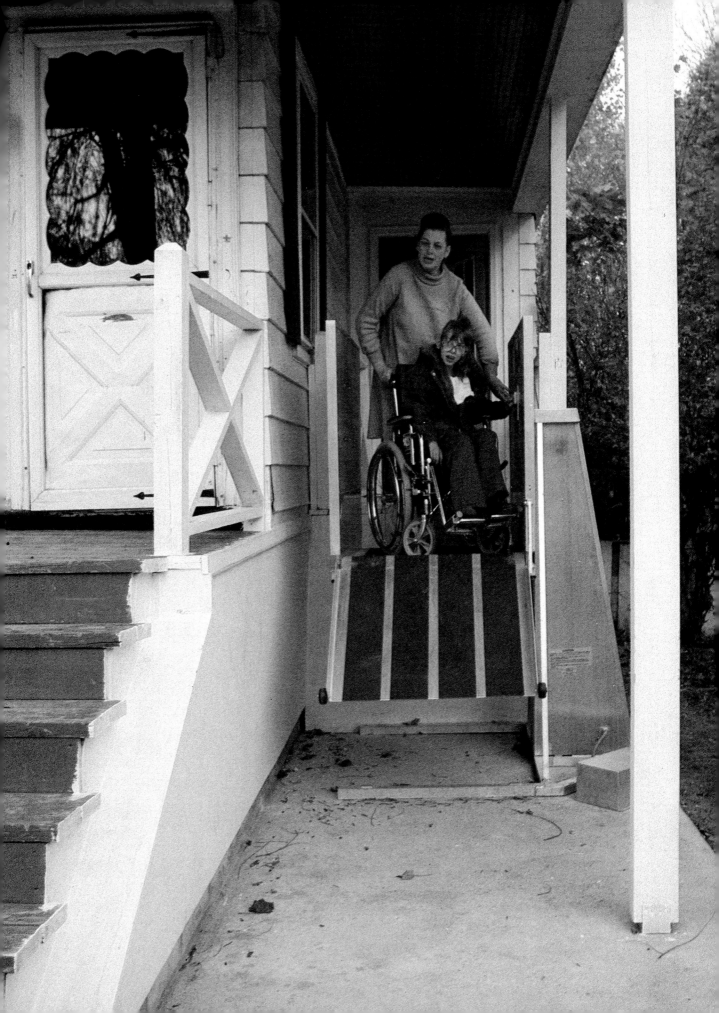

MOBILITY

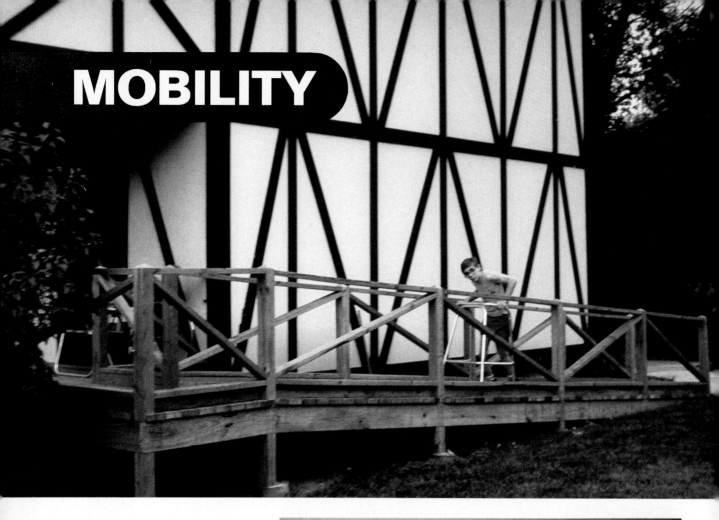

One of the major aims of the new designs for the disabled is to help the handicapped move about freely and independently in the community. Designers have created devices and equipment—like lightweight, easily maneuvered wheelchairs—to provide the disabled with greater mobility. At the same time, efforts have been made to make the environment itself more accessible.

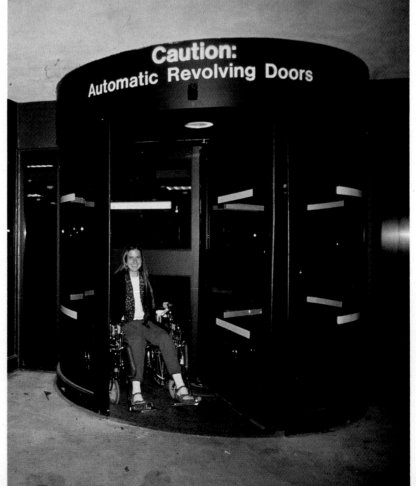

Caution: Automatic Revolving Doors

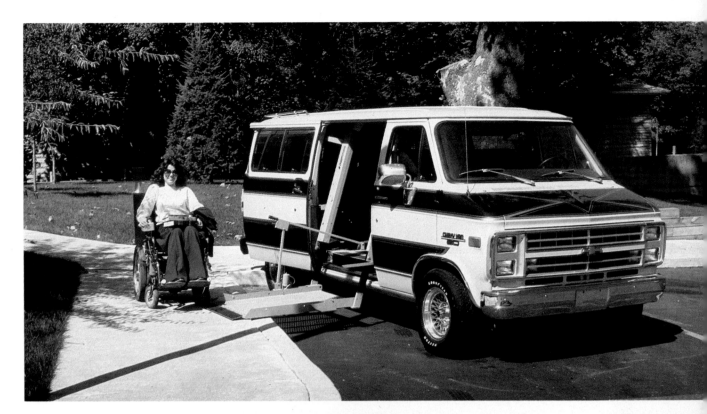

People who have problems getting around can take advantage of solutions as low-tech as the custom-designed wooden ramp (above left) or as sophisticated as the automated revolving doors (lower left) at Boston's Logan Airport, which have a reduced number of larger compartments. An automatic wheelchair lift (above) can be installed to fold out of and back into a van by remote control. The "Meldog" seeing-eye robot (right), developed by a Japanese professor of mechanical engineering, uses its sensors to guide a blind pedestrian safely.

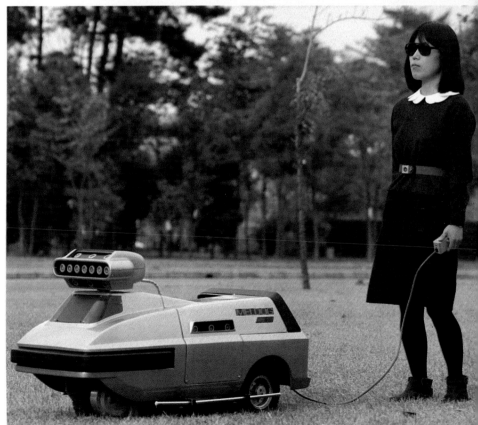

DAILY LIVING

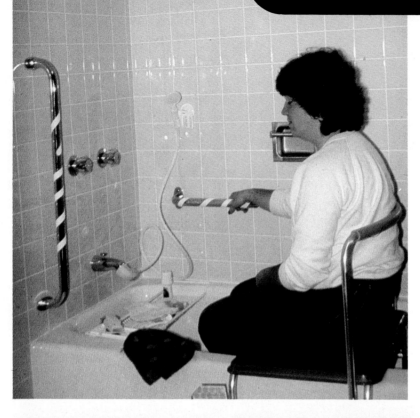

A wide range of products are available to make it easier for the elderly and disabled to cope with daily living. Many are based on the notion of universal design—that devices crafted for the least able can benefit and be used by everyone. Some of the newer adaptive aids are so beautifully designed that they were featured in a 1988 exhibit, "Designs for Independent Living," at New York's Museum of Modern Art.

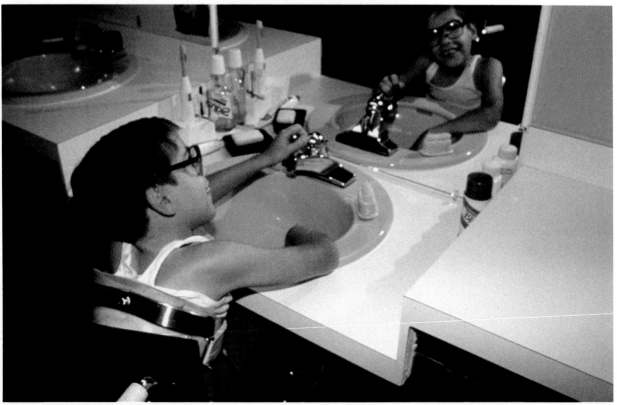

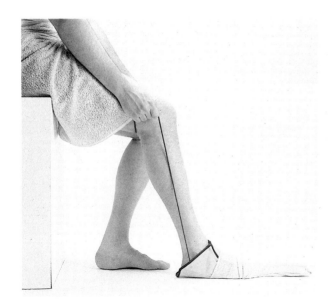

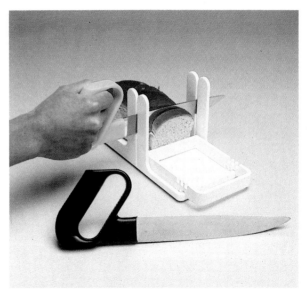

There are simple devices that can make the bathroom safer and more readily negotiable: here demonstrated are strategically placed grab bars to prevent falls, a tray to hold supplies, a hand-held shower, and a tub seat (above left). More elaborate is a custom-designed bathroom installation for a wheelchair user (lower left), featuring a low sink and mirror and a single-lever faucet. Common aids for daily living are a device to slide socks on without stooping (above); a cutting board that holds the bread and guides the knife, which is designed to transfer the cutting power efficiently from arm to blade (above right); and a pair of scissors with a spring band that reduces stress on the fingers and provides balanced pressure (right).

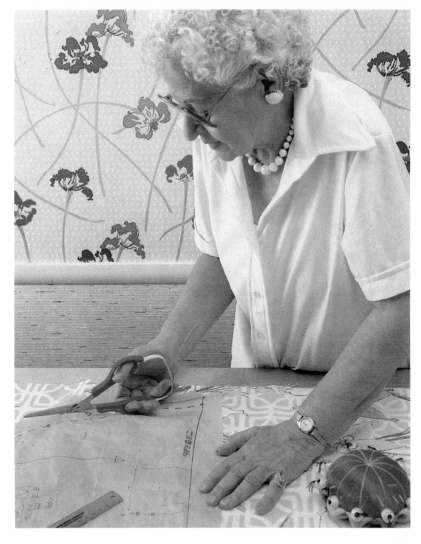

29

EDUCATION

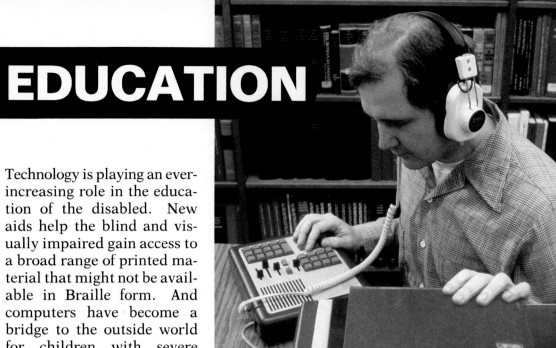

Technology is playing an ever-increasing role in the education of the disabled. New aids help the blind and visually impaired gain access to a broad range of printed material that might not be available in Braille form. And computers have become a bridge to the outside world for children with severe learning disabilities, whether they are caused by emotional, mental, or physical problems.

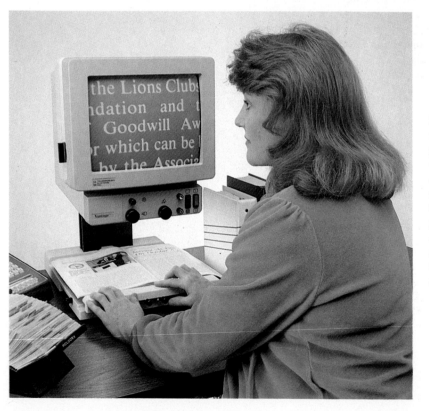

The Braille system of embossed dots is still in use, but the visually impaired can also read by making use of new technology. A blind student at the New York Public Library (above) uses a machine that recognizes printed characters and transforms them into synthesized speech that is heard over headphones. At left, a visually impaired woman reads magnified text off a closed-circuit TV monitor.

30

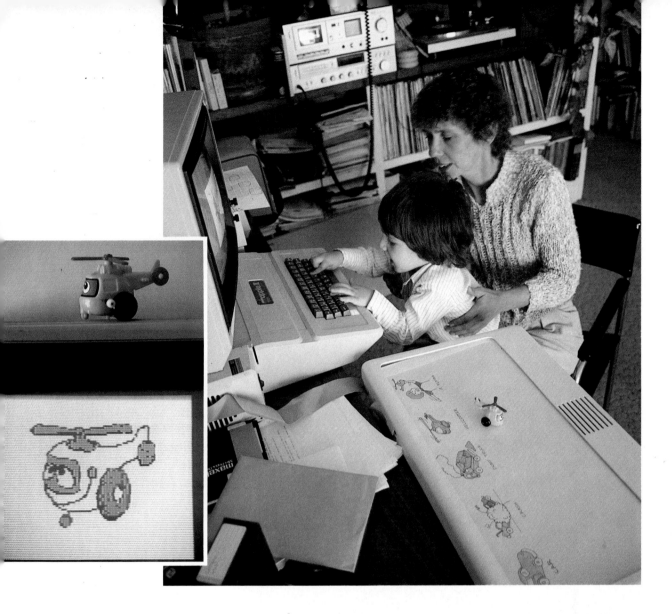

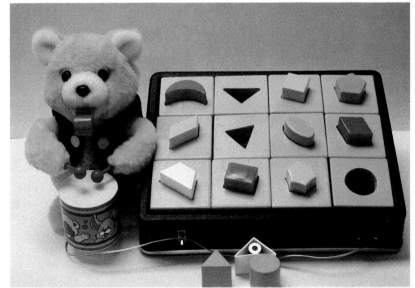

"Language-disabled" children who have difficulty communicating may find a voice through computers. Above, when a youngster touches a picture on a pressure-sensitive pad—in this case, a toy helicopter—the computer responds with a similar picture (inset), while a speech synthesizer pronounces the word. At right, another device provides positive reinforcement to help blind, deaf, or developmentally disabled children recognize shapes. When a block is inserted into the appropriate hole, the bear blows his whistle and beats his drum so that children, according to their capabilities, can hear, see, or feel a response.

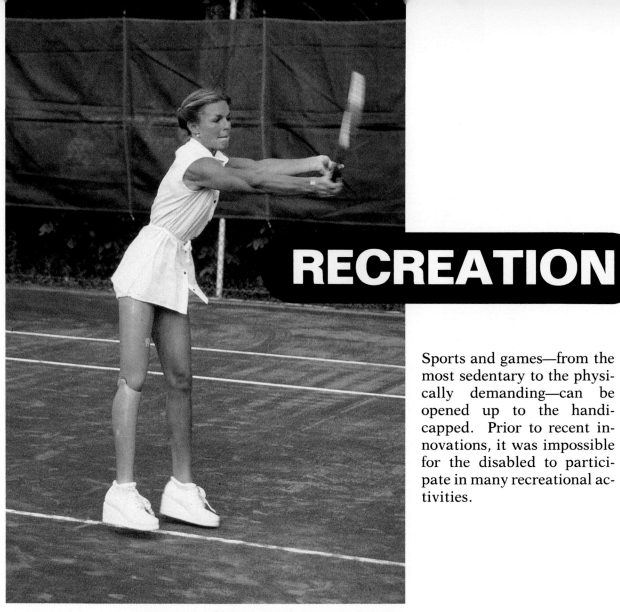

RECREATION

Sports and games—from the most sedentary to the physically demanding—can be opened up to the handicapped. Prior to recent innovations, it was impossible for the disabled to participate in many recreational activities.

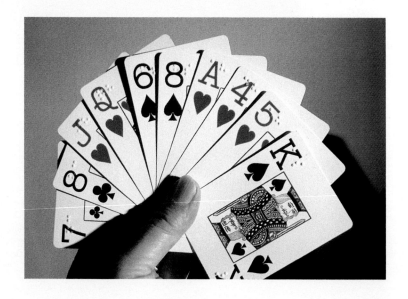

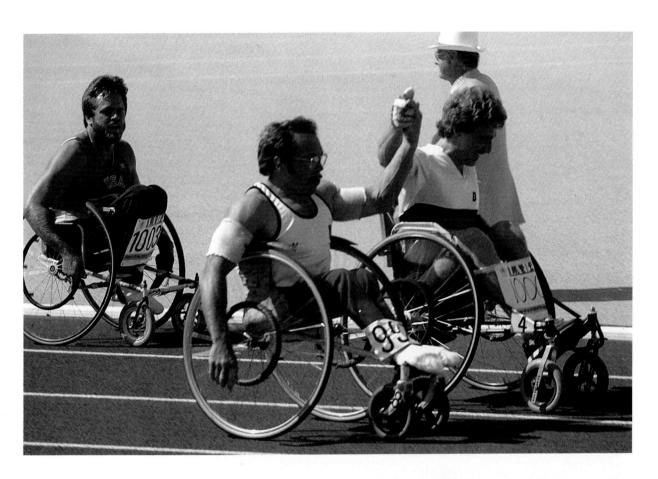

Among the activities the disabled can enjoy are (clockwise from top left): tennis, made possible in this case by a prosthetic leg; wheelchair racing, in which athletes use specially designed, lightweight chairs; skiing, using a special walker device to stay upright on the slopes; and a game of cards, with a deck featuring Braille marking and large type for the blind or visually impaired.

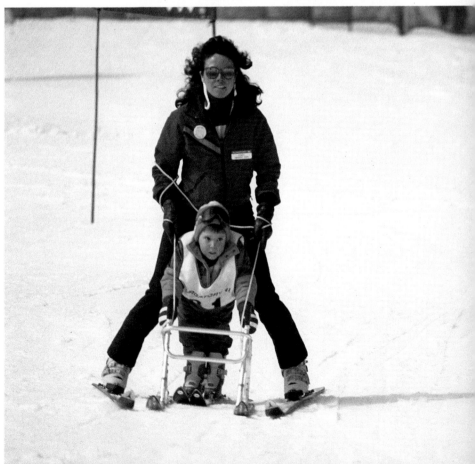

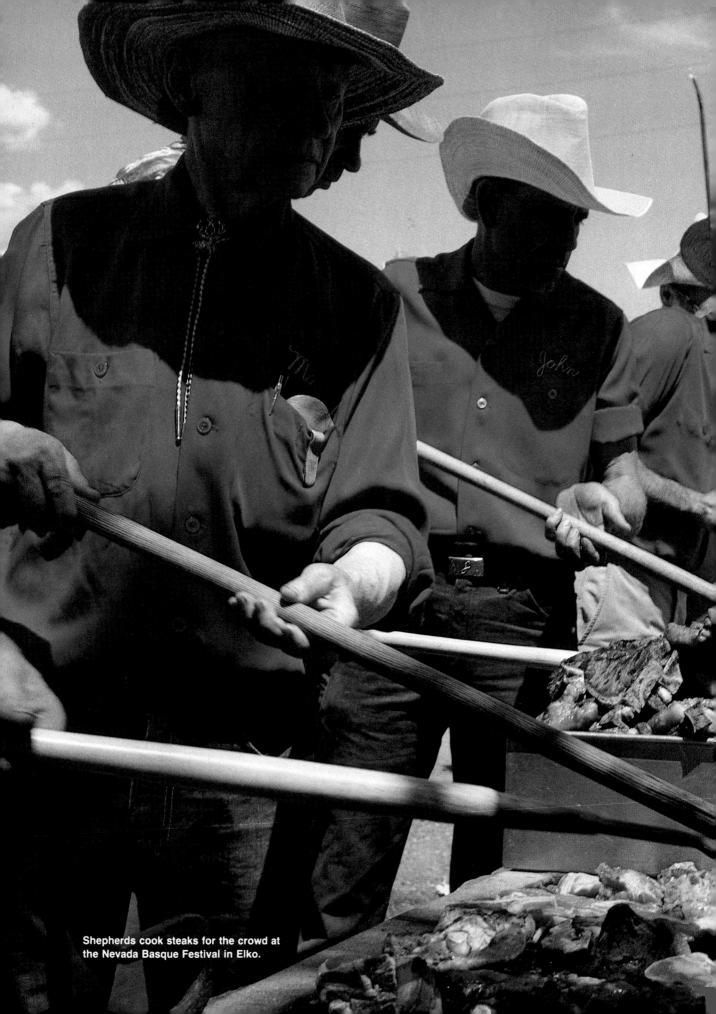

Shepherds cook steaks for the crowd at the Nevada Basque Festival in Elko.

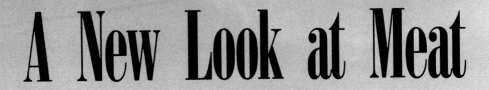

A New Look at Meat

Terrence Adolph

What Americans eat has changed considerably in the last decade. In particular, the amount of red meat—beef, pork, veal, and lamb—consumed each year in the United States has fallen dramatically. According to the U.S. Department of Agriculture, in 1977 the average consumption per person of beef, the most popular red meat, was 92 pounds. By 1987, that figure was down to a little over 70 pounds. Consumption figures for the other red meats have also declined.

Health experts view these changes in American eating habits as good; they have for years been warning people to cut back on red meat, largely because of its high levels of

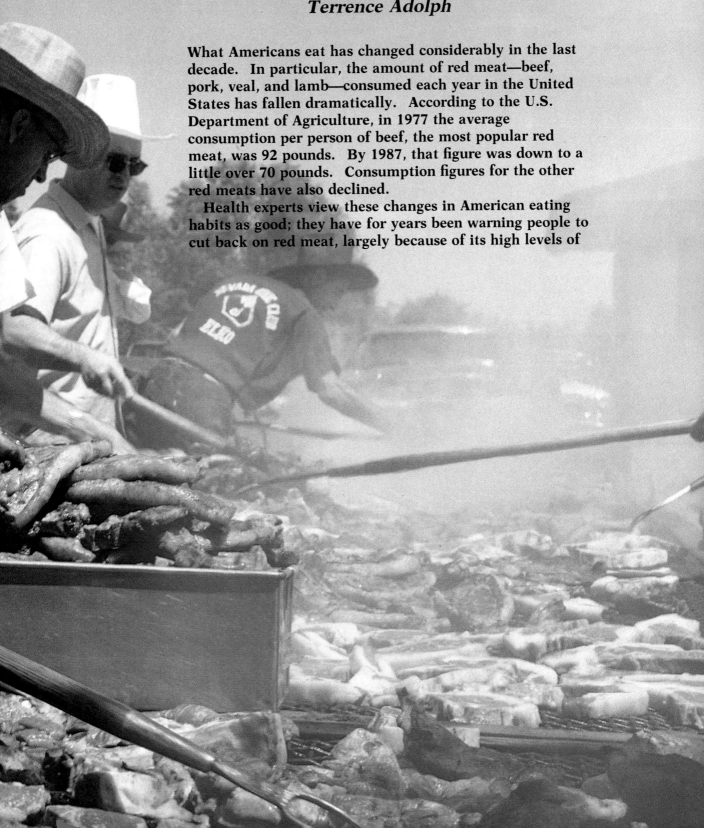

fat and cholesterol. An April 1988 report from the National Academy of Sciences, titled *Designing Foods*, emphasized that the overconsumption of fat and cholesterol contributes to a number of health problems. About 1 million Americans die each year from cardiovascular disease, which has been linked to high-fat and high-cholesterol foods. These foods have also been linked to several kinds of cancer, such as breast and colon cancer.

Few health experts, though, demand or expect that Americans completely eliminate red meat, since meat does contain essential nutrients and is a popular component of the traditional American diet. What they do suggest is that people eat less meat and choose and prepare it more carefully. Smaller portions and thorough trimming of fat can significantly reduce the total fat and cholesterol consumed. Also, in selecting meat in stores, consumers are advised to look for leaner cuts. Several new labeling systems have been developed to guide shoppers in choosing less fatty meat. Meat producers are even finding ways to make the animals themselves leaner.

Cutting Back on Meat

The American Heart Association and the federal government's National Institutes of Health state that Americans should reduce their total fat consumption to no more than 30 percent of their daily calories (from the current level of close to 40 percent) and their daily cholesterol consumption from the current 300 to 450 milligrams to less than 300.

A great deal of the fat in red meat is the type called saturated fat, which more than any other single dietary factor tends to raise blood cholesterol levels. Public health officials recommend that less than 10 percent of the fat in the daily diet be in the form of saturated fat. (A study released in May 1988 had some potentially heartening news. It suggested that one kind of saturated fat may actually lower overall cholesterol levels in the blood and may therefore moderate the cholesterol-raising effects of other types of saturated fat. However, medical experts stress that these findings are preliminary and people should still eat less of the foods that are high in saturated fat.)

If you eat a 3-ounce, well-trimmed portion of relatively lean beef, the fat in that serving might constitute some 40 percent of the meat's calories. But since the portion is relatively small, the total calories would be less than 200. The serving would also have only 75 to 80 milligrams of cholesterol; with that portion of meat, you could stay well within the fat and cholesterol guidelines of the American Heart Association and National Institutes of Health, if you eat sensibly for the remainder of the day. But if you eat a 12-ounce or 16-ounce T-bone, the amount of fat and cholesterol in that large serving would make it difficult for you to remain within the daily guidelines.

A Comparison of Nutrients

A 3-ounce serving of relatively lean beef provides about 15 percent of the National Research Council's Recommended Daily Dietary Allowance (RDA) of iron for women (about 25 percent for men) and

Health experts recommend that Americans eat less red meat to help them cut their fat and cholesterol intake.

more than 50 percent of the RDA of protein for women (about 40 percent for men). It also has more than 40 percent of the RDA of vitamin B_{12}, a nutrient not found in plant foods but essential for the growth of red blood cells, for nerve fiber development, and for the metabolism of fats and carbohydrates (deficiencies in it can cause pernicious anemia and nervous system damage). The beef serving contains other B-complex vitamins (such as thiamine and riboflavin) and phosphorus. But nearly 50 percent of its fat may be saturated. (The table on page 38 lists the amount of total fat, saturated fat, and cholesterol in different types of meat and poultry.)

By comparison, chicken has about the same amounts of protein, calories, and cholesterol as beef (a 3-ounce skinless serving has between 70 and 80 milligrams of cholesterol), but in general less total fat and less saturated fat. Only about 25 percent of the fat in chicken is saturated. (Chicken fried in highly saturated oils or in beef tallow—especially in fast-food restaurants—can have a considerably higher fat content, though.) Chicken also has less than half the iron of beef and only about 10 to 15 percent of the B vitamins.

About 30 percent of the calories in a 3-ounce serving of pork come from fat, and about 35 percent of that fat is saturated. Pork has more B vitamins and minerals than chicken, and a 3-ounce lean serving (with the fat trimmed away) has fewer than 200 calories. Because veal comes from young animals, which have not built up large stores of fat, it has less total fat than beef. Much of the fat can be saturated, however. Veal is a good source of protein and minerals. (Even though veal looks white compared to other meat, it is generally considered a red meat.) As for lamb, its nutritional figures are close to those of beef. About 50 percent of the fat is saturated. The cholesterol content of all meats is about the same (except for liver, which is much higher), since cholesterol is found in all animal tissues.

The Meat Producers Respond

The meat industry is a large one. In 1987 the U.S. meat and dairy industries had total sales of $114 billion. Enormous resources are devoted to bringing meat products to the market. The Worldwatch Institute, a Washington, D.C., environmental think tank, released a report in early 1988 that found that one-third of the land in North America is used for grazing livestock, more than one-half of U.S. cropland is planted with livestock feed (mostly intended for cattle), and more than half of all the water consumed in the United States is consumed by livestock (again, mostly by cattle). The report estimated that 5 pounds of grain and 2,500 gallons of water are required to produce every pound of steak cut from steers raised in feedlots.

With billions of dollars in annual revenue at stake, U.S. meat producers have not taken the drop in meat consumption lightly. They are searching for new ways of making meat more attractive to consumers. Their methods range from ad campaigns to new ways of

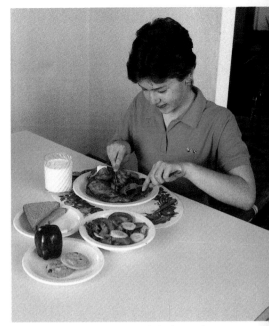

A teenage girl eats a well-balanced meal that includes, in addition to meat, a green salad, whole wheat bread, carrots, a baked potato, and an apple.

Terrence Adolph is a staff editor.

FAT AND CHOLESTEROL IN MEAT AND POULTRY

Type of Meat (3 ounces, cooked)	Total Fat (grams)	Saturated Fat (grams)	Cholesterol (milligrams)
Beef rib roast, choice			
fat well trimmed	11.4	5.6	78
fat untrimmed	33.8	16.2	81
Beef rump, choice, roasted			
fat well trimmed	8.0	3.8	78
fat untrimmed	23.4	11.3	81
Beef rump, select, roasted			
fat well trimmed	6.0	2.9	78
fat untrimmed	20.0	9.6	81
Pork loin, lean, roasted			
fat well trimmed	12.0	4.4	75
fat untrimmed	24.3	8.7	75
Ground beef			
regular	17.3	8.3	80
lean	9.6	4.7	80
extra lean	5.3	2.6	78
Beef liver, cooked with fat	9.0	2.6	372
Chicken liver, simmered	3.8	0.9	635
Chicken, roasted			
light meat, with skin	9.3	2.6	72
light meat, without skin	3.9	1.1	72
dark meat, with skin	13.5	3.8	78
dark meat, without skin	8.4	2.3	80
Turkey, roasted			
light meat, without skin	2.7	0.9	59
dark meat, without skin	6.2	2.1	72

Source: *Food 3,* published by the American Dietetic Association, based on material originally developed by the U.S. Department of Agriculture, 1982.

raising livestock to actually changing the genetic structure of the animals themselves.

Perhaps the easiest means of trying to improve meat's image is through advertising. In 1987 the National Pork Producers Council launched a $7 million ad campaign aimed at making pork more appealing to health-conscious consumers. The ads claimed that pork is "the other white meat"—an attempt to associate it with chicken, popularly perceived to be more healthful.

The Beef Industry Council devoted $29 million in 1987 to an ad campaign with similar ends—to convince consumers that beef isn't really as bad as they have been led to believe. Ads at one time featured celebrities such as Cybill Shepherd and James Garner extolling the virtues of beef, which became "real food for real people." Ads told consumers that beef, when trimmed of obvious fat, is as low in that pernicious substance as many chicken dishes.

While it may be too soon to tell how much effect such advertising campaigns will have on American buying habits, the ads have not passed without criticism. Some nutritionists have claimed the ads often confuse issues. For instance, an ad that featured Cybill Shepherd promoting hamburger failed to mention that hamburger is much higher in fat than other cuts of beef stripped of trimmable fat. And calling pork a white meat simply on visual grounds says nothing about its nutritional content. Though it has less fat than beef, pork—considered a red meat—in fact has more total fat and more saturated fat than chicken.

Raising Leaner Livestock

The U.S. Department of Agriculture announced changes (supported by the National Academy of Sciences) in the rules that have governed the grading of beef for more than 40 years. Nutritionists claimed, and USDA officials agreed, that the old rules actually encouraged ranchers to produce fattier meat. Ranchers have been paid for the total weight of the carcass, and meat could not be graded if fat was cut off the carcass. So ranchers sent cattle for months to feedlots where they were fattened on grains to add more weight before being slaughtered. The result was high fat content in the meat Americans have been buying in the stores.

In order to encourage ranchers to produce leaner animals, the USDA announced rules, to go into effect in April 1989, to allow external fat to be cut from carcasses before grading. Ranchers will then be paid only for the meat produced, not for the total weight of the carcass, and will have less incentive to fatten animals in feedlots.

In addition to suggesting that people cut back their fat and cholesterol consumption, the April 1988 National Academy of Sciences report also urged farmers to find ways to produce leaner animals—including having cattle spend less time in feedlots and a longer time on the range, where they eat grasses and remain leaner. Other methods of producing leaner animals are more complex and involve new technological processes.

Changing the Nature of the Beast

One way to grow leaner animals is to give them growth hormones. These drugs change the metabolism of the animals so that their muscles grow faster and the animals mature with less fat. They also require less feed to mature. A synthetic hormone that may soon go on the market is porcine somatotropin, or PST. Manufactured by Biogen Inc., PST is a genetically engineered version of the growth hormone that

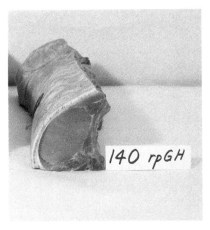

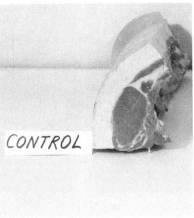

A pork loin from a pig treated with a synthetic growth hormone (top) has more muscle and less fat than a loin from a pig not treated with the hormone.

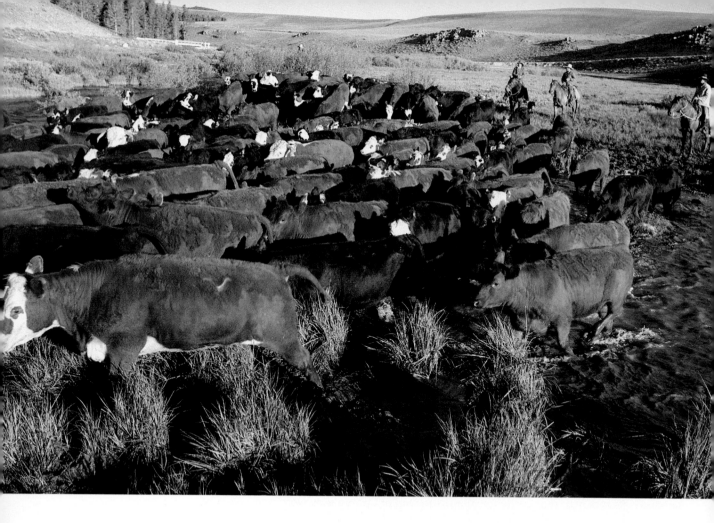

occurs naturally in pigs. In tests conducted at Pennsylvania State University during 1987, pigs treated with PST needed up to 30 percent less feed to mature and had up to 70 percent less fat content when ready for slaughtering. All that could be achieved for the relatively low price of $4 a pig.

The major fear livestock growers have about synthetic drugs is consumer response. Some parts of the United States have already witnessed protests against food products from animals that had been injected with genetically engineered hormones. The meat industry reminds consumers that every time they eat pork they are consuming porcine growth hormone, which occurs naturally in minute quantities in pigs; PST is merely an identical, though synthetic, copy. They also assure consumers that PST disappears from the pig's system almost immediately after it has been injected.

Another method of producing leaner livestock is by crossbreeding. When traditional American beef cattle are crossed with leaner breeds, they can yield meat with significantly less fat and fewer calories. (Cholesterol levels, unfortunately, remain the same.) Some crossbreeds are already on the market. The beefalo is a mixture of traditional cattle and the bison; the Chianina, a mix of traditional cattle and an Italian breed; and the zebu, a mix of traditional cattle and the humpbacked cattle of India and Brazil. Also on the market is beef derived from traditional cattle fed special diets and kept in feedlots

RAISING LEANER BEEF

Cattle raised for longer periods on the range (left), where they roam and feed on grasses, remain leaner than those fattened on grains in feedlots (right).

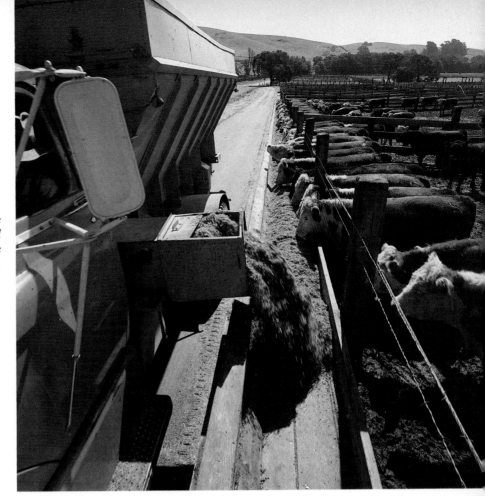

shorter periods of time to reduce their fat content. Brand names include Brae, Piedmonte, and Coleman Natural Beef.

Meat from animals bred to be lean or from cattle fed special diets is not always a bargain for consumers. For example, a top loin steak from the genetically lean Limousin cattle from France sells for $10 or more a pound in the United States. Brae and Piedmonte steaks sell for as much as $15 to $20 a pound. While it is true that these meats may have only 3 to 4 percent fat, much less expensive steaks from traditional cattle have only about 5 to 7 percent fat, when all the trimmable fat is removed.

A highly controversial method of producing leaner animals is through genetically altering the animals themselves. While creating animals with new traits in the laboratory raises ethical questions, many benefits are anticipated. Farmers look forward to the day when, through genetic engineering techniques, they can raise cattle or pigs with leaner meat, cows that produce more milk, or animals that resist infection.

Grading and Labeling

The U.S. Department of Agriculture is responsible for monitoring the safety of meat and any products that contain more than 3 percent meat by weight. USDA employees examine thousands of facilities where animals are slaughtered and their meat processed and packaged.

41

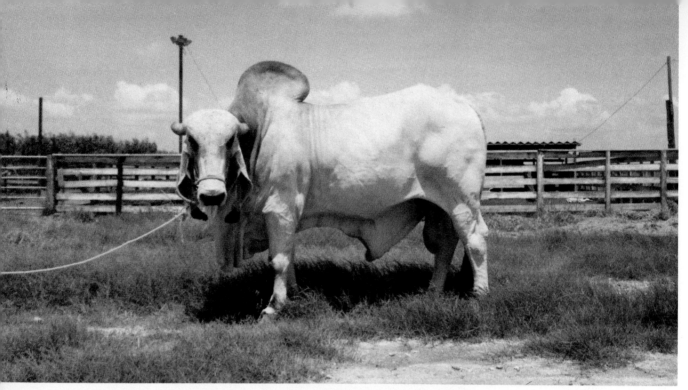

Crossbreeding American beef cattle with leaner breeds is one means of producing leaner meat. The zebu, above, is a mixture of traditional cattle and the humpbacked cattle of India and Brazil.

Virtually all meat sold in retail stores has been inspected for wholesomeness and safety by federal agents (or state agents, if the meat is processed and sold only within a state). Meat is graded by federal inspectors at the request of operators of the processing plants. This adds no extra cost to consumers, since the meat has to be inspected for safety anyway.

Grading is entirely voluntary. Plant operators decide which meat they want graded, but even so, supermarkets and butcher shops are not required to use those grades. They can repackage meat with or without the federal grades attached. Meat processors and retailers often desire the higher gradings, because they sell well in stores.

Pork is generally not graded in the United States. If veal or lamb is graded, most receive either a "prime" or "choice" rating, based partly on fat content and the age of the animal when slaughtered (the prime rating is the higher of the two).

For beef, USDA inspectors have for years used a grading system based on fat content—that is, how much marbling the meat has. Marbling, the white flecks of fat interlaced throughout the meat, lends the meat its juiciness, tenderness, and rich flavor. Thus, the highest grade, "prime," purportedly has the best taste—but it also has the highest fat content. The next lower grade—"choice"—has less fat. Since 1976 the lowest grade had been called "good," but in November 1987 the USDA changed that designation to "select." For the same cut, meat designated select has 5 to 20 percent less fat than choice (based on market averages) and about 40 percent less fat than prime.

The designation "good" was almost never used in stores. In 1986, 12 billion pounds of beef were graded by government inspectors: 94 percent was choice, and 6 percent was prime. Another 6 or 7 billion pounds could have been labeled good, but went unlabeled. Even though good meat had less fat and was better for consumers, few people bought it, since the label seemed to imply that the meat was inferior to other grades. The USDA hopes that "select" has a more appealing, even an enticing, ring to it.

Studies have shown that consumers do not understand the government grading system at all and have little idea of what the meat they buy contains. When asked which grade of meat is best for them, most consumers respond prime, possibly assuming that the highest grade should be for the most healthful meat. Perhaps in response to this confusion, the USDA in 1987 issued more specific guidelines for a separate system of beef classification. Under this new system, which is also voluntary, meat can now be labeled "extra lean" if it contains less than 5 percent fat by weight, and can be labeled "lean" or "low fat" if it contains less than 10 percent fat by weight. In addition, meat

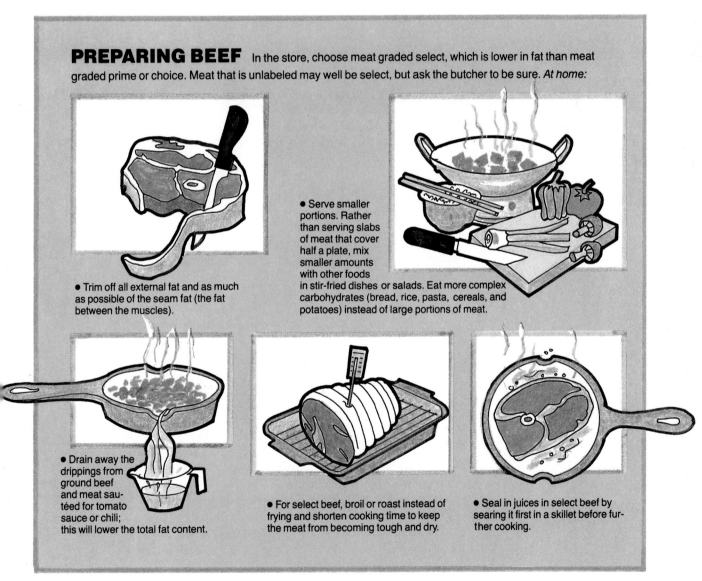

PREPARING BEEF In the store, choose meat graded select, which is lower in fat than meat graded prime or choice. Meat that is unlabeled may well be select, but ask the butcher to be sure. *At home:*

• Trim off all external fat and as much as possible of the seam fat (the fat between the muscles).

• Serve smaller portions. Rather than serving slabs of meat that cover half a plate, mix smaller amounts with other foods in stir-fried dishes or salads. Eat more complex carbohydrates (bread, rice, pasta, cereals, and potatoes) instead of large portions of meat.

• Drain away the drippings from ground beef and meat sautéed for tomato sauce or chili; this will lower the total fat content.

• For select beef, broil or roast instead of frying and shorten cooking time to keep the meat from becoming tough and dry.

• Seal in juices in select beef by searing it first in a skillet before further cooking.

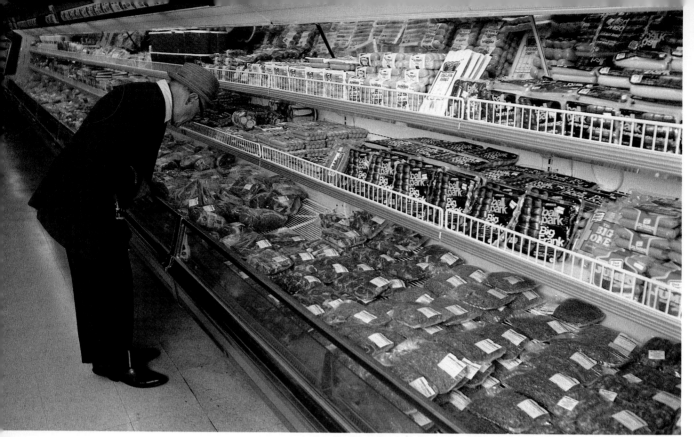

When buying meat, consumers should note its grade, which reflects the amount of marbling (the white flecks of fat) it contains. The leanest and healthiest meat is designated select; grades with more fat are choice and prime (with the most fat).

labeled "light" or "leaner" must contain 25 percent less fat than the standard market average (this category is used mostly for processed meats). The percentage of fat that a cut of meat has by weight, however, has little to do with the percentage of calories in that cut that comes from fat. For example, a well-trimmed top loin steak is 7.5 percent fat by weight, but the fat provides 36 percent of the steak's total calories.

One private, nonprofit organization has also taken on the task of trying to ensure standards for meat in the marketplace. The Nutritional Effects Foundation was organized in 1986 and plans to place seals of approval on meat for sale in stores. The two classifications the foundation will offer are NEF 1, for meat that contains less than 3.5 percent fat by weight, and NEF 2, for meat that contains less than 6 percent fat. The foundation also will refuse to approve any meat containing hormones or antibiotics that the U.S. Food and Drug Administration or the USDA considers to be of questionable safety, even if those agencies have not actually prohibited the use of such drugs. Antibiotics and various growth stimulants have been widely used by farmers since the 1950s to help cattle gain weight faster. The NEF hopes that it can help restrict the use of drugs of questionable safety and ensure that meats that reach the market have no drug residues. The meat industry, in cooperating with the NEF labeling, hopes that NEF seals of approval will bolster the image of meat as a healthful food.

The 1988 National Academy of Sciences report urged the Food and Drug Administration to require that foods be labeled to show the amount of fat and cholesterol in them. Currently, food companies are not required to provide such nutritional information on labels.

In recent years the meat industry itself has provided nutritional labels—not on individual packages of meat, but on meat counters. Its nutri-facts labels, found in some retail stores, list the amounts of fat, cholesterol, calories, and seven other nutrients in 3 ounces of well-trimmed cooked meat (about 4 ounces raw). Figures are based on USDA tests of the averages for all grades of meat of that particular cut.

Selecting and Preparing Meats

When buying beef, choose cuts with the smallest amount of marbling—the white flecks throughout the meat. A select cut of meat always has less fat than the same prime or choice cut. Because many of the calories in beef come from fat, select is also lower in calories than either prime or choice.

In buying meat remember that cut has as much to do with fat as grade. Some cuts are generally leaner than others. Thus, select beef has less fat than prime or choice beef of the same cut—but may have more fat than choice beef of a leaner cut. Select rib steak has less fat than choice rib steak, but more than choice top round or choice top loin steak. Even the leanest rib steaks are relatively fatty, while the fattiest top loin and top round steaks are comparatively lean. Among the leanest cuts are top round, eye round, sirloin tip, flank (from which London broil comes), and loin or tenderloin (from which filet mignon comes). Among the fattiest are brisket, rib roast, and short ribs.

Before cooking, trim all the external fat and as much of the seam fat (the whitish tissues between the muscles) as possible. Even though most people don't eat the fat anyway, it is important to cut it off before cooking. When meat is cooked with excess fat on it, the total fat content of the meat is up to 20 percent higher than if the fat had been trimmed off before cooking.

Remember that highly processed meats such as sausage and bacon are very high in fat (and more than 10 times higher in sodium—salt— than nonprocessed meats). Hamburger, too, can be very fatty. Ground sirloin is a relatively lean hamburger meat, though it is also more expensive than the meat generally sold simply as "ground beef" (which is not of any particular cut). If you cannot live without ground beef, try asking the butcher to trim all the excess fat from a top round or chuck steak and then grind it for you. To lower the total fat content of the cooked meat, broil hamburgers until they are well-done, and drain all drippings.

Studies have shown that although consumers prefer the taste of choice meat, they find the taste of select meat perfectly acceptable. To get the most flavor out of select beef, remember that since it has less fat, it should be cooked for shorter periods of time to keep it from becoming tough. To seal in juices, sear the beef in a skillet before cooking it, or marinate it for several hours. Or use select meat in a stew, where it is least likely to become tough and dry. □

Consumers can reduce the amount of fat and the number of calories they consume by taking care when preparing meats at home.

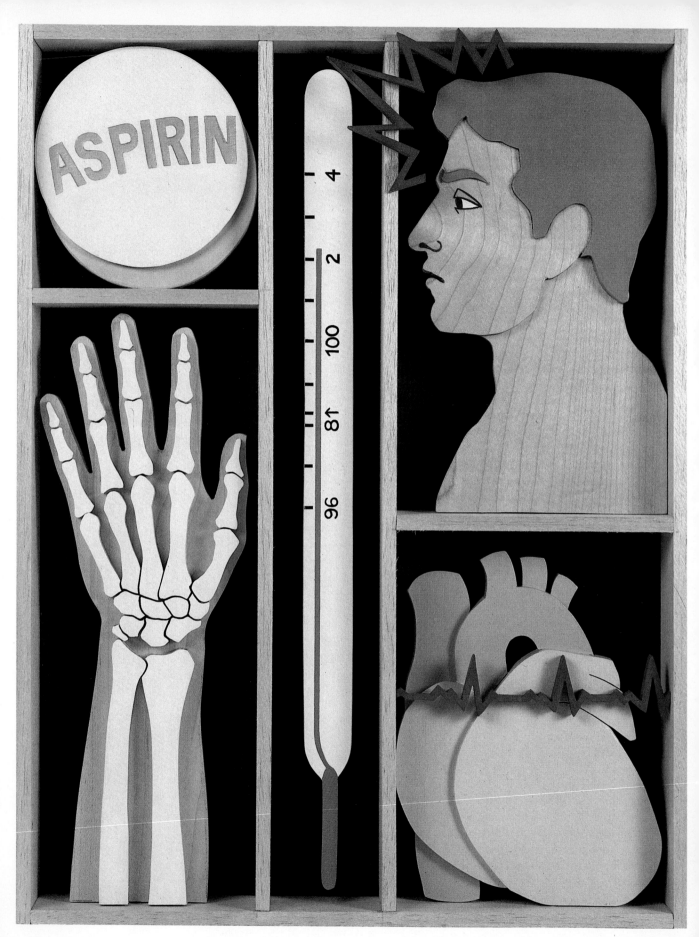

ILLUSTRATION BY LEE RENNER

ASPIRIN

Susan Carleton

Few medicines are as effective and reliable as the unassuming little tablet known as aspirin. It's surprisingly cheap—the standard dose costs no more than a few cents. It's readily available without a prescription under some 200 different brand names. And although side effects (sometimes serious) are possible, in general aspirin is extremely well tolerated when taken in normal doses by healthy people.

But perhaps the greatest wonder of this undisputed wonder drug is its amazing versatility. Aspirin has long been used to relieve headaches, toothaches, fevers, muscle soreness, arthritis pain, and similar afflictions. More recently, studies have found it beneficial in protecting against the life-threatening effects of cardiovascular disease. And still other uses may be on the horizon. Aspirin is being tested as a means of preventing certain serious complications of pregnancy, as well as curbing the eye and blood vessel problems associated with diabetes. Preliminary research suggests that aspirin may even help boost the immune system by increasing the body's production of key substances that help fend off infection.

Chance Development

Like many medical breakthroughs, the discovery of aspirin was somewhat serendipitous. Early 19th-century practitioners of the budding science of chemistry hit upon salicylic acid (aspirin's active ingredient) while casting about for a fever remedy. The substance was known to relieve pain, but it was so hard to extract from plants and so unpleasant to take that its usefulness was seriously limited. In 1853 an obscure Alsatian chemist named Charles Frédéric Gerhardt combined salicin, a plant-derived relative of salicylic acid, with acetic acid, producing a white powder he called acetylsalicylic acid. Little realizing the import of his finding, he shelved the experiment and went on to other things, thus depriving himself of fame and the world of a much-needed medication. Another 40 years would pass before the therapeutic value of Gerhardt's discovery came to light.

At the turn of the century, the combined efforts of an earnest young chemist and a savvy businessman brought aspirin to the mass market.

47

Both men were employed by what is now the company Bayer AG (headquartered in Leverkusen, West Germany). Felix Hoffmann, the chemist, had resurrected Gerhardt's old experiments in an effort to find a gentler form of salicylic acid. For Hoffmann the project was a personal quest: his own father had severe arthritis and was unable to tolerate the available forms of salicylic acid for treating his pain. He refined Gerhardt's method of synthesizing acetylsalicylic acid, tested the product on his father, and reported to his boss, Heinrich Dreser, on his success.

Dreser had the power to launch Hoffmann's discovery before an eager public or to sentence it to a quiet death in the laboratory. Several years earlier he had made his name with the discovery of heroin, which was at the time hailed as a powerful painkiller. Thus, Dreser could, if he chose, persuade the scientific community of the new drug's usefulness. At first, Dreser was skeptical of Hoffmann's enthusiastic claims, but his own experiments made him a believer.

Americans consume more than 40 billion aspirin tablets each year.

In 1899, when preparing to publish a paper describing the compound's discovery and extolling its clinical virtues, the two men realized that the drug still had no trade name. They combined abbreviated forms of the words "acetyl" and "Spirsaure" (an early name for salicylic acid, derived from the name of a salicin-rich plant, spirea) and added "-in" as a suffix. The result: aspirin.

In most parts of the world, aspirin is still a trademark only Bayer AG can use. (Sterling Drug Inc., however, has the trademark in Canada.) In the United States, aspirin is a generic name for acetylsalicylic acid, largely because a 1921 court decision denied the Bayer Company of New York (by then unrelated to its German predecessor) its request to extend the patent on the name and compound.

Aspirin's real history stretches back centuries before its formal scientific discovery. Hippocrates advised women in ancient Greece to use salicin-rich willow extracts to relieve labor pains. Plants containing salicin are prominent ingredients in many folk medicine remedies. North American Indians, for example, used juice from willow bark in an anti-fever medication.

From these humble beginnings emerged the drug that, in the years following World War I, became the preeminent analgesic, or painkiller, of the Western world. Despite the inroads newer drugs have made into its territory, aspirin remains the pain reliever that a majority of Americans prefer; they consume more than 40 billion tablets each year.

How Aspirin Works

By the 1940s, aspirin's efficacy as a remedy for pain, fever, and inflammation was well established. Only in the past 20 years, however, have researchers begun a serious exploration of its potential value for other uses. Not coincidentally, new ideas about aspirin's therapeutic potential paralleled increasing knowledge about a group of hormonelike substances called prostaglandins that are produced in minute amounts

---

Susan Carleton writes on a variety of healthcare topics.

by nearly all types of cells in the body. Although prostaglandins were first discovered in 1930, the technology required to study them closely was not developed for more than 30 years.

Then, in a virtual explosion of research, scientists found that these substances play a role in almost all biologic processes—sometimes with beneficial effects, sometimes with harmful ones. For instance, prostaglandins regulate blood pressure and induce and resolve the body's inflammatory response to injury or bacteria. Prostaglandins even appear to take part in the earliest stages of life; not only do they initiate the uterine contractions that result in childbirth, but some researchers believe that the high concentrations of prostaglandins in semen may help make conception possible.

Sir John Vane, a British researcher studying prostaglandins, began exploring a possible link between aspirin and these powerful, multipurpose substances in the late 1960s. In 1971 he published a landmark paper establishing the link once and for all. Aspirin, he found, inhibits the activity of cyclo-oxygenase, an enzyme needed by cells to synthesize prostaglandins. Thus, aspirin indirectly inhibits the synthesis of prostaglandins, which seem to be responsible for many of the symptoms that aspirin relieves. After more than a century enshrouded in mystery, the key to aspirin's effectiveness was finally revealed.

Vane shared the 1982 Nobel Prize in physiology or medicine for his work with prostaglandins. Meanwhile, scientists in all parts of the world followed up on the implications of the aspirin-prostaglandin link. Because aspirin works by preventing prostaglandin synthesis, and because it relieves symptoms such as fever and inflammation, prostaglandins are likely to be fundamental to the processes that produce these symptoms. Although many researchers have devoted their careers to elucidating these complex processes, questions remain about exactly how prostaglandins are involved. The following paragraphs describe the known mechanisms and leading theories about how aspirin's ability to block prostaglandin synthesis relieves the common symptoms for which the drug is used.

Fever. Body temperature rises above normal in response to pyrogens, chemicals released by white blood cells in the process of fighting infection. Pyrogens elevate the setting on the body's "thermostat"—the hypothalamus, a structure at the base of the brain. They do this with the help of prostaglandins generated in the hypothalamus. Aspirin, by blocking the production of those prostaglandins, lowers body temperature. It also increases blood flow to the skin, causing sweating and further cooling. These effects begin about one hour after aspirin is taken.

Pain. The types of pain aspirin is most effective against are those caused by injury or inflammation. Injured, inflamed tissues release a pain-causing chemical called bradykinin. Prostaglandins seem to sensitize nerve endings to bradykinin, thus magnifying its effect; aspirin, by blocking the prostaglandins, diminishes bradykinin's effect. Aspirin may also affect the perception of pain in the brain.

Inflammation. The highly complex process of inflammation is imperfectly understood, but prostaglandins seem to be involved. It has

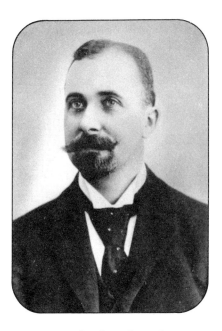

Aspirin was first brought to the mass market through the efforts of chemist Felix Hoffmann (above) and his boss, Heinrich Dreser (below), of what is now the Bayer company.

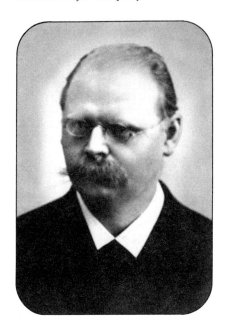

49

been suggested that white blood cells in tissue undergoing an inflammatory response produce certain enzymes that, in turn, cause the release of prostaglandins. The prostaglandins then cause some of the signs of inflammation (such as redness and swelling) and attract more white blood cells, perpetuating the process. Eventually, however, prostaglandins build up in large enough amounts to reverse the process.

One explanation for the chronic, joint-destroying inflammation of rheumatoid and other inflammatory forms of arthritis (such as juvenile rheumatoid arthritis and the crippling spinal disorder known as ankylosing spondylitis) is that in these conditions prostaglandin levels never get high enough to "turn off" the process. Instead, they are released in minute amounts, perpetuating the influx of white blood cells and the destruction of tissue.

Aspirin's ability to suppress the synthesis of prostaglandins, particularly early in the inflammatory process, is the key to its effectiveness. (This anti-inflammatory effect is absent in acetaminophen, aspirin's chief rival in the over-the-counter analgesic market; ibuprofen, another popular rival to aspirin, has an anti-inflammatory effect equal to that of aspirin.) Arthritis sufferers require a constant, high level of salicylate (a chemical closely related to salicylic acid) in their bloodstream to keep inflammation under control, so they may have to take from 12 to 20 aspirin tablets each day.

Helping the Immune System?

Aspirin also has potential value in several other areas, the most intriguing of which is helping the immune system. Preliminary research suggests that suppression of prostaglandin synthesis with aspirin may enhance this vital system's ability to fight off disease. Researchers at George Washington University have found, in test-tube experiments, that aspirin boosts the action of thymosins, which are hormones produced by the thymus gland, the control center of the immune system. Researchers think that certain prostaglandins may prevent thymosins from inducing cells to manufacture naturally occurring immune system stimulants such as interleukin-2 and interferon. When aspirin inhibits prostaglandins, cells can manufacture these stimulants. Although this research is still quite preliminary, it has the potential for great importance. If aspirin does prove to boost immunity, it could one day play a role in the treatment of disorders in which the immune system is suppressed, including AIDS and many kinds of cancer.

The Cardiovascular Connection

Aspirin's greatest potential value could be in the prevention of the deadly complications of cardiovascular disease, America's number one killer. According to the American Heart Association, each year 1.5 million Americans suffer heart attacks, more than 500,000 of which are fatal. Hundreds of thousands more die from strokes, which also leave a high proportion of their surviving victims permanently disabled. Based on 20 years of testing and studying aspirin in cardiovascular disease,

---

A Powerful Drug

Aspirin has been shown to be effective against many different conditions. When used properly (in some cases under a doctor's direction), it can:

- relieve pain from such common problems as headaches, menstrual cramps, and toothaches
- lower fever
- control inflammation and associated swelling and tenderness, as in the inflammatory types of arthritis
- possibly lower the risk of death and disability from stroke
- prevent the recurrence of "warning strokes" (transient ischemic attacks)
- cut the risk of heart attacks in people with unstable angina
- help prevent second heart attacks in people who have survived one
- help prevent first heart attacks in healthy individuals
- improve the chances of survival when given shortly after a heart attack

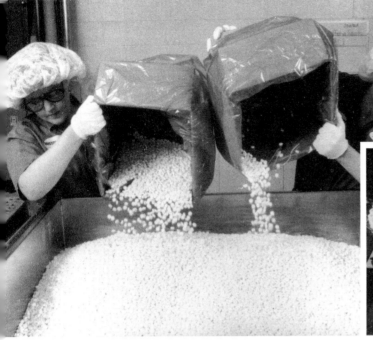

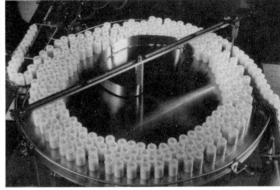

Vast quantities of aspirin are manufactured under controlled, hygienic conditions. Here, workers produce Bufferin at a Bristol-Myers plant in North Carolina.

however, some researchers estimate that proper preventive use of the drug could save as many as 100,000 lives a year.

The idea that aspirin could help prevent the formation of blood clots that lead to heart attacks and strokes has been knocking around for some time, but the scientific rationale for such an effect did not exist until Sir John Vane's discovery of the aspirin-prostaglandin link. In the 1940s a California doctor named Lawrence L. Craven, hypothesizing that because aspirin increases bleeding time it might also prevent heart attacks, began prescribing one or two aspirin tablets a day for patients whom he considered likely heart attack candidates.

In 1956, Craven announced dramatic results of this treatment: of 8,000 aspirin-taking patients, all male, none had suffered heart attacks or strokes. The scientific community met his claims with skepticism. Craven's study had several glaring flaws. First, he studied only men receiving aspirin, without looking at a similar group of men who did not take aspirin. Such a comparison group (called a control group) is essential for a test of a drug's efficacy to be considered valid. Second, he conducted the research alone, with no outside observers to confirm his findings. And third, he had no way of knowing whether his patients were, in fact, taking aspirin regularly, or whether they took other steps that could also have reduced their risk of heart attacks and strokes. Even so, his observations made an impression, and the debate was launched on whether aspirin protects against heart disease and stroke.

Answers were slow in coming because accurate evaluations of a drug as widely used as aspirin in a condition as common as cardiovascular disease are, at best, difficult and expensive to obtain. To be sure their results were reliable, scientists in the various studies had to recruit thousands of volunteers and painstakingly divide the subjects into two groups that had virtually the same medical histories. One of those groups would receive aspirin and the other would receive a placebo, or inactive substance, on the same schedule and under the same conditions. In some cases, researchers even went so far as to disguise the flavor of aspirin and imbue the placebo with a similar taste so that none of the participants would know what they were receiving. Finally, both groups had to be followed long enough for results to become evident. Here are the highlights of recent research on the effect of aspirin in preventing different manifestations of cardiovascular disease.

Strokes. Most strokes occur when the blood supply to an area of the brain is cut off by partial or total obstruction of an artery. Generally, the cause of the obstruction is a blood clot—usually one lodged in an artery narrowed by a plaque (a buildup along the arterial wall of fatty material and platelets, colorless particles in the blood that are necessary for clotting). In 1980 investigators from the Canadian Cooperative Study Group, which conducted one of the largest studies of aspirin and strokes to date, reported a 31 percent reduction in death and disability from stroke in patients treated with aspirin.

There is another type of stroke called a hemorrhagic stroke that involves the rupture of an artery within the brain. Recently, the Harvard-based Physicians' Health Study Research Group found slightly more hemmorrhagic strokes in men treated with aspirin than in those treated with a placebo—possibly because of aspirin's ability to inhibit blood clotting. This finding indicates that the indiscriminate use of aspirin may be unwise. However, most physicians believe that unless a

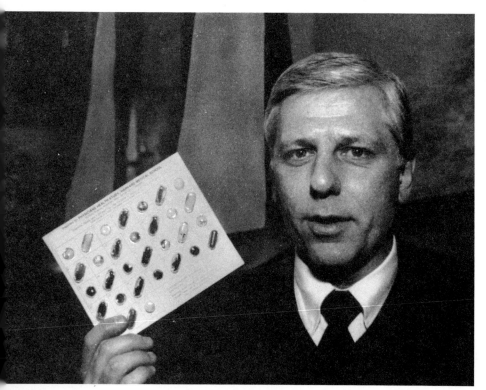

Dr. Charles H. Hennekens, who headed the Harvard-based Physicians' Health Study Research Group, displays the monthly packs of pills distributed to study participants. The study showed that taking a buffered aspirin every other day could help reduce the risk of a first heart attack in healthy men.

person has a tendency to bleed, the possible benefit of aspirin in preventing strokes caused by clots outweighs the risk of a hemorrhagic stroke.

Transient ischemic attacks. TIAs, or brief episodes of symptoms such as weakness on one side, vision or hearing loss, dizziness, and difficulty speaking, often precede full-blown strokes. A TIA occurs when the blood supply to an area of the brain is briefly but drastically reduced. Because of convincing evidence from the Canadian Cooperative Study Group and a similar large study based at the University of Texas Medical Center, the U.S. Food and Drug Administration (FDA) in 1980 approved the use of aspirin, following a doctor's recommendation, to prevent recurrent TIAs in men. (Women were excluded because the data failed to show a similar benefit for them.) In numerous studies, aspirin has significantly reduced the incidence of subsequent TIAs in men who have already suffered such episodes. Many of the same studies also show a reduction in stroke death and disability in aspirin-treated men with a history of TIAs.

Unstable angina. Deep, crushing chest pain, or angina, signals the presence of an arterial plaque obstructing the flow of blood to an area of the heart. In unstable angina, this pain occurs without the provocation of exercise, emotional upset, or some other strain upon the heart. Unstable angina is often a prelude to a heart attack. A Veterans Administration study completed in 1983 found that men with unstable angina who received aspirin suffered 50 percent fewer heart attacks than a similar group of unstable angina patients who received a placebo. As a result, in 1985 the FDA approved new labeling for aspirin stating its effectiveness in preventing heart attacks in people with unstable angina.

Second heart attacks. In 1985 the FDA also approved aspirin, taken on a doctor's instruction, to prevent second heart attacks in patients who have survived one heart attack. This decision was based on data from six studies conducted in the United States and the United Kingdom between 1974 and 1981. The six studies combined involved more than 10,000 heart attack survivors in whom aspirin therapy produced an overall 21 percent reduction of further heart attacks. (It should be noted that several of the individual studies did not show a significant effect of aspirin on heart attack patients and that aspirin's effect was made clear only after the studies were combined.)

First heart attacks. In perhaps the most dramatic results reported to date, the Physicians' Health Study—designed to determine whether aspirin has any effect on the incidence of first heart attacks in a large group of male physicians with no history of heart disease—was ended ahead of schedule in late 1987 because of a startling finding. After less than five years of what was intended to be an eight-year study, the investigators found that the physicians taking a buffered aspirin every other day experienced 47 percent fewer heart attacks than the controls who were taking a placebo.

Treating heart attacks. A British study reported in August 1988 found that aspirin could significantly improve the chances of survival following a heart attack if taken within hours of the attack and daily for a month afterward. When given orally along with the clot-dissolving

Aspirin is surprisingly cheap—the standard dose costs no more than a few cents.

53

drug streptokinase (administered intravenously shortly after the attack), aspirin helped reduce the mortality rate in thousands of heart attack patients by 42 percent compared with patients receiving neither treatment. When given alone, aspirin reduced the number of deaths by 23 percent compared with patients receiving only a placebo.

Preventing Platelet Buildup

Studies show that low dosages of aspirin may prevent the development of some serious disorders.

In preventing cardiovascular problems, aspirin works because of its distinct effect on platelets. When a blood vessel is injured, platelets immediately adhere to the edge of the wound and begin to produce various chemicals that within minutes attract other platelets to the area and create a plug to prevent bleeding. Later, white blood cells initiate a second process that dissolves the plug and ultimately rebuilds the vessel. In most situations, this action of platelets, known as aggregation, is highly desirable—in fact, essential. But when the injury occurs in the wall of a plaque-lined artery, platelet aggregation is detrimental, leading to thickening of the plaque and the development of potentially deadly blood clots.

The buildup of platelets upon injured blood vessels depends on a prostaglandin called thromboxane A_2. The main functions of thromboxane A_2 are to promote platelet aggregation and constrict blood vessels, so suppression of this particular prostaglandin should curtail the destructive process. But the picture gets complicated when other prostaglandins, also subject to suppression by aspirin, enter it. Specifically, a prostaglandin called prostacyclin is important in preventing platelet aggregation and dilating blood vessels. A reduction in prostacyclin could cause heart attacks instead of preventing them. Very large doses of aspirin given to animals have had just that effect.

Current thinking holds that for aspirin to be effective in preventing heart attacks and other cardiovascular problems, the dose should suppress thromboxane A_2 while preserving prostacyclin. A small aspirin dose, such as the single tablet (325 milligrams) every other day used in the Physicians' Health Study, may achieve this balance. Some researchers even believe that other studies of aspirin and heart disease showed little or no aspirin efficacy because the doses were too large.

Interestingly, an imbalance between thromboxane A_2 and prostacyclin in the blood supply to the uterus is also thought to be involved in the development of preeclampsia, a dangerous condition marked by high blood pressure in the final months of pregnancy. Preliminary studies in Europe indicate that low doses of aspirin may protect against this disorder, as well as against a similar disorder in which fetal growth is slowed drastically for no apparent reason. Larger studies of this possibility are now under way; until they are concluded, it is inadvisable for pregnant women to use aspirin.

Cautions on Aspirin Use

The day after the report on the Physicians' Health Study was published in the *New England Journal of Medicine* (on January 28, 1988), aspirin manufacturers launched an advertising campaign promoting their

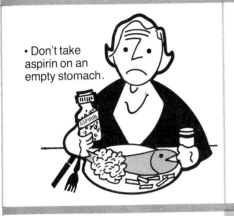

• Don't take aspirin on an empty stomach.

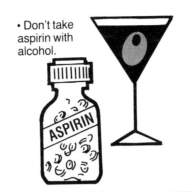

• Don't take aspirin with alcohol.

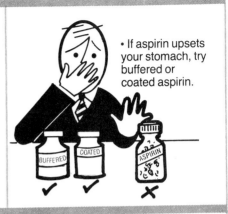

• If aspirin upsets your stomach, try buffered or coated aspirin.

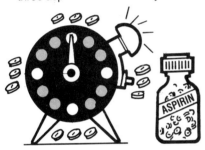

• Unless advised otherwise by your doctor, never take more than three aspirin four times a day.

TAKING ASPIRIN SAFELY

Aspirin is a powerful drug that should be used carefully to prevent possible unwanted effects.

• If your doctor prescribes another medication or a particular treatment, ask if aspirin will interact with it.

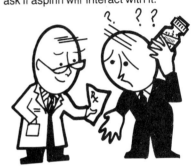

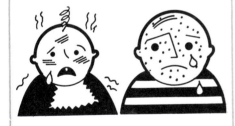

• Don't give aspirin to children suffering from chicken pox or influenza.

• Do not take aspirin without a doctor's approval if you have any of the following: liver disease, kidney disease, a bleeding disorder like hemophilia, a history of asthma, a bleeding ulcer, chronic hives, nasal polyps.

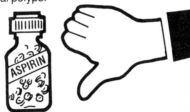

• If aspirin smells like vinegar, it is too old and should be discarded.

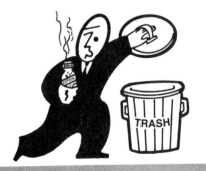

product's ability to prevent first heart attacks. This bold action came on top of early publicity of the report, which put watered-down versions of the study's results into the hands of laypeople before their doctors had a chance to evaluate the evidence.

As a result, both the manufacturers and the news media came under fire for gross irresponsibility. The premature publicity, said Representative Henry Waxman (D, Calif.), chairman of the House Subcommittee on Health and the Environment, was a "disservice to consumers and a public health hazard." Many prominent physicians emphasized that taking aspirin was no substitute for exercising, losing weight, stopping smoking, lowering blood cholesterol levels, or controlling high blood pressure, all of which substantially reduce an individual's risk of heart disease. The Federal Trade Commission and FDA warned aspirin makers to stop their campaign until more information was available.

These reactions were justified. Despite aspirin's nonprescription status and the public's perception of it as being innocuous, it is a powerful drug with more than a few potential dangers. Its anti-platelet effect makes it hazardous for anyone with a bleeding disorder such as hemophilia. Its tendency to cause gastric irritation makes it unsafe for anyone with a bleeding stomach ulcer. Furthermore, it can interact dangerously with certain other drugs, including anticoagulants, oral medications to control diabetes, and drugs to treat gout. (Large doses of aspirin may relieve gout, but newer drugs are more effective, and small amounts of aspirin actually exacerbate the disease.) In general, unless a doctor has specifically prescribed it as an adjunct, people taking other arthritis medications should not take aspirin as well.

In pregnant women, aspirin can prolong gestation and labor and cause increased bleeding at the time of delivery. It is also associated with low birth weight in newborns. And because it passes through the liver and is excreted by the kidneys, aspirin is unsafe for anyone with liver or kidney disease.

Despite its innocuous reputation, aspirin can be dangerous for certain people.

Stomach Problems and Aspirin Intolerance

The most common side effect of aspirin is stomach upset, which most likely occurs because aspirin suppresses prostaglandins that otherwise cause the secretion of substances that protect delicate stomach tissue from irritants. Stomach upset occurs in up to 25 percent of users and can range in severity from mild heartburn (the most frequent complaint, present in about 23 percent of aspirin users) to sharp pain and vomiting (in fewer than 2 percent of users). Endoscopic studies, in which the inside of the stomach is visually examined through a device passed down the throat and esophagus, found that one 650-milligram dose of aspirin—two standard tablets—causes minor bleeding (usually insignificant in healthy people) and irritation in the stomach lining in almost all patients. Irritation worsens with larger and more frequent doses of aspirin and can be minimized with enteric-coated aspirin (tablets with a special coating to prevent them from dissolving until they pass through the stomach into the intestines) or with buffered aspirin (coated to lessen stomach irritation).

Ordinarily, the stomach lining adapts to aspirin so that regular doses do not lead to bleeding or ulcers. This adaptation is best exemplified by arthritis patients, only a quarter of whom have visible injuries to the stomach lining after taking large doses of aspirin for long periods. In some people, however, aspirin continues to cause damage; in these individuals, continuous aspirin use may cause ulcers or chronic blood loss leading to iron deficiency anemia.

Aspirin has also been linked to serious episodes of heavy bleeding in the stomach, but the connection remains tenuous. Some doctors think the association only appears to exist because of the frequency of aspirin use in the general population; in any group of people with any disorder, they reason, you are bound to find a preponderance of aspirin users, but that doesn't mean aspirin causes the disorder. A recent study that attempted to overcome this statistical problem, however, found that the risk of acute bleeding in the upper gastrointestinal tract was 15 times greater in frequent aspirin users than in those who used no aspirin.

A small number of people suffer an outbreak of hives, an asthma attack, burning eyes, or nasal congestion when they take aspirin. This aspirin intolerance is most common in people with preexisting conditions such as chronic hives, nasal polyps, and severe asthma. Individuals who have these problems with aspirin are usually also sensitive to similar drugs such as ibuprofen and naproxen (a prescription anti-inflammatory drug sold as Naprosyn).

Risks in Children

Aspirin use in children and adolescents who have chicken pox or influenza appears to lead to a frightening and often fatal disease called Reye's syndrome. The syndrome, first described in Australia in 1963, manifests itself late in the course of a seemingly minor illness. The symptoms include vomiting, fatigue, disorientation, and belligerence, and patients often lapse into comas before the syndrome is diagnosed. In the early 1980s several studies suggested that the common denominator in most Reye's syndrome cases was ingestion of aspirin or aspirin-containing drugs in the preceding illness. A large pilot study reported by the U.S. Public Health Service in 1985 confirmed this connection.

In light of these findings, health officials issued public warnings against giving aspirin to children, and aspirin manufacturers placed similar warnings on package labels. In the years since Reye's syndrome first came to public attention, sales of children's aspirin have declined, while sales of children's acetaminophen have increased. Paralleling those changes, the number of reported U.S. cases of Reye's syndrome decreased from 555 in 1980 to 101 in 1986.

Although scientists have yet to prove definitively that aspirin causes Reye's syndrome, it is generally agreed that children and adolescents up to age 19 should take acetaminophen instead. If a child must take aspirin for a condition such as juvenile rheumatoid arthritis, close medical supervision is necessary.

However, perhaps a greater threat to children (and adults) is the risk of an aspirin overdose. As few as 30 adult-strength aspirin have been known to cause death in adults; a fraction of that number can be fatal to a child. Of the 10,000 cases of aspirin poisoning reported each year, a substantial number are in children under age five. Symptoms of aspirin overdose are vomiting, fever, sweating, and hyperventilation. In extreme cases, the respiratory system shuts down, resulting in death.

A milder form of aspirin toxicity, marked by ringing in the ears, dizziness, and disorientation, can result from long-term ingestion of large doses of aspirin. This reaction can be reversed by reducing the aspirin dosage. ☐

Children and adolescents should usually take acetaminophen instead of aspirin, which has been linked to Reye's syndrome.

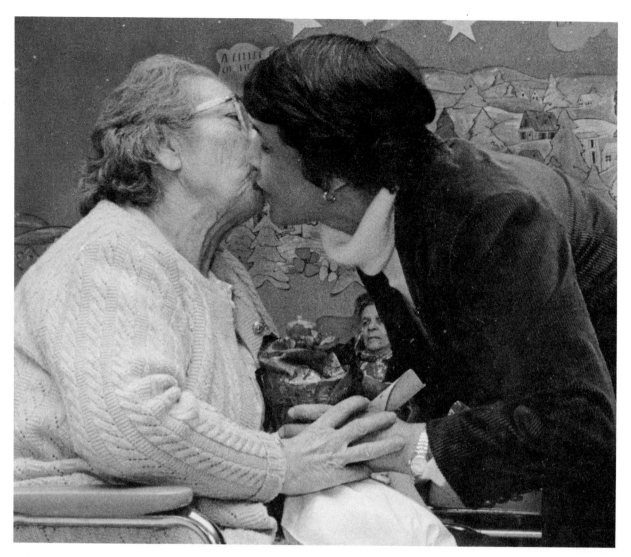

Choosing Long-Term Care

Barbara Scherr Trenk

To provide the special care many older people need, a variety of services and facilities are available. Options range from at-home assistance to full-time medical attention in a nursing home.

Millions of Americans are faced with the problem of how to provide the best possible care for aging parents and other relatives or friends. People are living longer and, with old age, often need special custodial or medical attention. Who is to provide this, and where is it to be provided?

Some younger people take on at least part of this care themselves. A survey by Travelers Insurance Company of Illinois found that 20 percent of its employees over the age of 30 provided at least some care for an elderly parent. One researcher estimates that in the United States, 27 million days of unpaid, informal care are provided each week for chronically ill or disabled elderly people, either in their own homes or in those of relatives.

For those who want professional care for an elderly person, several options exist—from hiring part-time healthcare workers who go into the individual's home to placing the individual in a full-care nursing home. The trick is in selecting the right alternative. The American Association of Retired Persons suggests that the key to obtaining optimum care lies in exploring various options before there is a crisis that requires hasty decision making. People can get help in making sensible choices from a number of sources. Government offices for the aged, private and voluntary social service agencies, public libraries, and friends and neighbors who have faced similar decisions can all provide useful information.

The Luxury of Living at Home

Often those who must arrange for care for ill or disabled elderly people start out by investigating ways of enabling them to remain in their own homes. Surveys show that most older people prefer to remain at home, and this is often the most comfortable choice for children as well.

Many older people who need assistance but not around-the-clock care benefit from an adult day-care center. Here they may receive hot meals, nutritious snacks, assistance with medication, rehabilitation services, and counseling (and also take part in recreational activities). A medical expert devises a specific, structured program for each participating individual. Hospitals, nursing homes, city and county governments, religious organizations, and privately owned centers provide this form of care. Adult day-care centers are usually open five days a week, roughly during regular business hours. Many are extending service to weekends. Participants can usually attend any number of days during a week. The centers give family and friends a much-needed break in responsibility for an older person's care.

Home health aides can be hired through home health agencies on an hourly basis to help older people with bathing, preparing meals, shopping, and light housekeeping. In some states these nonmedical services may be covered by Medicaid for low-income elderly people.

Skilled nursing care, as well as speech and physical therapy, is available through home health agencies. Because Medicare—the U.S.

Barbara Scherr Trenk is a free-lance writer who specializes in health subjects.

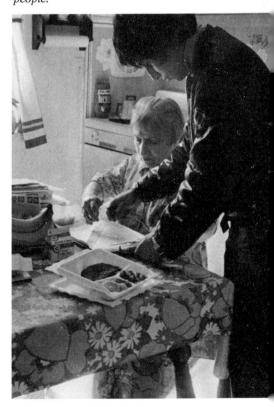

A woman signs a receipt for her dinner from Meals on Wheels, one of many services for housebound elderly people.

government's health insurance program for those over age 65—and Medicaid—the joint federal-state health insurance program for the poor—pay for some physician-ordered home healthcare services, it's a good idea to be sure that an agency considered for home healthcare participates in these government programs. The agency that supplies such professionals should work with the patient's physician to develop a written plan for services.

Before contracting for nursing care or care by home health aides, check the references of both the agency through which the help is hired and the individuals themselves. The American Association of Retired Persons advises that the agency should be insured against injury to its employees working in patients' homes and should be responsible for paying workers' Social Security and withholding taxes.

A Difficult Decision

Despite the availability of these services, some older people cannot live independently. Relatives or friends may, then, consider inviting these people to live with them. While providing such care may be satisfying and rewarding, it can also cause social, emotional, and financial problems. It is important for potential caregivers to be realistic about the problems as well as the benefits and to weigh the needs of the older person against those of the entire family. A study by the Duke

Adult day-care centers and neighborhood centers offer hot meals, recreational activities, and rides to and from the facilities.

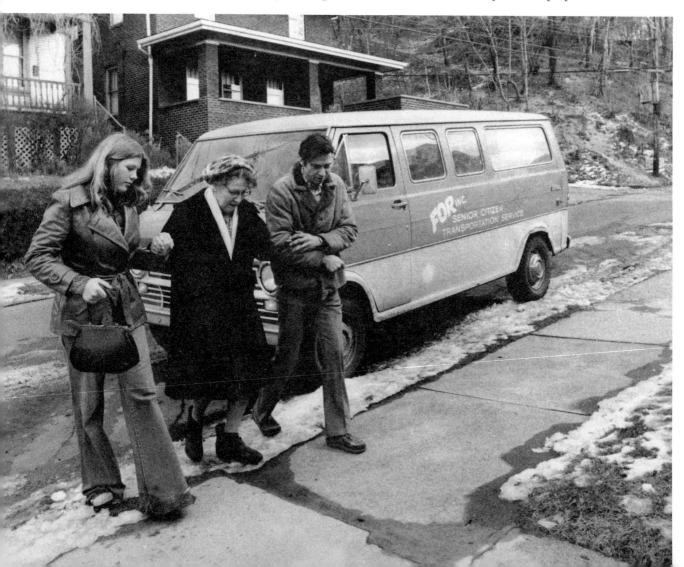

University Center for Aging found that people caring for relatives with Alzheimer's disease, a major disabling disease of the elderly, used prescription drugs for depression, tension, and sleep disorders over three times as much as the general population. In addition, 22 percent of the caregivers used alcohol every day to relax or get to sleep.

Nursing home care is sometimes the best answer for both elderly individuals and their families. While not advocating nursing home care for all older people, the American Association of Retired Persons advises that a nursing home may be appropriate for those who need "continuous healthcare for an extended period of time." Even with such assurances, however, people often feel guilty about arranging for someone, especially a parent, spouse, or close friend, to stay in a nursing home, rather than in their own home. They also fear that the person will not be well cared for. Beyond these concerns, there is the reality of paying for nursing home care.

The weight of these concerns is often compounded by the need to make a fast decision, during a period of great stress, about placing someone in a nursing home. For example, after a parent has been hospitalized for an acute illness, the doctor might say that the patient's medical condition no longer warrants hospital care—but needs more attention than can be provided at home. Or perhaps family members are exhausted or frustrated from the responsibility of caring for the patient at home. Before trying to decide which nursing home is best, it is important to be realistic about the need for making such a choice. A person haunted by guilt or overwhelmed by new responsibilities will not be able to appraise any facility fairly.

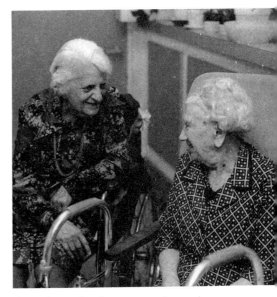

A good nursing home can give residents a communal environment and the opportunity to make new friends.

What Nursing Homes Offer

There are 1.6 million people in nearly 20,000 nursing homes in the United States. While some residents of these facilities are young adults and men and women of middle age, the vast majority of residents are over 65. About 5 percent of all Americans over the age of 65 live in nursing homes; one-fourth of those over 65 spend at least some time in a nursing home. The average age of nursing home patients is now 80, up from 77.9 in 1977.

Different types of nursing homes provide different levels of care. A skilled nursing facility provides 24-hour care, rehabilitation programs, and other specialized services under the supervision of a registered nurse. The cost ranges from $65 to $140 or more a day.

An intermediate care facility (also known as a health-related facility) offers personal care and help with daily living activities, plus less intensive nursing care than that available at a skilled nursing facility. Residents are not well enough to live independently, yet do not need 24-hour nursing care or supervision. This kind of care generally costs between $40 and $70 a day.

Custodial nursing home care is for people who need assistance with personal care (such as with dressing, bathing, and eating) in addition to room and board, but who don't require regular healthcare services. This type of care typically costs $35 to $55 a day.

Some facilities offer all three kinds of care, with patients grouped on floors or wings according to the kind of assistance they require.

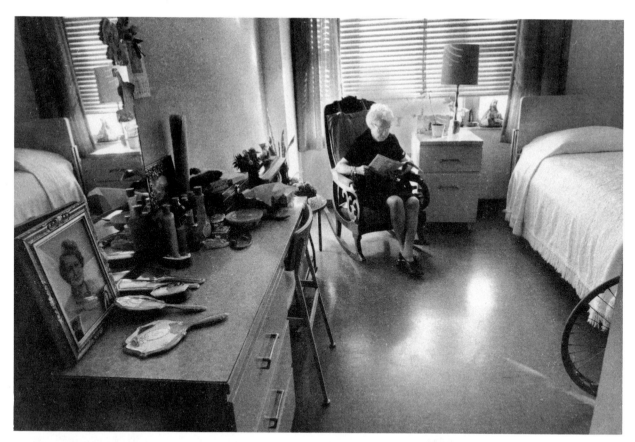

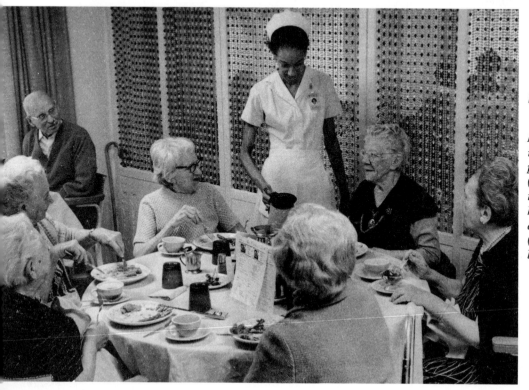

Levels of Care

Nursing homes provide varying levels of care. Some have private rooms for people (above) who do not need full-time healthcare but may need help with personal care, such as meals (left) and grooming (above right, a nursing home beauty parlor).

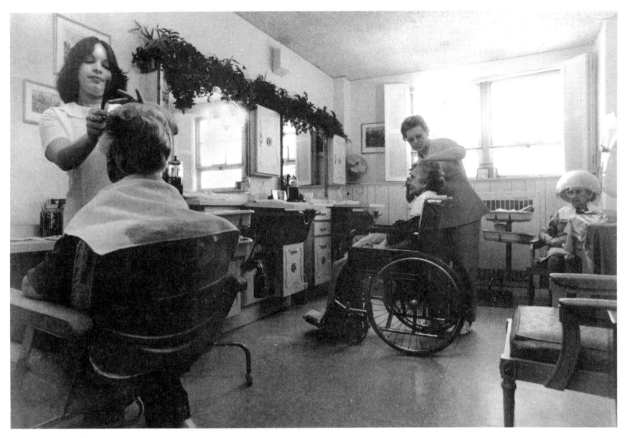

Sources of Information

Often the best way to begin looking for a nursing home is to talk to people who know nursing home residents and have recently visited homes in the area where your relative or friend would like to live. Talk with the physicians who are currently treating the patient to find out whether they have other patients living in nursing homes. Ask where your person's specific medical needs would best be met. For instance, some homes may have special facilities for stroke victims; others may be better prepared to meet the special needs of Alzheimer's patients. If the patient is hospitalized at the time the decision is made, talk with the hospital social worker. If you are happy with the care provided at that hospital, find out which nursing homes transfer their patients to that hospital for acute care.

Members of the clergy frequently visit people in nearby nursing homes and often counsel those who are dealing with the stress of an older person's illness. They may be good sources of information about facilities that would meet the patient's needs.

Local mental health associations, Ys, and community centers sometimes hold programs on choosing nursing homes. These programs provide an opportunity to share experiences with other people facing the same decision. Such organizations may also have ongoing group meetings for people with parents in declining health.

Voluntary social service organizations—the National Conference of Catholic Charities, the Federation of Jewish Philanthropies, the

63

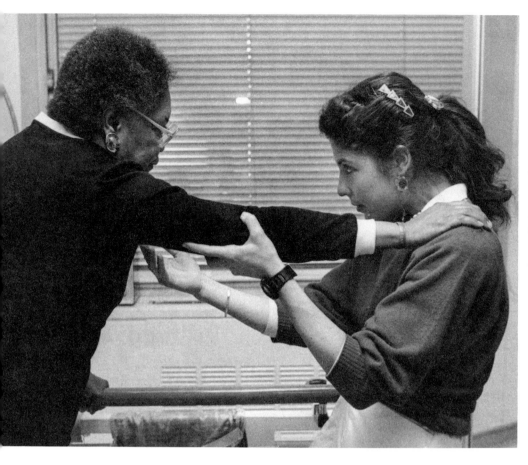

Medical Attention

At a skilled nursing facility, residents in need of more serious medical attention can receive physical therapy (left) and intensive care (right).

Federation of Protestant Welfare Agencies, and the United Way, to name a few—may be able to recommend agencies that can provide advice on nursing homes. Other resources include reference staff at public libraries and state and county offices on the aging.

Consumer groups in some communities publish evaluations of nursing homes, and in 1988 the U.S. Health Care Financing Administration published a comprehensive guide to all nursing homes nationwide that participate in Medicare and Medicaid. While such guides may be useful, Toby Edelman of the National Senior Citizens Law Center warns that because the quality of nursing homes can change, the information can become outdated by the time it is distributed. "It can be misleading in both directions, making some homes look better than they really are, and others look worse," she said.

Factors to Consider

Just as no one college is best for all students, no single nursing home is best for all patients. A variety of factors need to be considered before a final choice is made.

Geography should be one factor. If the elderly person lives in a home that is near family and friends, visits can be frequent and casual. This is often more satisfactory for both the resident and visitors than long

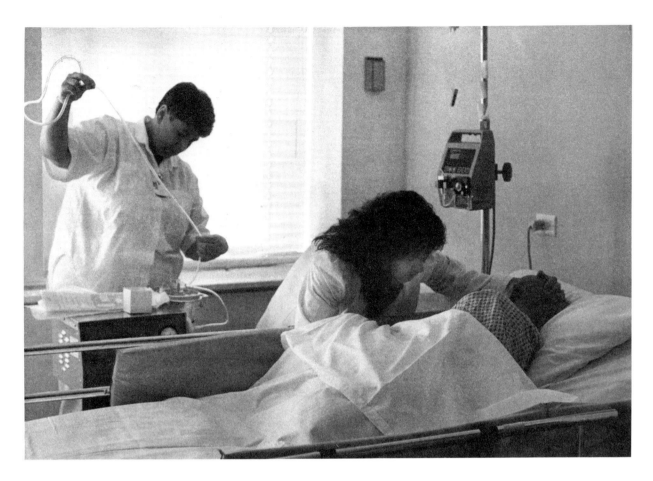

weekly or monthly trips and extended visits. Consider also the convenience of visiting hours. Can people who work during the day visit in the evening?

Sometimes moving to a nursing home in the community where the person has lived provides an opportunity for reunions with friends. When an 82-year-old New York City woman moved to a nursing home after a broken hip left her unable to live at home, she was pleasantly surprised to learn that the home's residents included former neighbors from her apartment building. Moving to a facility near home may also allow outings to familiar spots—trips to a favorite restaurant or a chance to sit on a familiar park bench.

Nursing homes operated by religious groups may appeal to some people, especially if they have been active church or synagogue members. The opportunity for daily worship offers religious comfort as well as social benefits for people who share a common bond. People whose first language is not English may be more comfortable in a residence where patients and staff also speak their native language.

Getting a Firsthand Look

You will probably want to visit several nursing homes before deciding which is most appropriate. Besides looking for such physical qualities as cleanliness, convenience of bathrooms, and compliance with fire safety regulations, pay attention to the general feeling of the place, its ambience. Is the paint fresh—not just in the entry lobby, but in the residents' rooms? Do residents hang pictures on the walls and keep photos of grandchildren on their night tables, or is the atmosphere sterile and impersonal? Do staff members address patients by name and with respect, or is attention less than warm and caring?

When you go to see the home, ask what kinds of facilities are available for family visits. Can furniture be moved into conversational groupings? Are private rooms available for times when confidential family matters must be discussed? One Long Island, N.Y., family arranged to have their Thanksgiving dinner at the nursing home where the wife's mother lives. The facility allowed them to use a private room, and the family supplied the turkey and trimmings.

Paying for a Nursing Home

Economics often play a role in the choice of a nursing home. The cost of nursing home care is high—averaging $22,000 a year in 1988.

For nursing home residents whose social interaction might otherwise be limited to other elderly people and staff, some facilities make efforts to bring young visitors into the home, such as the high school girl below.

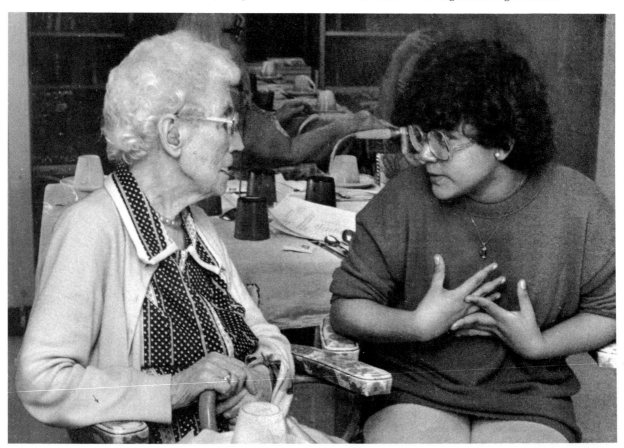

According to *Caring for the Disabled Elderly*, a study by the Brookings Institution (a nonprofit scientific and educational public interest corporation in Washington, D.C.), more than half of all nursing home patients ultimately depend on public payments for their care.

Under the 1988 catastrophic health insurance act, which took effect January 1, 1989, and greatly revised the Medicare program, Medicare pays for a greater share of nursing home stays. Although it does not cover custodial care, it does pay for up to 150 days of skilled nursing home care a year. (Patients pay 20 percent of the average daily cost of the first eight days.)

For the "medically indigent," Medicaid pays for intermediate and custodial nursing home care. It is not unusual for people who never expected to need a social service program to use up most of their financial resources on nursing home care and become eligible for Medicaid. Because many people who enter nursing homes will eventually qualify for Medicaid benefits, it may be desirable to choose a home that is certified for Medicaid, even if residents will be paying for their own care initially.

The new catastrophic health insurance law also reduces the threat of poverty for spouses of nursing home patients who qualify for Medicaid. The amount of assets that at-home spouses may retain will be increased to $12,000 (this provision takes effect after September 30, 1989); until 1989, a nest egg of only $1,800 was allowed.

When Problems Arise

Relatives and friends of nursing home patients should be alert to the kind of care they receive. Sometimes older people may be reluctant to speak up if they are not getting proper treatment. They may not question doctors or nursing home staff if they do not receive the physical therapy prescribed for them, or they may not know that they can request substitutions for certain foods served at meals.

New regulations for nursing homes that accept Medicare and Medicaid were proposed in early 1989 by the U.S. Department of Health and Human Services. When finalized and put into effect, these regulations would require nursing homes to ensure, among other things, that patients enjoy privacy, are allowed visitors, and are free from physical or verbal abuse. Facilities providing nursing care would be required to have some type of nurse on duty 24 hours a day.

Patients and families should also be aware that each state has an ombudsman program to handle questions and complaints about long-term care. These programs were mandated by Congress in 1978 as a way of curbing widely publicized nursing home abuse. Many states have a separate long-term-care ombudsman's office. In some states the program is part of the agency on aging; in others it may be part of the human services department or attached directly to the governor's office.

About 9,000 paid and volunteer advocates for elderly nursing home residents work in more than 700 state and local ombudsman programs throughout the United States. Representatives of these programs can help to resolve a wide range of potential problems. They can go to the nursing home and negotiate when there are misunderstandings between patients or their families and nursing home administrators over the

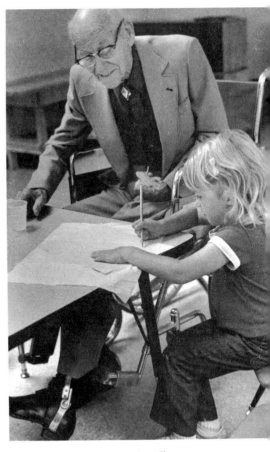

An innovative program in Albuquerque, N.M., combines a nursing home with a day-care center, with benefits to both the elderly and the children.

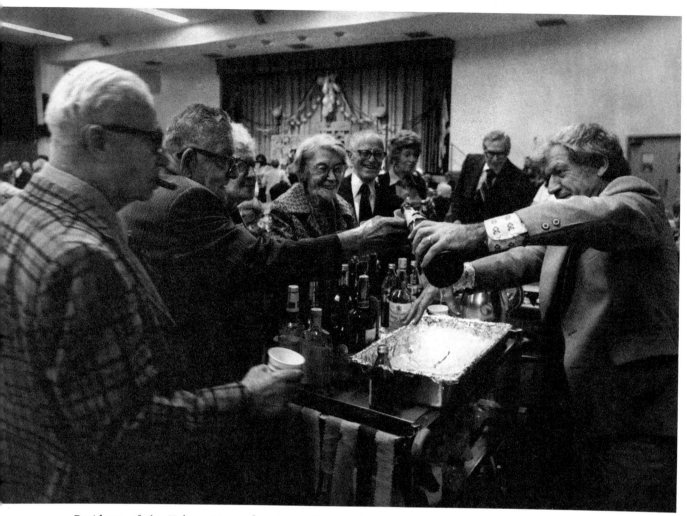

Residents of the Hebrew Home for the Aged in New York City celebrate their monthly cabaret night.

kind of care to be provided. They can see that violations of the health code are corrected. The office in some states may have information that will help in selecting a nursing home.

Planning for the Future

What can be done to plan ahead for the care of parents or other older people who are still healthy? Some experts recommend long-term-care insurance policies. While these policies are expected to pay for more nursing home care in the future, in 1985 they covered only about 1 percent of expenditures for long-term care.

By 1989, more than a million long-term-care policies were in force in the United States, with over 100 different companies marketing them. But Consumers Union and other experts warn shoppers to consider these policies carefully before buying. Some policies exclude mental illness from coverage, some limit the types of nursing home care paid for, and some provide coverage only for patients who have first been hospitalized. Some policies will not pay for the care of patients who have or develop Alzheimer's disease. Some of the best policies, warns

Consumers Union, are available only to healthy people, with rejection rates running as high as 30 percent.

The cost of long-term-care insurance increases with the age of the purchaser; for example, it may run less than $100 a month for a person 65 years of age, but be substantially more expensive for older people. In May 1988, *Consumer Reports* recommended that people under 60 should not buy such insurance unless benefits rise periodically with inflation. Many policies offer between $25 and $60 a day in benefits, but offer no adjustment for inflation. By the time 60-year-old policy purchasers needed their coverage, nursing homes costs could average $200 a day.

Another way of planning ahead for long-term care is for an older person to join a continuing care community. But these facilities, which combine the benefits of an insurance policy and a retirement community, are expensive. There is an initial entrance fee (which can range from $15,000 to $250,000), and monthly charges may be between $250 and $1,500. Residents have private apartments or cottages and share dining and recreational facilities. Such services as housekeeping and meals may be provided as part of the basic fees or may be billed separately. Prepaid healthcare is provided as part of the contract when a person moves into a continuing care community, but the kinds of care and extent of coverage may vary. These communities usually have nursing homes on-site to which a person may move if necessary. But financial arrangements may change if a person moves from an apartment or cottage to a facility that provides more services.

It's important to investigate thoroughly the background of the managers of such a community, as well as the operating organization's financial status. Prospective residents should ask for information on the community's reserve funding and learn whether their prepaid fees will be placed in an escrow account. Attention to the facility's financing and business operation is important, because if it were to become bankrupt, residents could end up without a place to live after having invested their life savings in the community. ☐

It is important to make plans for an older person's future living arrangements while the person is still healthy.

SOURCES OF FURTHER INFORMATION

American Association of Retired Persons, 1909 K Street NW, Washington, DC 20049.
National Citizens' Coalition for Nursing Home Reform, 1426 16th Street NW, Washington, DC 20036.

SUGGESTIONS FOR FURTHER READING

American Association of Retired Persons. *The Right Place at the Right Time: A Guide to Long-Term Care Choices.* Washington, D.C., AARP, 1985.
MANNING, DOUG. *The Nursing Home Dilemma: How to Make One of Love's Toughest Decisions.* New York, Harper & Row, 1986.
RICHARDS, MARTY, et al. *Choosing a Nursing Home: A Guidebook for Families.* Seattle, University of Washington Press, 1985.
RIVLIN, ALICE, AND JOSHUA WIENER. *Caring for the Disabled Elderly.* Washington, D.C., Brookings Institution, 1988.

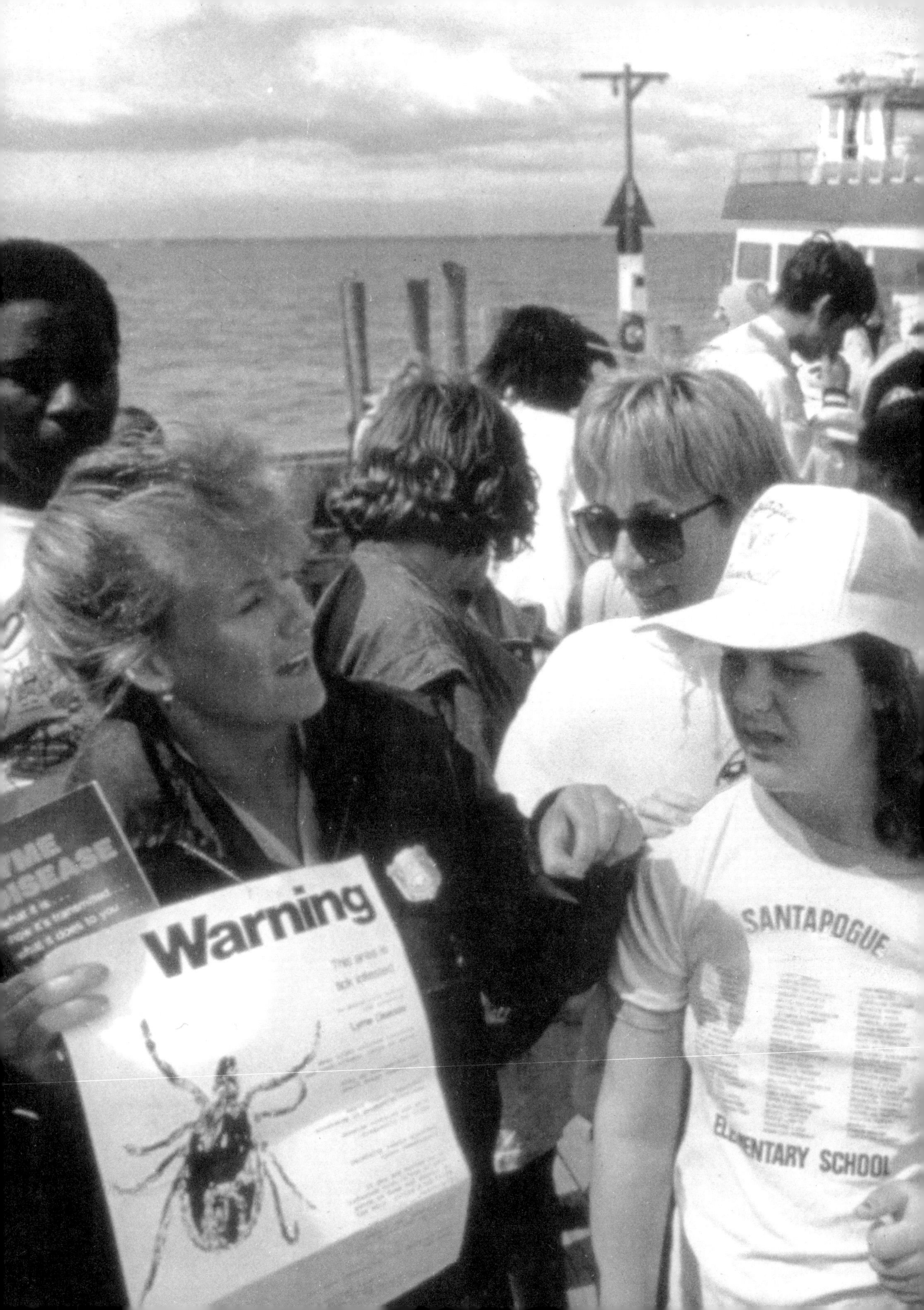
Warning
LYME
DISEASE
SANTAPOGUE
ELEMENTARY SCHOOL

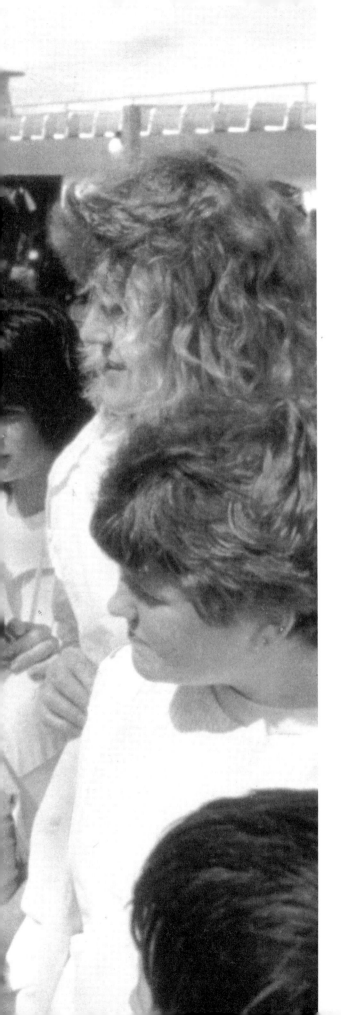

Lyme Disease

James F. Jekel, M.D., M.P.H.

Fifteen years ago no one had heard of Lyme disease. Today it is the most common tick-borne illness in the United States and continues to spread. The tick that carries it flourishes in grassy areas and woodlands, often suburban or semirural in character. People who live or work in such areas, or who go there for recreation, need to take precautions.

Lyme disease has been called a "great imitator" because of the variety of symptoms it can produce, including skin rash, arthritis, and problems of the heart and nervous system. The symptoms can mislead a physician trying to make a diagnosis. The disease is not usually fatal and generally can be effectively treated with antibiotics—if the treatment is begun soon after infection. But if not treated quickly, Lyme disease can condemn its victim to years, perhaps even a lifetime, of painful, debilitating ills. Were it not for AIDS, Lyme disease would be studied and talked about much more than it is at the present time.

"Watch out for ticks!" a park ranger warns people arriving at the Fire Island National Seashore, east of New York City. The area is one of many now infested with ticks carrying the bacterium that causes Lyme disease.

Discovery of a New Disease

There is evidence that Lyme disease has been around for some time. Its hallmark—a spreading, red "bull's-eye" rash—was described in Sweden as early as 1909. An instance of what may have been Lyme disease was reported as long ago as 1887 in Australia.

But in a sense the discovery of the disease may be said to have begun in 1975, when two concerned mothers in the Lyme, Conn., area alerted the Connecticut State Health Department to the existence of an unusual pattern of arthritis cases. One woman, a resident of Old Lyme, a village with a population of about 5,000, reported that 12 children, including her own daughter, had been diagnosed as having juvenile rheumatoid arthritis, which is ordinarily rather rare. The other woman was a Lyme artist who was sometimes unable to paint owing to arthritis in her hands and who for years had suffered a variety of ailments of unknown origin. By 1975 her husband and two sons had symptoms of what would later be called Lyme disease. One of her sons was diagnosed as having juvenile rheumatoid arthritis. This alarmed her, because she knew that a number of area children were thought to have the disease; she was particularly disturbed that an "epidemic" of arthritis seemed to be occurring in her very own family.

A team of specialists from the Yale University School of Medicine, headed by Dr. Allen C. Steere, a rheumatologist, investigated the situation. In the towns of Lyme, Old Lyme, and East Haddam, with a combined population of about 12,000, they found 39 children and 12 adults showing the symptoms of what they called Lyme arthritis. The researchers were struck by the fact that the cases were clustered in a wooded area, occurred within families, and typically began in summer or early fall. This suggested that the illness was caused by a microorganism carried by an insect or perhaps by a tick. Of the 51 patients, 13 showed the spreading red rash, which decades before had been named erythema chronicum migrans (ECM for short; the name means chronic migrating red rash). A major break in the search for the carrier of the disease came in 1977 when nine patients remembered having been bitten by a tick at a place on the skin where the rash later developed. One of the nine had even saved the tick.

Each year brought new cases. These and the original cases were carefully studied over several years. The researchers saw, of course, arthritis. It was migratory—that is, the arthritis would affect one or two joints for a few days or weeks, then get better, only to reappear later somewhere else. But nervous system problems also showed up; some patients developed meningitis (inflammation of membranes surrounding the brain) or suffered pain or weakness due to nerve damage. And there were heart problems, mostly abnormal heart rhythms. Because the illness in the long run clearly involved many body systems, the name "Lyme arthritis" gave way, by 1979, to the more general "Lyme disease."

James F. Jekel is professor of epidemiology and public health at the Yale University School of Medicine.

Were it not for AIDS, Lyme disease would receive much more public attention than it has.

72

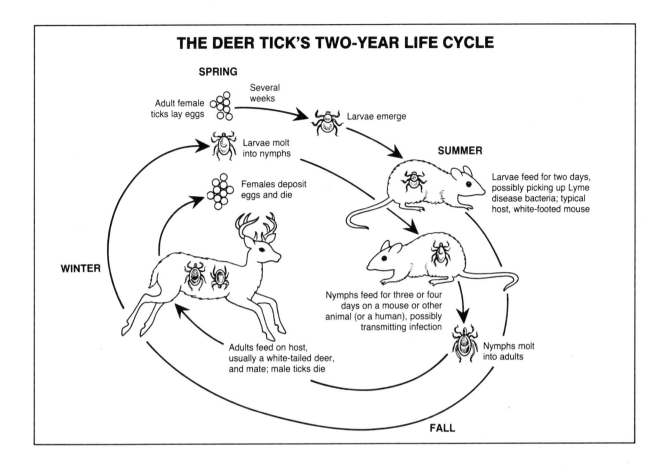

THE DEER TICK'S TWO-YEAR LIFE CYCLE

SPRING

Adult female ticks lay eggs

Several weeks

Larvae emerge

Larvae molt into nymphs

Females deposit eggs and die

SUMMER

Larvae feed for two days, possibly picking up Lyme disease bacteria; typical host, white-footed mouse

WINTER

Nymphs feed for three or four days on a mouse or other animal (or a human), possibly transmitting infection

Adults feed on host, usually a white-tailed deer, and mate; male ticks die

Nymphs molt into adults

FALL

The Cause, a Bacterium

Initially it was widely thought that the cause of Lyme disease would prove to be a virus. But Steere and his colleagues found that penicillin was effective against ECM and sometimes prevented the development of arthritis in new patients from Connecticut. This antibiotic was known to combat bacteria.

European studies of ECM discovered suggestive evidence that the microorganism being sought was a spirochete. Spirochetes are small corkscrew-shaped bacteria that cause diseases like syphilis and relapsing fever. European researchers showed that ECM is infectious in origin with a series of experiments using scientist-volunteers: it was found that the rash could be passed from one person to another through inoculation with tissue taken from the edge of an active rash. Early studies in Europe also suggested that antibiotic treatment was effective against ECM.

The tick responsible for spreading the disease in the Connecticut area was identified as the tiny deer tick, *Ixodes dammini*. In 1982 the spirochete responsible, a new species, was discovered by Willy Burgdorfer and his colleagues in ticks collected on Shelter Island, a major Lyme disease area in New York State. Burgdorfer, a specialist in tick diseases, worked at the Rocky Mountain Laboratories in Hamilton, Mont., part of the National Institute of Allergy and Infectious

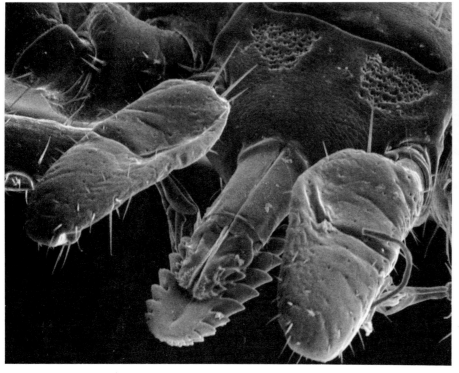

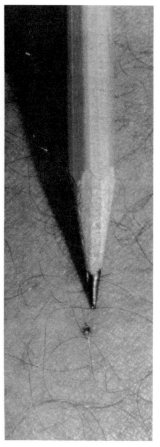

The Deer Tick Up Close

The fearsome object above is the head of an adult tick; the jutting "proboscis" drills into the host's skin and draws out blood. In actuality, the adult is only slightly larger than the nymph, seen at right on a man's leg.

Diseases. His group injected the spirochete into rabbits and produced a rash like ECM. The bacterium was eventually named *Borellia burgdorferi*.

Lyme disease was found to be spread by other types of *Ixodes* ticks as well. *Ixodes dammini* was the main cause in the Northeast United States, but on the West Coast there was *Ixodes pacificus*, and in Europe, *Ixodes ricinus*. The spirochetes in ticks from California and Europe are very similar, if not identical, to *Borellia burgdorferi*.

The Tick

Ticks, like spiders and mites, generally have eight legs, while insects have six. Many ticks do not carry any disease at all. But others do. Before Lyme disease burst into prominence, pride of place among tick-borne diseases in the United States belonged to Rocky Mountain spotted fever, which is potentially more dangerous—it can be fatal if not treated. Other diseases caused by microorganisms borne by ticks include relapsing fever and babesios, a mild (in most cases) malaria-like disease that can be carried by the same kind of tick as Lyme disease. There also is the condition called tick paralysis, apparently caused by a poison produced by some ticks.

The ticks that spread Lyme disease are much smaller, and less common, than the familiar dog tick. The deer tick is about the size of a pinhead and, except when it is engorged with blood after eating, is very difficult to see. It usually feeds on white-tailed deer and white-footed mice; it may also be found on several species of birds and, occasionally, on raccoons.

The deer tick's life cycle lasts two years. After hatching in the spring or summer, the young ticks, six-legged larvae, attach themselves to small animals or birds. They treat themselves to a blood meal and then rest until the following spring, when the larvae molt, becoming eight-legged "nymphs." The nymphs, looking for a blood meal, attach themselves typically to small rodents, notably the white-tailed mouse, but sometimes a nymph takes a human for a host. With the end of summer, the ticks, now adults, attach themselves to deer, but dogs or humans can also be hosts. The adult ticks mate and then die—first the males and then, the following spring, the females, after they lay their eggs.

If a tick's host is infected with Lyme disease bacteria, the tick may ingest them when it takes its blood meal. People commonly pick up ticks on their bodies as they walk through infested wooded or grassy areas. Exactly how the bacteria are transmitted from tick to human is not well understood. In most of the ticks studied the spirochetes were in the middle part of the digestive tract, from which they would not ordinarily be transmitted by the act of biting. A few ticks, however, had a generalized infection, with spirochetes found, among other places, in the storage area for the blood taken during feeding. Perhaps only the rare ticks with a generalized infection spread spirochetes to people when they bite. It is possible, however, that if the tick regurgitates or defecates while biting, spirochetes in the tick intestines may be transmitted to people through contamination of the bite wound.

Lyme's Spread

After the ECM rash was described in Sweden in 1909, it became known throughout Scandinavia and most of Eastern and Western Europe, including England and Scotland. By now, cases of Lyme disease have been reported on every inhabited continent, in at least 19 countries. A few cases have been reported in Canada. The fact that cases have been reported in Australia, where no ticks of the expected varieties occur, makes it probable that other carriers may be involved on occasion.

As to the United States, in 1975 fewer than 60 cases were recorded, and they were all in Connecticut. In 1986, a little over a decade later, about 1,500 new cases were reported, according to the U.S. Centers for Disease Control, and they were distributed in various areas of the country. The number of U.S. cases has grown each year since. The disease has been reported in well over 30 states. Of course, there may be many more cases than those actually reported, not only because diagnosed cases are not always reported to health officials, but also because the varying symptoms, along with the inconclusiveness of blood test results, can easily cause Lyme disease to be mistaken for some other disorder. Until more adequate laboratory diagnostic

Since 1975, Lyme disease has spread from Connecticut to more than 30 other states.

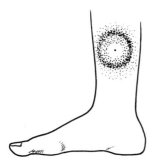

Phase 1

Most victims of Lyme disease develop a spreading, red, bull's-eye rash 3 to 32 days after infection from a tick bite. The rash may be accompanied by flulike symptoms and stiff neck.

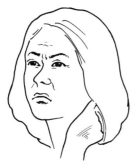

Phase 2

Several weeks or months after the rash, some persons experience heart problems or neurological complications, such as meningitis or pain and paralysis in head and neck nerves.

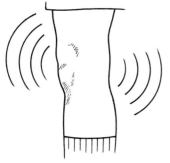

Phase 3

Several weeks to two years after the initial symptoms, many people develop arthritis, which may move from joint to joint but is particularly likely to affect the knees.

techniques are developed, scientists' knowledge of the true incidence of the disease will remain incomplete.

There are three "endemic" areas in the United States, regions where the ticks and spirochetes are found in abundance. Two are the Northeast and the upper Midwest, where the tick involved is *Ixodes dammini*; the third is the California-Oregon region, where the responsible tick is *Ixodes pacificus*. The areas most heavily infested with the ticks in the Northeast are southeast Connecticut, New York State counties just to the north and to the east (Long Island) of New York City, north coastal Massachusetts, Cape Cod, Nantucket, Martha's Vineyard, and rural southeast New Jersey. A quarter of the cases in one New Jersey study were due to exposure to the ticks in outdoor occupations. The states in the Midwest with the most Lyme disease are Wisconsin and Minnesota.

The increase in the spread and number of reported cases over the past decade may be partly due to improved detection and reporting. But the ticks' range does seem to be expanding, and as residential development of the countryside proceeds, increased human contact with ticks may also be playing a role. Some experts speak of a recent population explosion of the ticks. It has been suggested that the growth in the country's deer population may have contributed to the spread of the ticks, which may also have been furthered by migrating birds. Another possibility is that new restrictions on the use of pesticides may have facilitated the ticks' spread.

Symptoms

The symptoms of Lyme disease occur in three phases. Most (but by no means all) infected individuals first develop ECM. The spreading, red, circular rash is centered where the tick bite occurred. The rash tends to be less bright in the center than at the spreading rim, and it appears from 3 to 32 days after the tick bite. It can become as large as 20 inches across. Several such skin lesions may develop over time, and some may not look typical. The rash may be accompanied by headache, fatigue, chills and fever, and aching muscles—it may seem rather like the flu. In addition, there may be a stiff neck and enlarged lymph nodes. These symptoms tend to lessen or disappear within three or four weeks, although the skin rash may reappear.

Several weeks or months after the initial symptoms, some people may experience the second phase, involving the nervous system and/or heart. About 15 percent of patients develop nervous system complications, including meningitis (characterized by head pain and stiff neck) and pain and paralysis in head and neck nerves, such as the facial paralysis called Bell's palsy. These symptoms may last for months but generally go away without causing permanent damage.

Approximately 8 percent of patients develop heart abnormalities, usually producing heart block, a problem with the conduction of electrical impulses in the heart. Other possible problems include inflammation of the heart muscle and outer membrane and, occasionally, enlarged heart. These also tend to disappear, after three to six weeks.

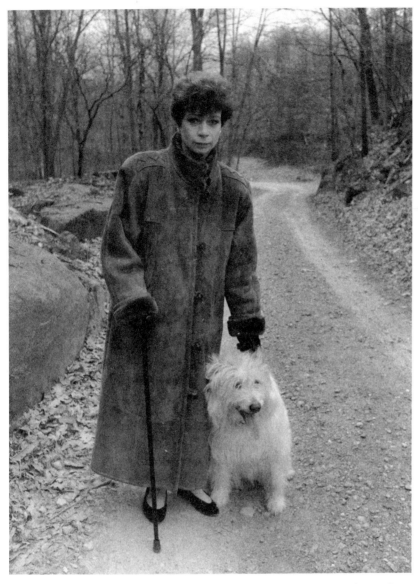

Both Claire Palermo and her dog, Mabel, have Lyme disease. Palermo lives near parkland that is filled with mice and deer—two favorite hosts of disease-bearing ticks.

The third phase begins several weeks to two years after the initial symptoms, when about 60 percent of patients develop arthritis, with pain and swelling of the joints. During this stage many patients often experience fatigue. The arthritis typically moves around from joint to joint, but the knees are especially susceptible. The arthritis becomes chronic in about 10 percent of patients, and bone and cartilage may be worn away, in a manner that somewhat resembles rheumatoid arthritis.

Patients' symptoms often do not clearly point to Lyme disease, and the physician may face a difficult choice in deciding whether or not to treat vague symptoms as though they represent it. ECM is regarded as a good indicator of the presence of Lyme disease, but it does not appear in all victims. The blood tests most commonly available so far are not always accurate, often giving a negative result for people who actually have the disease. Such tests seek to detect antibodies to the Lyme bacterium, but antibodies do not usually appear in the bloodstream until a few weeks after a person is infected. Some authorities consequently recommend that persons with symptoms compatible with Lyme disease who may have been exposed to the ticks be treated as though they have the disease.

It is unclear to what extent Lyme disease in pregnant women poses a hazard to their infants, but some stillborn or newborn infants whose mothers had the disease have been found to be infected with the bacterium causing it. Doctors think that the hazard to the fetus is greatest when the mother is in the early stages of the disease.

Treatment

In the early stages of Lyme disease, such antibiotics as tetracycline, penicillin, or erythromycin, taken orally, appear to give satisfactory results for most, but not all, patients. Tetracycline may be the best antibiotic for such early cases. There may be a one-day increase in symptoms upon treatment, because of toxins and antigens released from the dead spirochetes.

Antibiotics are generally effective against Lyme disease, if treatment is begun soon after infection.

In the later stages of the disease, when heart, joint, or nerve problems have developed, antibiotic treatment is more complicated. Prolonged treatment may be required, with the antibiotics given intravenously, and the treatment sometimes fails. It is far better for the patient's health, and far less expensive, to treat Lyme disease early.

Prevention and Control

Tick bites can usually be prevented by a few simple measures. People walking in a possibly infested area should wear shoes, a long-sleeved shirt, and long pants, tucked into their socks. Both shirt and pants should have tight cuffs. Light-colored clothes will make the ticks easier to see. Tick repellent containing the chemical deet will help if applied to clothing, particularly around the ankles, and exposed areas of the skin. Repellents with a high level of deet should be used only on clothing. (For children, it's best to avoid using repellents stronger than 50 percent deet even on clothing.) On returning home, one should change clothes, and the clothes worn outside should be washed. To reduce the risk of infection, it is a good idea to take a shower. Certainly the body should be checked for ticks. The checking must be done carefully because the ticks are so small. Since the tick bites can be painless, it's easy not to be aware of the danger that may have struck.

Any ticks embedded in the skin should be removed with tweezers. To guard against shooting the bacteria into the body, the tick should be squeezed as little as possible. The tick should be saved in a bottle; it may prove helpful in the diagnosis of any suspicious symptoms that later develop. If a spreading red rash or such general symptoms as fatigue, aching, and/or fever appear, a physician should be consulted.

Lyme disease is more common in families with pets, perhaps because members of such families are more likely to walk, with their pets, in fields or woods and because pets may bring ticks home on their fur. Some authorities recommend that the animals wear flea and tick collars and be checked frequently for ticks. Daily combing or brushing, with the pet on a light-colored cloth, is a help. Evidence is accumulating that Lyme disease can cause a variety of symptoms in cows, cats, and dogs, including lameness.

Control measures directed against ticks may seem an obvious way to halt the advance of Lyme disease, but there are no easy solutions here. Brush can be burned, but that can be done only in small areas, and the brush will grow back. Broad-scale application of pesticides raises environmental concerns, and even if used, a pesticide will likely not penetrate under the vegetation to reach tick nymphs. A pesticide aimed at adult ticks in the autumn, after leaves have fallen, may be a more promising approach.

Another possibility is to focus on tick hosts, notably deer and mice. In some areas fear of Lyme disease has translated into opposition to deer, seen as carriers of the ticks. "To coexist with deer has become a nightmare," commented one Massachusetts resident. But elimination of all deer and mice from an area is not generally practical. Anyway, the ticks might very well find other hosts.

One ingenious approach that has gained the approval of the U.S. Environmental Protection Agency is aimed at killing larvae and nymphs. It involves the use of a product called Damminix, which takes advantage of the fact that mice like to use cotton in building their nests. Cotton balls treated with the pesticide permethrin are placed in biodegradable cardboard tubes, which are scattered in areas where mice live. After a filling meal on a mouse, ticks fall off their host. Ordinarily, larvae that drop off a mouse may remain in the nest for as long as eight months—abundant time in which to be exposed to the poison. The pesticide does not hurt the mouse. The U.S. Army has used on clothing a tick-repellent based on permethrin, but the repellent has not yet been approved by the EPA for general use. (Over 25 states have approved it for special local use.)

Much remains to be learned about Lyme disease and its tick carriers. In the meantime, people should not be afraid to go on outings in woods and fields or to relax on their lawns, even in endemic areas—as long as they remember to take appropriate precautions, especially in the late spring and summer in the upper Midwest and Northeast, when the tick nymphs are active. People in California should be on their guard most of the year, as the tick season is longer there. □

Tick bites can usually be prevented by wearing appropriate clothing and using a tick repellent.

SUGGESTIONS FOR FURTHER READING

HABICHT, GAIL S., GREGORY BECK, AND JORGE L. BENACH. "Lyme Disease." *Scientific American*, July 1987, pp. 78-83.

RICCIUTI, EDWARD R. "Something Scary Lurks Out There." *Audubon*, July 1988, pp. 88-93.

ROUECHÉ, BERTON. "Annals of Medicine: The Foulest and Nastiest Creatures That Be." *The New Yorker*, September 12, 1988, pp. 83-89.

Dancing for Fun and Fitness

Barbara Scherr Trenk

"A time to weep, and a time to laugh; a time to mourn, and a time to dance." Ecclesiastes 3.

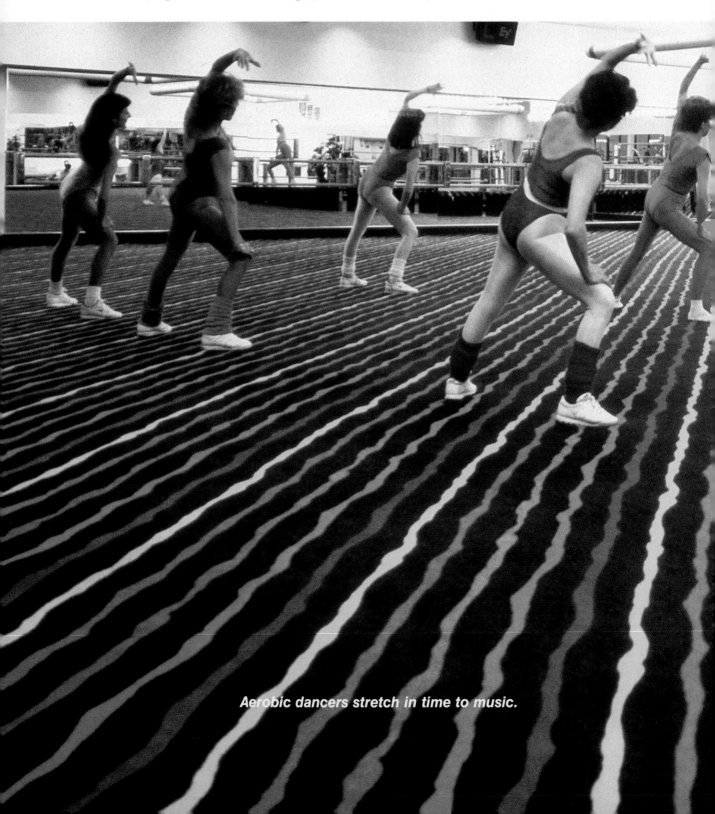

Aerobic dancers stretch in time to music.

In the world of the Old Testament, dance was a means of expressing joy. Today, dancing is still a part of many celebrations. It can also be a way of maintaining ties to one's culture, an exacting art form, a means of self-expression, or a social experience.

Dance can be a healthful experience as well, good for both body and mind. It can lead to strengthened muscles, cardiovascular fitness, better posture and coordination, and improved quality of sleep. And if these benefits are not enough, dance in its many variations can be fun!

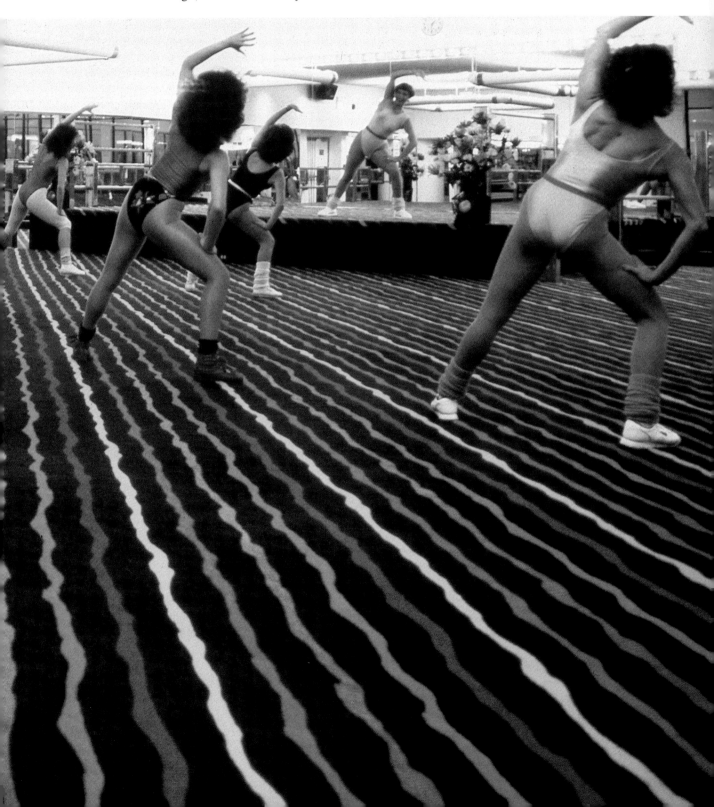

There are many kinds of dance to choose from, among them ballroom, Latin, tap, ballet, and modern. There is also a variation known as aerobic dance, designed for the specific purpose of conditioning the heart.

Aerobic Dance

Twenty million Americans—mostly women, but a substantial number of men—participate regularly in aerobic dance. The concept was developed in 1969 as a series of exercises choreographed to popular music. While purists may argue that this is not really dancing, the name has become accepted.

Like other forms of aerobic exercise, aerobic dance improves the functioning of the cardiovascular system. By increasing the body's maximal oxygen intake, it enables the heart to function more efficiently, possibly reducing the risk of heart attack. To provide this benefit, aerobic exercise should involve continuous physical activity for a minimum of 20 to 30 minutes and should be done at least three times a week. (Sedentary people, however, need to work up to that amount of exercise, and anyone over 40 should consult a doctor before beginning a program.)

Participants in aerobic dance programs learn to warm up and cool down, measure their pulse rate, and dance to the beat. They learn about working heart rates and resting heart rates (for an explanation of these terms, see the accompanying box). According to the American Heart Association, the benefits of aerobic exercise, in addition to cardiovascular fitness, can include increased energy and resistance to fatigue, improved self-image, and release of tension. The National Dance Association cites still other benefits: loss of body fat along with increased muscle tone and strength; weight loss and/or maintenance, including appetite control; retardation of bone mineral loss; and reduced blood pressure and lower cholesterol levels.

Aerobic dance classes are given in Ys, adult education centers, church recreation halls, and health clubs. Aerobic dance has also entered the age of video. Tapes by celebrities like Jane Fonda and Debbie Reynolds, as well as aerobic dance pioneer Jackie Sorenson, give instructions for stretching and reaching right in your own home.

One variation of aerobic dance is low-impact aerobics, in which one foot is on the floor most of the time and bouncing and jumping are eliminated. Low-impact aerobics began as a way to help the elderly, the obese, and beginners enter the world of exercise and enjoy the benefits of a conditioning program. Today, advocates of low-impact aeorbics claim that the specially designed dances are appropriate for everyone, since they are less likely than jumping and hopping to result in painful shinsplints—inflammation and swelling of connective tissue around the main bone in the calf. Some exercise authorities argue that knee, ankle, and lower-back problems are the price for avoiding shinsplints; such injuries are, however, quite rare.

Barbara Scherr Trenk is a free-lance writer specializing in health subjects.

What Is Your Target Heart Range?

Your "working heart rate" should remain within a target range during exercise. To determine your own target range, follow this formula: Subtract your age from 220 to get your maximum heart rate. Then find your heart rate while you are at rest by counting the number of pulses at your wrist or neck in 60 seconds. Subtract this result—your "resting heart rate"—from your maximum heart rate, then multiply the resulting number by 0.7 and by 0.85 (or, if you are over 50, by 0.6 and 0.75). Add the resting rate to each of these numbers to get the lower and upper limits of your target range.

Still others say that with aerobics, as with any other form of exercise, the expertise of the instructor, the design of the exercises, and the physical condition of the participants are the most important factors in preventing injuries. Aerobic dance should be done on a well-padded, carpeted floor, or else on wood flooring, and not, says the Aerobics and Fitness Association of America, on a concrete floor, even if covered with carpet.

Other Kinds of Dancing

Ballroom dancing as we know it today began in the courts of European royalty in the 18th century. This form of dance continues to be enjoyed at parties, in nightclubs, and in dance studios. Ballroom dance is increasing in popularity, according to the United States Ballroom Branch of the Imperial Society of Teachers of Dancing, headquartered in London, England. Many people sign up for ballroom dance lessons because they want to learn to dance for a special occasion—their wedding, perhaps, or a cruise. For others, the waltz, fox-trot, tango,

Whether the steps are simple or as fancy as the ones shown off by these champions, ballroom dancing can provide pleasurable exercise.

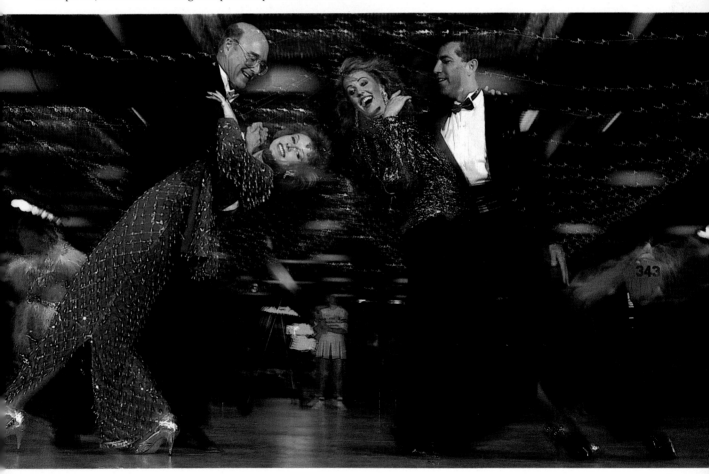

83

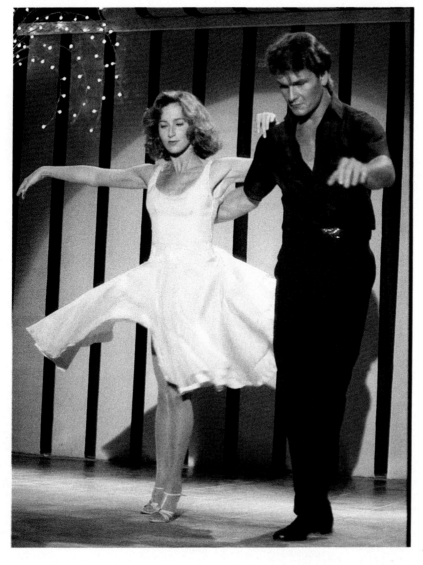

Even social dancing can provide vigorous exercise. At left, in the popular movie Dirty Dancing, *Patrick Swayze teaches neophyte Jennifer Grey to step out. At right, the middle-aged cast of the hit show* Tango Argentino *performs a lively tango.*

and cha-cha are serious pursuits. In July 1988, over 600 dancers participated in the North American Championship dance competition, held in Cherry Hill, N.J. The competition, sponsored by the U.S. Imperial Society of Teachers of Dancing, awarded medals and money to both professional and amateur dancers.

Sometimes a particular dance that is featured in a motion picture or play captures the popular imagination. When *Dirty Dancing* was in the movie theaters, dance studios received calls asking for mambo lessons, according to Lorrain Hahn of the Imperial Society. *Newsweek* magazine credits the movie *School Daze* for the popularity of the song— and accompanying dance—"Da Butt," which caught on in clubs across the United States. The stage show *Tango Argentino* aroused an interest in Latin dance. And the popularity of 1950s and 1960s music has also added to the interest in ballroom dancing.

A 1983 revival of the Depression-era Broadway play *42nd Street* brought renewed interest in tap dance. Lessons were offered in Ys,

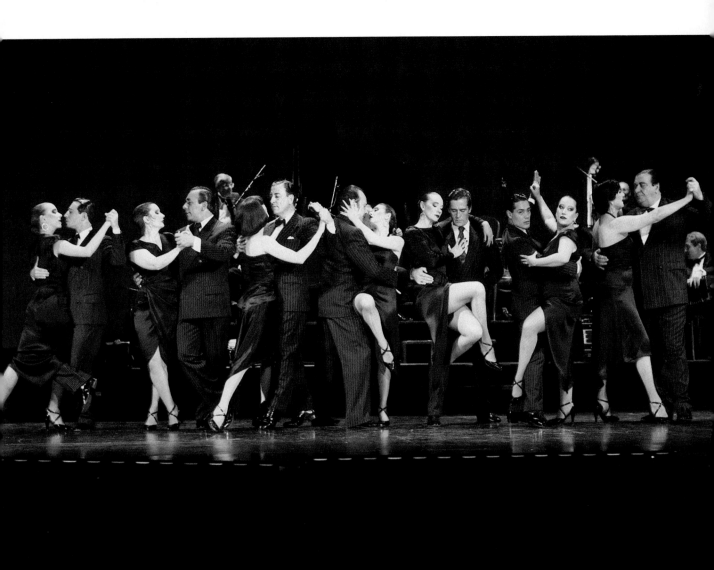

health clubs, and dance studios, and instructional videotapes became available. Tap has been described as the only kind of dance where the dancer follows the exact beat of the music.

Ballet began in the 17th century in France, during the reign of Louis XIV. When the king founded l'Academie Royale de Danse in 1661, the opportunity was created for dancers to study and become professionals. Modern dance is a less structured 20th-century relative of ballet; it was developed in the 1920s and 1930s by Isadora Duncan and Martha Graham, and it continues to be popular today.

While millions of Americans enjoy watching ballet or modern dance on the stage, others like to participate. In 1985 more than 200,000 Americans over age 18 took part in either amateur or professional ballet performances, according to the National Endowment for the Arts. Many more danced for their own pleasure or for the exercise, without appearing in public performances. And ballet lessons continue to be popular among school-aged children, especially girls.

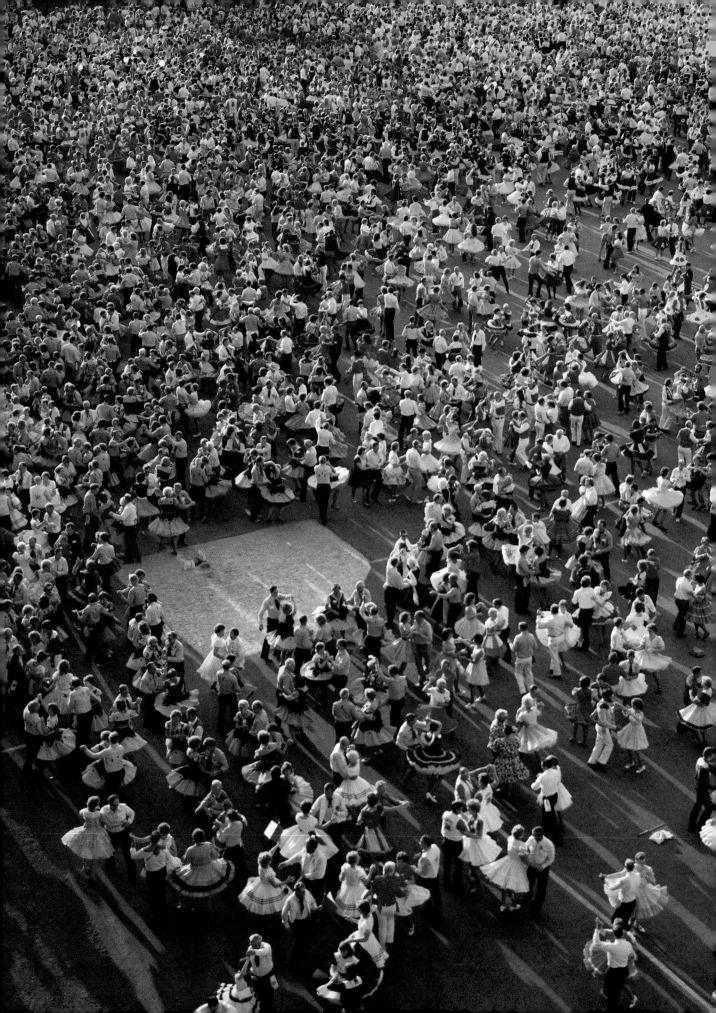

Just Plain Folk Dancing

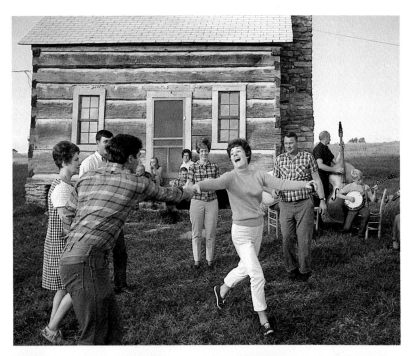

Besides being good exercise, dancing reduces stress and makes people feel better about themselves. Here, folk dancers have a good time at a get-together in Marshall, N.C. (right) and at the Marietta Festival in Lancaster, Pa. At left, a square dancers convention in Louisville, Ky.

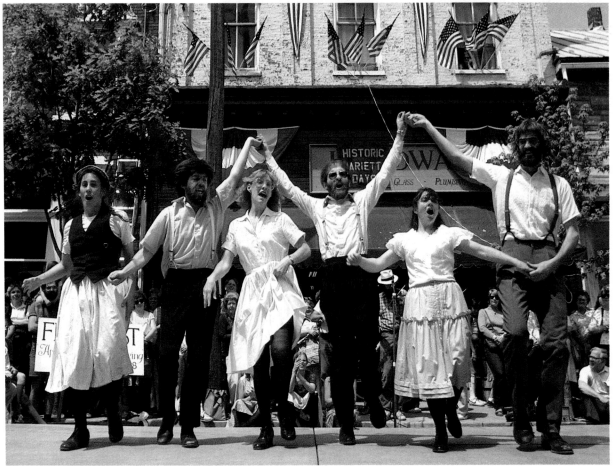

Folk and ethnic dancing are also extremely popular, according to pollster Louis Harris. Harris's research indicates that in 1984, 30 million Americans enjoyed doing folk or ethnic dance. This type of dance gives participants an opportunity to preserve part of their cultural heritage and to share it with others. No Jewish wedding would be complete without a hora, an Italian family would expect its guests to join in a tarantella, and people of Polish descent would surely plan at least one polka during the course of a celebration.

Many classes and clubs are formed to do the folk and ethnic dances of a specific nationality—Israeli or Greek, for instance. Others are international in scope and are geared to the skill level of the participants and the extent of their interest. And because many folk dances are performed in lines or circles, without partners, they can provide social opportunities for single people.

An estimated 3 million Americans participate in square dancing on a regular basis, according to the *Wall Street Journal*. Some square dance callers hold regular classes at adult education centers, Ys, and other recreation facilities. Sometimes a group of dancers will form a club, then hire a caller to lead its events.

Stepping Out for Fitness

Almost any form of dance provides physical and psychological benefits.

According to Lynne Emery, Ph.D., of the Department of Health, Physical Education, Recreation and Dance at California State Polytechnic University at Pomona, virtually all forms of dance "have the potential of providing physiological, psychological, social and aesthetic benefits." Exercise experts agree that whatever activity is chosen for the purpose of improving fitness, it should be both enjoyable and convenient. Participants are more likely to stick with a program if they choose one close enough to home so that transportation will not be a problem, and one that looks as if it would be fun.

Aerobic dance programs are designed with specific health and fitness benefits in mind. Nevertheless, more traditional kinds of dancing can provide similar results if an adequate pace is maintained. If folk, ballroom, and square dancing have sets (known as "tips" in square dancing) that last more than 20 minutes, their effect can be aerobic. "Surely anyone who dances in the lively style of Fred Astaire, Ginger Rogers, or Gene Kelly is getting aerobic benefits from dancing," says Boston-based physical therapist Cynthia Zadai, a specialist in cardiopulmonary rehabilitation.

Ballroom dancers do not usually check their pulse rate after each set. But two physical education specialists from California State University at Long Beach did study the aerobic benefits of a set of dances. The set consisted of a warm-up cha-cha followed by a samba, a polka, two swings (jitterbug or lindy), and a Viennese waltz; it concluded with a cool-down cha-cha. The researchers found the program so beneficial that they have marketed it on videotape under the title "Social Dance Aerobics."

Another affirmation of the fitness benefits of ballroom dancing came from instructor Lorrain Hahn, who reported on the visit of a cardiologist to one of her dance society's competitions. "He measured

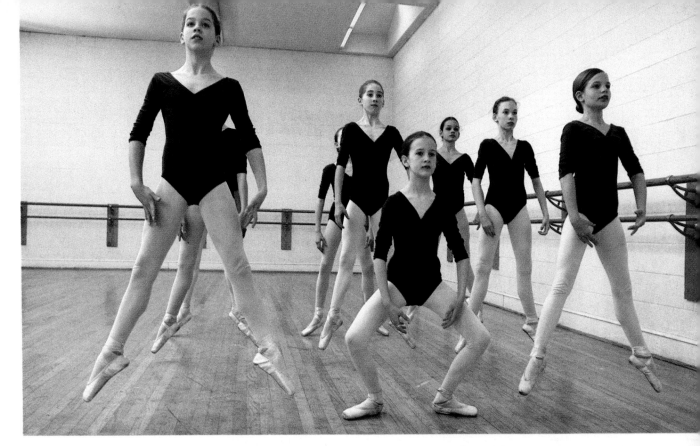

the pulse rates of dancers leaving the floor after the rumba and declared the dance to be definitely aerobic," Hahn said.

Tap dancing can be an aerobic activity if it is done in an active, athletic style, with lots of hopping and jumping. Ballet and modern dance are also aerobic exercises when the dancer remains active for a sufficient period of time. Often, however, these dance styles are characterized by periods of intense movement that are too short to provide aerobic benefit.

Starting young, millions of people enjoy the vigorous exercise of formal ballet classes.

Less Vigorous Programs

Regular participation in less vigorous dance programs—including those that have too many breaks to be aerobic—can still provide physical and emotional benefits, according to exercise expert Lynne Emery. These include improved posture and body alignment, a heightened sense of well-being, improved coordination and balance leading to more efficient movement and reduced likelihood of injury, increased flexibility, and improved quality of sleep.

Virtually any dance program will strengthen leg muscles. The type of dancing done on a regular basis will determine which muscles become the strongest. Ballet dancers tend to have strong feet and legs as a result of their long warm-ups at the barre, while modern dancers have stronger backs and torsos because of their reliance on floor exercises to warm up.

Dancing may also help to prevent osteoporosis, the bone loss that affects many people as they age, especially postmenopausal women. Lawrence E. Schulman, director of the National Institute of Arthritis and Musculoskeletal and Skin Diseases, recommends three to four hours

89

a week of moderate weight-bearing exercise—and dancing qualifies as such—for people of all ages as a way to prevent the bone loss that can result from inactivity.

People who are interested in weight loss will be happy to know that any kind of dancing will burn calories. Various studies have found that ballet is likely to burn 300 calories per hour for men, and 200 for women. During a typical three-hour evening of square dancing, men burned 425 calories, and women about 390. Vigorous disco dancers can burn 400 calories per hour; ballroom dancers between 360 and 600 calories per hour. A study of aerobic dance participants found that 600 calories could be burned per hour, and one aerobics expert estimated that another 600 calories are burned during the six-hour period following a vigorous aerobics session.

Besides burning calories, dancing can help dieters by keeping their thoughts away from food. One business executive told *Fortune* magazine he lost 40 pounds as a result of his interest in ballroom dance. He was too busy dancing to eat and drink as much as he had during his more sedentary past.

While it is difficult to measure the psychological benefits of dance, there is wide agreement from participants and health professionals that

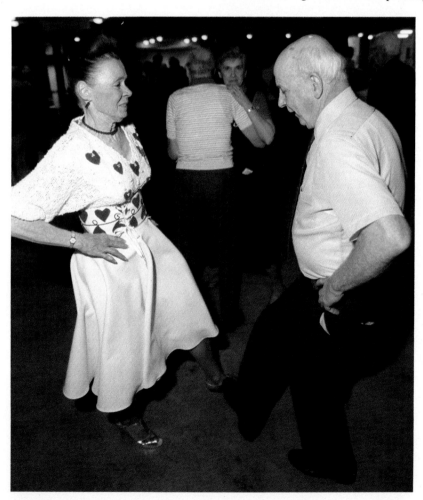

You're never too old—or too heavy— to benefit from dance. At left, senior citizens celebrate Valentine's Day. At right, Women at Large stretch a leg in Key Largo, Fla.

they exist. "We know that exercise releases endorphins, and they make you feel good," says Lynne Emery, who emphasizes the stress-reduction benefits of all kinds of dance. Endorphins are natural opiates that originate in the brain.

Cliff Lothery, associate director for program services of the YMCA of the USA, is enthusiastic about all forms of dance because dance can help people look and feel better and—at the same time—have a good time as well.

Improved self-esteem is often mentioned as a benefit of dance. Andrea Maddox Dallas, a doctoral candidate at St. Louis University (and a regular dancer at local ballet studios), reported to the 1987 convention of the American Psychological Association on her study of a group of women who were not overweight but who had negative feelings about their bodies. Dallas found that after eight weeks of participating in an aerobic dance class, the women became measurably happier with their appearance—even though their bodies had actually changed very little.

The U.S. National Institute ot Mental Health says that appropriate exercise can help relieve emotional stress—anger, tension, hostility, and aggression. When an English psychologist compared the anxiety-reduction effects of dance, music, and sports for a group of college students, dance was found to be the most effective.

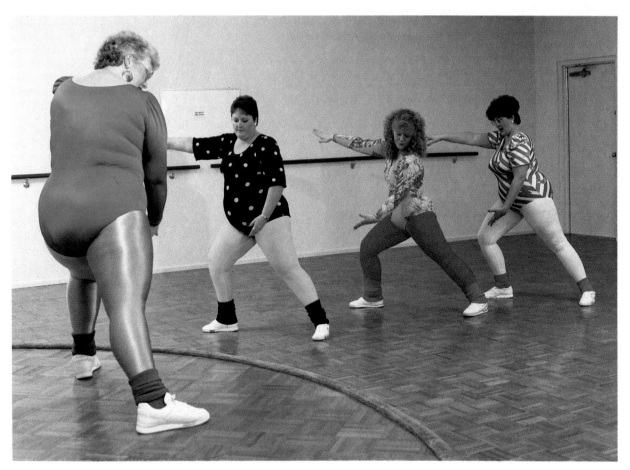

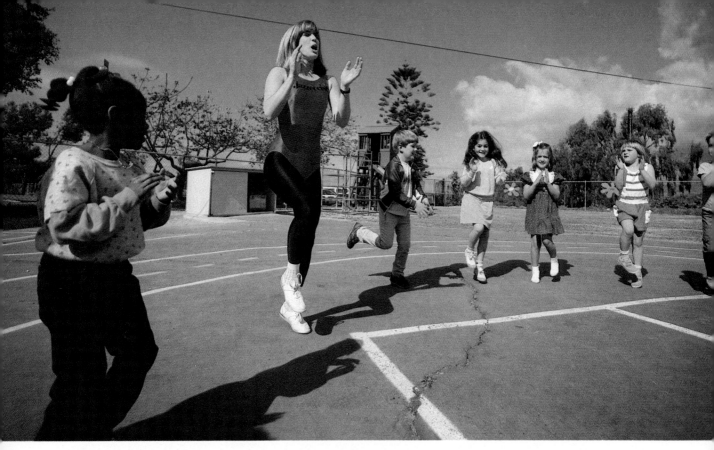

Kids clap their hands to the beat of a Jazzercise class in Mission Viejo, Calif.

Dance as Therapy

Dance can serve as a form of therapy to help people who have a variety of physical and psychological disabilities. The American Academy of Pediatrics describes folk dancing as an activity that can give mentally retarded children and adolescents a sense of participation, as well as social contact and physical exercise. The National Institute of Mental Health suggests that dancing is an effective recreational activity for psychiatric patients because it can be done in small groups and can help promote relaxation, cooperation, self-expression, and creativity.

A specialized group of health professionals known as dance/movement therapists combine dance and psychotherapy in their work with people who have social, emotional, or physical problems (such as the effects of stroke or Parkinson's disease). These specialists work in a variety of settings, including psychiatric hospitals, community mental health centers, correctional facilities, special schools, and rehabilitation facilties.

Dance/movement therapy is often effective with people who have difficulty expressing themselves verbally because it gives them the opportunity to express their feelings through movement. This treatment "furthers the emotional and physical integration of the individual," according to the American Dance Therapy Association.

A properly conducted dance program can also be a beneficial activity for the disabled or physically limited. Jean Rosenbaum, who heads the American Aerobic Association, has adapted aerobic dance programs for obese members of Weight Watchers and Overeaters Anonymous. Dr. Rosenbaum has also run special classes for people whose physical problems include asthma, arthritis, heart disease, and lower-back pain.

Guidance from a physician is, of course, essential for anyone with an injury or chronic disease. It is important for people with acute or chronic health problems to know their limitations before starting any kind of exercise program, and their instructor should be aware of their medical condition. "People with known or suspected heart disease should ask their doctor what their [working] heart rate should be," advises the American Heart Association.

Carefully developed dance classes may help people with arthritis to remain active and maintain their movement capabilities. A team of New York physical therapists who monitored such a class reported that the participants found in it an enjoyable physical and emotional outlet. For these participants, the class helped develop a positive self-image, provided a group support network, and improved daily functioning.

It is not unusual for people who take up dancing as a way to improve fitness to continue the activity simply because they enjoy it. And for a few, dance can become a life's work. The late Robert Joffrey began to tap dance as a young boy as a form of relaxation exercise to help control his asthma. By the time he was 17, the talented young man was studying with George Balanchine in New York. In 1956, at age 25, he founded his own dance company, the Robert Joffrey Ballet. □

SUGGESTIONS FOR FURTHER READING

AMERICAN HEART ASSOCIATION. "Dancing for a Healthy Heart." Available from the Association. See Sources of Further Information below. Or contact your local heart association.

GRIFFITH, BETTY ROSE, AND PHIL MARTIN. "How a Night on the Town Can Keep Your Fitness Program in Step." *Shape* magazine, January 1988, p. 66.

IMPERIAL SOCIETY OF TEACHERS OF DANCING. *Dancing: Ballroom, Latin American, and Social.* London, Hodder and Stoughton, 1977. Available from the Imperial Society. See Sources of Further Information below.

JACOB, ELLEN. *Dancing: A Guide for the Dancer You Can Be.* Reading, Mass., Addison-Wesley, 1981.

JOHNSON, SUSAN. "Head Over Heels." *Shape* magazine, January 1988, p. 68.

OPSATO, MARGARET. "Don't Be a Square—Dance." *50 Plus* magazine, September 1986, p. 65.

SOURCES OF FURTHER INFORMATION

American Dance Therapy Association, 2000 Century Plaza, Suite 108, Columbia, MD 21044. Tel. (301) 997-4040.

American Heart Association, 7320 Greenville Avenue, Dallas, TX 75231. Tel. (214) 373-6300.

National Dance Association, American Alliance for Health, Physical Education, Recreation and Dance, 1900 Association Drive, Reston, VA 22091.

United States Ballroom Branch of the Imperial Society of Teachers of Dancing, 68 Centennial Road, Warminster, PA 18974. Tel. (215) 674-0340.

All About Allergies

Mark Deitch

ILLUSTRATION BY MORDECAI GERSTEIN

Surely, allergies are nothing to sneeze at.

An estimated 40 to 50 million Americans have some type or degree of allergy and suffer symptoms ranging from seasonal sniffles to chronic discomfort; extreme cases can even lead to life-threatening collapse.

The straight facts about the scope and swath of allergic disease are compelling enough—yet many people want to see more than what's really there. Encouraged by self-styled health and nutrition experts and by popular book authors, there is a tendency afoot to blame every headache, mood shift, and upset tummy on "an allergy" of some kind or other. Worse, some people have been led to believe that their (or a loved one's) rheumatoid arthritis, mental illness, or even cancer is really a product of hidden allergies.

Why such dark suspicions surrounding a typically moderate and eminently survivable disorder? Lack of knowledge is part of the answer. Scientists still have a lot to learn about the causes and ultimate effects of allergic reactions, which leaves plenty of room for speculation, both informed and otherwise. Also, allergies involve the body's immune system, which these days occupies approximately the same position for health paranoids as the CIA does for conspiracy theorists.

Mark Deitch is a medical writer and editor.

Be that as it may, the good news about allergies is that there is no convincing evidence that they wear down resistance to disease or lead to any major illness, physical or mental. Furthermore, allergies today are better understood and can be better controlled than ever before. Where past remedies often seemed either too strong, too weak, or too fraught with side effects, a new wave of safer, more effective, and better targeted treatments has emerged in recent years to improve dramatically the level of allergy care.

Allergy Facts

No one knows precisely why some people have allergies while others don't. Some kind of genetic component seems to be involved, since the children of allergic parents (especially those with two allergic parents) have a much better than average chance of developing allergies themselves. But bloodlines guarantee neither susceptibility to nor protection from allergic disease. And even when allergies do run in a particular family, parent and child will not necessarily have the same type of allergy.

The fact that family members don't share the same allergies is hardly surprising when you consider that an individual may not suffer the same allergies as an adult that he or she did as a child. Generally speaking, food allergies and allergic eczema (skin inflammation) are more likely to occur

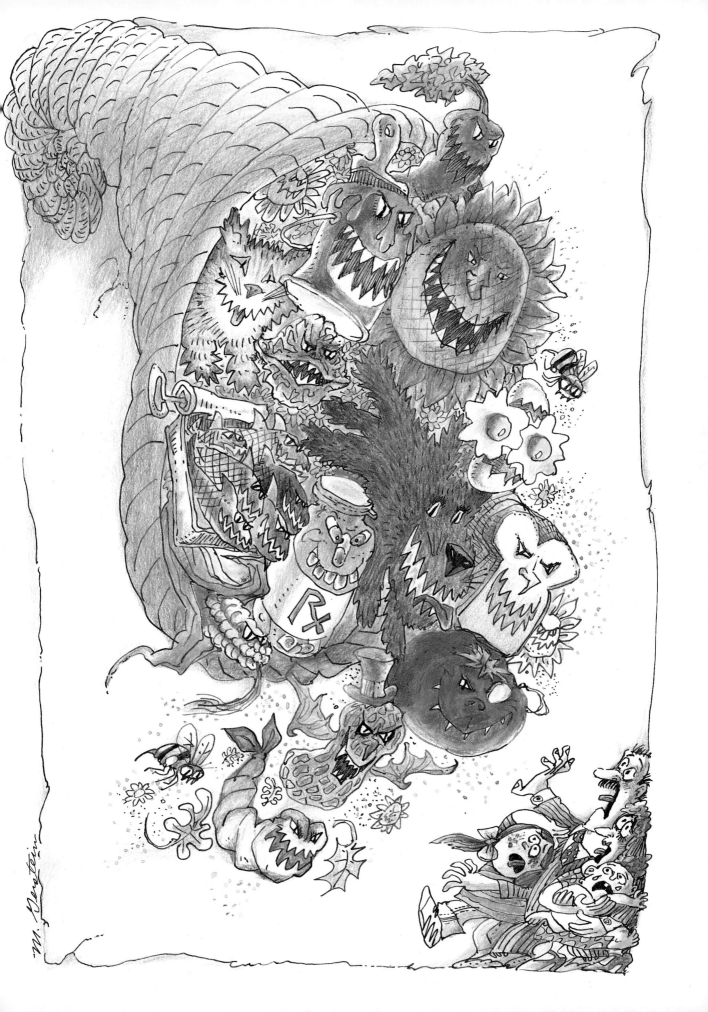

in very young children and to fade away by adulthood, while cases of hay fever and insect bite allergies usually appear before the end of the teen years. Overall, 70 percent of allergy cases show up before age 30. Allergies can emerge at any age, however, and people who have had one type of allergy stand a good chance of developing another (or several more) later on.

Ragweed allergy, the primary cause of hay fever, is almost certainly the most common variety of allergy in the United States. Also quite widespread are dust allergy (usually a reaction to tiny insects called mites imbedded in the dust) and "rose fever," which is actually triggered not by spring flowers but by the trees and grasses that produce pollen in the spring. At the other end of the spectrum are some rare and occasionally bizarre sensitivities, such as allergy to dental braces or to male sperm (leading to infertility problems in some women).

Priming the Pump

If you have an allergy, you have a minor defect in your immune system, which boils down to overproduction of the antibodies known as immunoglobulin E, or IgE. Antibodies are proteins employed by the immune system to seek out foreign particles—"antigens"—that invade the body; if the antigens are dangerous, antibodies start the process of destroying them. In most cases, the more antibodies you have, the better off you are. With IgE, however, it's a different story. That's because IgE responds primarily not to disease-causing bacteria or viruses but to otherwise harmless antigens like pollen, dust, molds, and animal dander. In some people IgE reacts to certain foods, most commonly fish, shellfish, milk, eggs, peanuts, tree nuts, and wheat. Other individuals may have "IgE-mediated" responses to any of a wide variety of medicines.

The first time one of these allergy-causing antigens, or allergens, enters a susceptible person's system, it may encounter only a handful of IgE molecules programmed specifically to react to it. Nothing much happens on this initial exposure, aside from an increase in the number of these antibodies. With each succeeding exposure, the antibody level rises, until the individual is "sensitized" to that antigen, which means that the pump is primed and the dam is ready to burst.

The sensitized person has a critical mass of IgE molecules dotting the surfaces of two kinds of cells: mast cells (found primarily in the membranes lining the inner surfaces of the nose, throat, lungs,

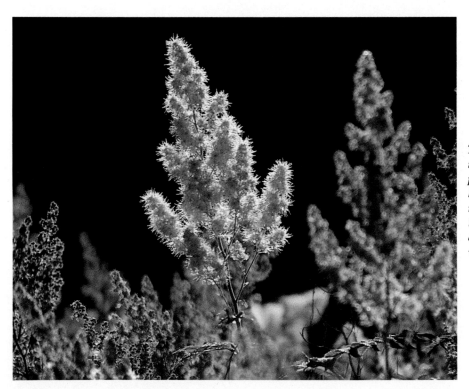

The innocent-looking but ubiquitous ragweed is the prime culprit for sufferers from hay fever. In late summer, as ragweed releases its pollen into the air, the allergic can be easily identified by their wheezes and sneezes.

intestines, and skin) and basophils (a type of white blood cell). Aside from providing a home for IgE, mast cells and basophils are noteworthy in that both contain reservoirs of chemical "mediators," such as histamine, that play a leading role in the body's allergic response.

The next time that particular antigen finds its way into the person's system, all hell breaks loose. As soon as antigen-antibody contact is made, the massed ranks of IgE molecules set off a chain reaction that causes their mast cells to unravel—"degranulate" in medical terminology—and release loads of histamine and other potent chemicals into the surrounding tissues.

After the Mast . . .

On the loose, histamine and its cousins may cause several kinds of trouble. Perhaps the major effect is to make blood vessels leaky, so that nearby tissues become swollen with excess fluid. In addition, histamine and the other chemicals seem to draw various blood components to the affected area, which is part of the process of inflammation. They also increase mucus production and trigger contraction of the involuntary muscles that regulate air passage through the lungs.

The resulting symptoms may vary according to the part of the body under siege. If the offending substance rubs against the skin and causes histamine to be released there, the outcome may be an itchy rash or outbreak of hives. If airborne antigens like dust or pollen land on the moist linings of the eyelids, there may follow itchy, watery eyes and inflamed eyelids (conjunctivitis). Inhaled into the nose or throat, such particles may produce the familiar congestion, runny nose, scratchy throat, and sneezing of hay fever. And in the lungs of some people, they may set off the struggle for breath and wheezing characteristic of asthma.

Asthma and allergies are often—but not necessarily—related conditions. Asthma, technically defined as hyperreactive (or "twitchy") airways in the lungs, appears most frequently in young children and teenagers. Most kids with asthma have allergies that can set off their wheezing and gasping attacks. But a host of nonallergic triggers may also induce asthma, including cold air, exercise, and respiratory infections. Furthermore, when asthma makes its first appearance in a previously unaffected adult, the condition is usually

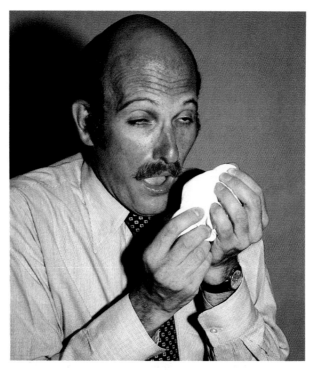

An allergic person has an overly sensitive immune system, producing too much of certain antibodies. When the offending pollen or other substance is inhaled and comes into contact with the antibodies, the result is an explosion—a sneeze—as special cells release strong chemicals like histamines.

more severe than childhood asthma and is seldom allergy-induced.

Anywhere from five to ten hours after an initial asthma or allergy attack, some people may undergo a second assault of symptoms unprovoked by antigens or any other external trigger. This "late-phase response" may be milder than the original reaction, but it may also be more resistant to standard treatment. Scientists suspect that basophils drawn into the affected area and somehow induced to release their mediators are at least partly responsible for the late-phase response, which has become one of the hottest areas of allergy-asthma research.

Not all allergic reactions occur at the body site where the antigen touches down. Food allergies, for example, may cause hives or redness and swelling in just about any part of the body—or all over. The most potentially dangerous allergic reaction involves the entire body and is called systemic anaphylaxis. Such a reaction tends to come on suddenly and, in the most severe instances, may

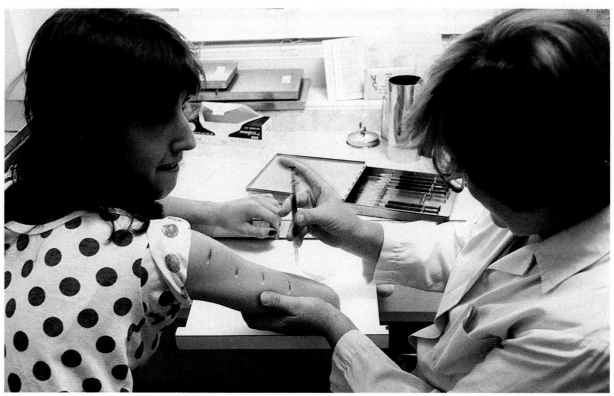

A skin test can be given to help identify allergies. When various substances are applied to the skin through scratches or pricks, or injected into it, a redness or swelling will indicate that the person has already developed antibodies.

induce a precipitous drop in blood pressure leading to collapse, shock, and even death. Allergies to foods, penicillin, and bee stings are the most common causes of systemic anaphylaxis. Fortunately, anaphylactic reactions are easily and effectively treated with a shot of epinephrine (also called adrenaline). People who know they are at risk for this condition often carry small quantities of epinephrine in a self-injecting dispenser, to be used in case of an insect sting or food reaction.

Tracking the Culprit

Thanks to advances in medical technology, an array of useful testing procedures—and a few unproven or dubious techniques, as well—are available to verify the existence or pinpoint the cause of allergies. Still, the first and most important step in diagnosing and treating allergies is a physical examination and thorough discussion with your doctor. For many people with allergies, a careful description of the symptoms and the setting in

which they occur may go a long way toward nailing down the culprit and staking out a course of prevention or therapy.

If the problem is severe or if more detailed information is needed, the doctor may suggest a visit to an allergy specialist, or allergist. Following are some of the testing procedures generally recognized as helpful in diagnosis.

• *Skin Testing.* The most reliable and popular test for allergies involves scratching, pricking, or injecting the skin (usually on the forearm) with a series of substances suspected of causing a reaction. If the person tested has antibodies to a given allergen, the site of the scratch or injection will become red and swollen within a few minutes. (This does not, however, necessarily mean that the individual is allergic to that substance; the allergist must interpret the test in the light of other data.) Scratch or prick forms of skin testing are extremely safe and practically painless; they do, however, occasionally miss a sensitivity because of the small amount of allergen used. Injection skin tests, on the other hand, sometimes err on the side of excess by provoking reactions that are not allergic in origin.

• *Patch Testing.* This procedure is used for identifying the cause of a common skin allergy, called contact dermatitis, that often results from exposure to chemicals found in cosmetics or in other household or workplace products. A sticky patch containing suspected irritants is affixed to the skin (usually on the back); the test is considered positive if a rash appears at the patch site within two to four days.

• *RAST.* With RAST (for radioallergosorbent test), a blood sample is taken and then analyzed in a laboratory to measure the amount of IgE molecules specific to a given allergen. RAST is convenient in that a single blood sample is enough for several tests, but the procedure is far more expensive than skin testing and offers no practical advantage in accuracy. It may come in handy, nevertheless, for infants or for people with severe skin problems who cannot tolerate scratch or prick testing, as well as for older people whose skin is not "reactive."

• *Nasal Smears.* A simple microscopic examination of nasal mucus, this procedure is typically performed when there is no clear sign whether a person's constant runny nose is the result of allergies or some other cause.

• *Inhaled Challenge.* The allergist may have an individual inhale controlled concentrations of pollen, cat dander, molds, or other airborne allergens, to see what effect they have on breathing capacity. Inhaled challenges with histamine or with the drug methacholine are often used to test for asthma.

• *Oral Challenge.* This is the most effective method of determining the cause of potentially serious food allergies. It is ideally performed in a hospital setting, in case immediate care is needed to counteract a severe reaction. The person is given very small quantities of a suspected food substance, and the amount is gradually increased until a clear-cut reaction (such as hives or wheezing) occurs. In the most rigorous form of the test, the individual is fed unmarked gelatin capsules containing either the suspect food extract or a placebo, that is, a substance known to be harmless. To rule out subjective responses, the procedure should be "double-blind": neither the person being tested nor the doctor or nurse administering the test knows which capsules contain the food extract and which the placebo.

Some allergists use another, controversial type of challenge testing called provocation and neutralization both to diagnose and to treat allergies to foods and, occasionally, inhaled substances. The provocation part typically consists of injecting progressively smaller concentrations of a suspect substance into or beneath the skin until symptoms appear. At that point, advocates of this method claim, still smaller concentrations of the offending substance will neutralize the symptoms and prevent their recurrence. A 1987 report by the American Medical Association's Council on Scientific Affairs found no convincing proof of the effectiveness of provocation-neutralization testing, while acknowledging that more research was needed in order fairly to test the test.

The AMA council came out strongly against "cytotoxic" testing, a much-ballyhooed blood analysis procedure purported to identify food allergies. The test is regarded as unproved, unreliable, and scientifically unfounded. Anyone to whom this test is recommended should consider getting a second opinion. The U.S. Food and Drug Administration (FDA) has moved to ban the marketing of cytotoxic self-test kits.

Prevention Tips

Despite the development of sophisticated new antiallergy medications and safer and more effective drug delivery systems, the best way to overcome allergies remains the simplest (and cheapest): when possible, avoid the allergen.

If allergy testing or harsh experience tells you that a specific item in your diet or environment triggers symptoms, then prevention should not pose much of a problem. Unfortunately, some of the most common allergens, like pollen, molds, and dust, are pretty tough to avoid altogether. If you are sensitive to them, minimizing your exposure is the most reasonable goal. During heavy pollen seasons (spring for grasses and trees, midsummer to early fall for ragweed), keep home and car windows shut and use air conditioning if possible; air conditioners help to filter airborne allergens. If you can, get someone else to rake leaves and mow the lawn—activities likely to stir up a microscopic storm of molds and spores. Stay out of damp, mildewy basements, attics, and tool sheds.

Before finalizing vacation plans, check ahead to find out if local plants to which you are allergic will be pollinating during your stay. Packing up and leaving town permanently to avoid allergies is not recommended, however. Aside from the financial and emotional tolls of relocation, there may well be a whole new set of environmental irritants waiting for you at your new homesite. No allergy-free regions may be found in North America today. Places that once were, like Arizona, have long since been overrun by settlers who brought their old allergy sources with them.

Inside the home, dust control is a never-ending battle, but the effort may pay off in decreased symptoms and improved sleep. The ideal decor for an allergic person is simple and stark: basic wood and metal furnishings, without dust-catching carpets, drapes, venetian blinds, or upholstery. Stuffed toys and knickknacks can be stored in the closet, with the door shut tight. Clothes can be kept in dust-free garment bags. Mattresses, box springs, and cushions can be lined with zippered plastic covers. High-efficiency air filter units may also help—and *everything* should be dusted (with a damp cloth) and vacuumed frequently.

If a family member is allergic to animals, the cold hard fact is that you are better off finding a new home for Rover or Tabby (especially Tabby: cats' constant self-cleaning leaves a highly allergenic trail of saliva particles wherever they go). A compromise solution may be keeping pets outdoors or at least out of sleeping rooms.

Medications

Once you get past avoidance and prevention, there are two main categories of allergy treatment: drugs and allergy shots. Drugs may help ease or control symptoms; the shots may actually eliminate some types of severe allergy. Here are the chief types of drugs available:

• *Antihistamines.* The most widely used allergy medications, these drugs work by blocking the effects of histamine, the primary mediator of allergic reactions. There are seven different classes of antihistamines; some are more effective against skin allergies, some are better at controlling hay fever symptoms, and some aren't used for allergies at all. The popular antiulcer drugs cimetidine (trade names, Tagamet, Novocimetine, Peptol) and ranitidine (Zantac, Apo-Ranitidine) are actually a special type of antihistamine that lowers stomach acidity.

For allergy treatment, antihistamines are available in both prescription and over-the-counter formulations, the latter sometimes combined with a decongestant. From their development in the 1940s antihistamines were dogged by a major drawback—unpleasant side effects, most notably drowsiness. This limited their effectiveness, because as dosage strength increases, so do the sedative side effects. People using standard antihistamines are advised not to drive or drink alcohol.

The advent several years ago of terfenadine (Seldane), a nonsedating antihistamine, was a considerable boon to many allergy sufferers, who previously had to choose between constant sniffling or nodding off at their desks. It also signaled the opening of a lucrative new drug market, with new nonsedating competitors seeking FDA approval; one of them, astemizole (Hismanal), already available in Canada, was recently approved for marketing. Because terfenadine and company can be tolerated at higher dosage levels than standard antihistamines, researchers are exploring their use against allergic asthma.

• *Decongestants.* These are drying agents that work by shrinking the swollen mucous membranes of the nasal passages. They come in tablet, liquid, nasal spray, and drop forms, whose active ingredients are pseudoephedrine or phenyl-propanolamine. Decongestants may provide effective temporary relief. But since the effect doesn't last, there may be a tendency to use the sprays, especially, more frequently and over longer periods than the package instructions recommend. Decongestant abuse may then lead to "rebound congestion," a condition in which the original problem returns in a more severe form. Jitteriness and increased heart rate are among the possible side effects of decongestants; these drugs are not recommended for people with high blood pressure, an irregular heartbeat, or glaucoma.

• *Cromolyn Sodium.* One of the newest and most promising antiallergy agents, cromolyn sodium is a mast cell stabilizer, which means it works to prevent the disintegration of mast cells and the subsequent release of histamine and its companion chemicals. Unlike other antiallergy drugs, cromolyn sodium may be taken preventively, before an anticipated allergy or asthma attack, rather than being used merely to ease symptoms after the fact. It also appears to be useful in warding off late-phase responses. Cromolyn sodium is available by

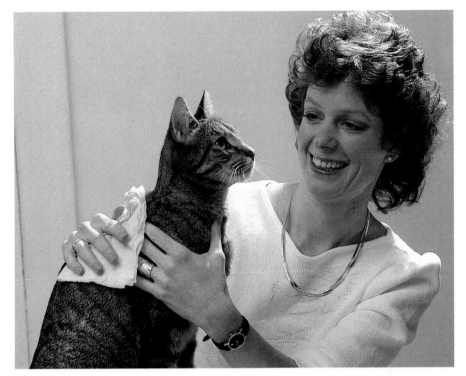

A domestic crisis can occur when a cherished pet is found to cause allergic reactions in a family member. Here the offending animal is being carefully rubbed down with damp paper towels.

prescription in nasal spray (Nasalcrom, Rynacrom), eye drop (Opticrom), and inhalant (Intal) forms.

• **Corticosteroids.** These are potent anti-inflammatory drugs used to control severe allergy or asthma attacks. If taken orally or by injection on a regular basis, they can cause serious side effects throughout the body, which limits their long-term use. The development in recent years of "topical" corticosteroids, which are sprayed into the nose or inhaled into the lungs, with greatly reduced side-effects potential, has been hailed as a breakthrough. Examples are flunisolide and beclomethasone.

• **Bronchodilators.** Usually prescribed to treat asthma, these drugs may also be used when allergies or respiratory infections interfere with breathing. They come in liquid or inhalant forms and work by relaxing the smooth muscle of the air passages in the lungs. Bronchodilators are chemically similar to adrenaline and may cause jitteriness or difficulty in sleeping. Among the better-known bronchodilators are theophylline, taken orally, and albuterol and metaprotenorol, both available in oral and inhaled forms.

Allergy Shots

Allergy shots, or immunotherapy, offer a court of last resort for people whose allergies won't respond to any other form of treatment. Immunotherapy is an expensive, long-term, and often inconvenient undertaking, but it does work: up to an 85 percent success rate in significantly reducing and sometimes wholly eliminating symptoms of ragweed and other pollen allergies. Immunotherapy is also very effective in preventing insect sting reactions and has demonstrated usefulness in easing asthmatic response to dust, mites, and cat dander. It does not appear to work as well against mold allergies.

The basic principle behind immunotherapy is gradually to build up the person's tolerance of the allergy-causing substance. This is done through a series of injections containing increasingly larger doses of allergen extract; an initial series may require a shot a week for up to two years. Depending on how well the treatment works, the frequency of shots may then be reduced to once a month or so. The average patient is treated for three to five years.

Immunotherapy has a very good safety record, although there is a small risk of anaphylactic reaction to the allergy shots. Such reactions are easily controlled if treated immediately by trained health workers. For this reason, people on immunotherapy are (or should be) routinely advised to remain in the doctor's office or waiting room for

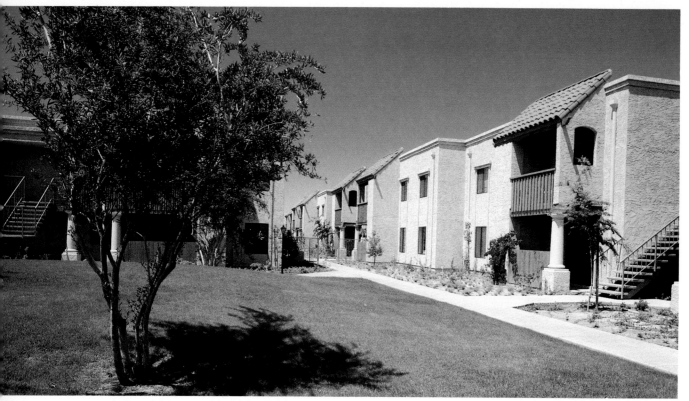

Newly planted lawns and trees in Phoenix, Ariz., have changed this once pollen-free area into a hay fever capital. Shrubs, plants, and grasses have been imported by allergy sufferers who could not resist bringing to the dry, cactus-sprinkled landscape the very same types of greenery that they were fleeing from.

20 to 30 minutes after a shot, just in case a reaction does occur.

Food Allergies: Facts and Follies

Food allergy is one of the more controversial areas in medicine, and also one in which the gap between popular belief and orthodox professional opinion looms largest. While surveys indicate that 43 percent of the general population think they have or have had food allergies, laboratory tests show at most a 6 or 8 percent incidence of food allergies in infants (the most vulnerable group) and a steadily declining rate with increasing age. There are, however, maverick specialists who contend that their personal observations are more telling than laboratory results and that food allergies are a widespread and pernicious health problem. Most allergists and other medical authorities tend to frown on these claims, but in the absence of definitive research, the debate rages on.

A big reason for the confusion among the public is that many people fail to distinguish between allergy and intolerance. Start with the fact that the food we eat constitutes the largest source of different antigens introduced into our systems. A variety of adverse reactions may result, including food poisoning (caused by bacteria like salmonella); chemical mismatches between different foods or between food and drugs or medical conditions; and reactions caused by digestive defects, such as lactose intolerance, a common inability to break down the milk sugar found in dairy foods. Comparatively speaking, true food allergy, which must involve the immune system (IgE antibodies, in particular), is not very common, while food intolerance, which embraces just about anything you eat that doesn't agree with you, happens all the time.

Symptoms often overlap. Both food allergies and other food intolerances may cause gastrointestinal upset, such as nausea, vomiting, cramping, and diarrhea. Food allergies, however tend also to produce hives; redness and swelling of the lips, face, or other areas of the skin; or wheezing (occasionally in children, rarely in adults).

Diagnostic Difficulties. Another problem is the absence of a simple, convenient, and reliable test for food allergies. Standard allergy tests (scratch, prick, or injection variety) are not nearly as sensitive to allergy-provoking foods as they are to airborne provocateurs, such as pollen and dust. Other procedures touted specifically for food allergies—such as provocation-neutralization testing, and cytotoxic blood analysis—are unproven at best and highly questionable at worst. Removing suspect items from the diet one by one may help to identify the cause of a food reaction, but it can't determine whether or not the problem is an allergy.

The best method for detecting food allergies is a rigorous oral challenge test. Based on the results of such challenge tests, researchers have found that adults' most common food allergies are to milk, eggs, peanuts, tree nuts, shellfish, and fish. For infants and young children the list also includes soy products and gluten, which is found in wheat flour and some other grain products. It may come as a surprise to learn that true allergies to chocolate, strawberries, or citrus fruits are so rare as to be virtually nonexistent, although some people may well have trouble tolerating these items. On the encouraging side, allergies to specific substances often subside after an interval of abstinence—which means that you may have to forgo that lobster salad for only a few months.

Infancy is the most vulnerable age for food allergy because a newborn's digestive tract is more porous than an older person's and thus more likely to allow large, allergy-causing proteins to pass into the bloodstream. A major source of these large proteins is the cow's milk found in many infant formulas. Recent research shows that soy-based formulas, often recommended in the past as a substitute, may also cause allergic symptoms (hives, eczema, wheezing, colic, excessive fussiness). The best protection against food allergies is breast-feeding for at least the first six months of life. Women who cannot or choose not to breast-feed can ask their pediatricians to recommend a "hypoallergenic" infant formula—a formula carrying a low risk of causing allergy.

Food Allergy and Disease. Part and parcel of the misconception that food allergies are a common problem is the equally mistaken notion that they cause an assortment of chronic physical and mental disorders. The general drift of the argument is that repeated exposure to allergy-causing antigens in the diet produces subtle and cumulative changes in the body that ultimately result in arthritis, cancer, depression, migraine, hyperactivity, or—in the absence of a clear diagnosis—a vague, lingering malaise called tension-fatigue syndrome.

In reality, allergic reactions to food are almost always immediate and obvious, with little mystery attached. People who are truly allergic to foods tend to know what foods set them off. Furthermore, there is no conclusive evidence that food allergy can produce behavioral disturbances or depression.

As for food allergy involvement in arthritis—particularly rheumatoid arthritis, potentially the most severe form—anecdotal reports abound of flare-ups of joint pain and inflammation occurring after consumption of a given food. Although objective proof is lacking, such claims make some sense. Allergies or other food reactions are sources of physical stress, and stress of any kind can set off rheumatoid flare-ups. But doctors have no reason to believe that allergies, intolerances, or dietary factors of any kind are responsible for causing arthritis.

Migraine headache presents a somewhat similar situation. It, too, may be triggered or worsened (but not originally caused) by a variety of environmental factors, including certain foods and beverages. But specifically allergic reactions do not seem to play a role in migraine.

Finally, the most alarming claims of all: that constant exposure and reaction to foods to which one is allergic wears down the immune system and renders the allergic person more susceptible to cancer and perhaps AIDS (acquired immune deficiency syndrome). The basic flaw in that argument is that a person with allergies actually has an overly active immune system, which if anything might confer an extra dash of protection. □

SOURCES OF FURTHER INFORMATION

American Academy of Allergy and Immunology, 611 E. Wells Street, Milwaukee, WI 53202.
Asthma and Allergy Foundation of America, 1717 Massachusetts Avenue N.W., Suite 305, Washington, DC 20036.

Wellness in

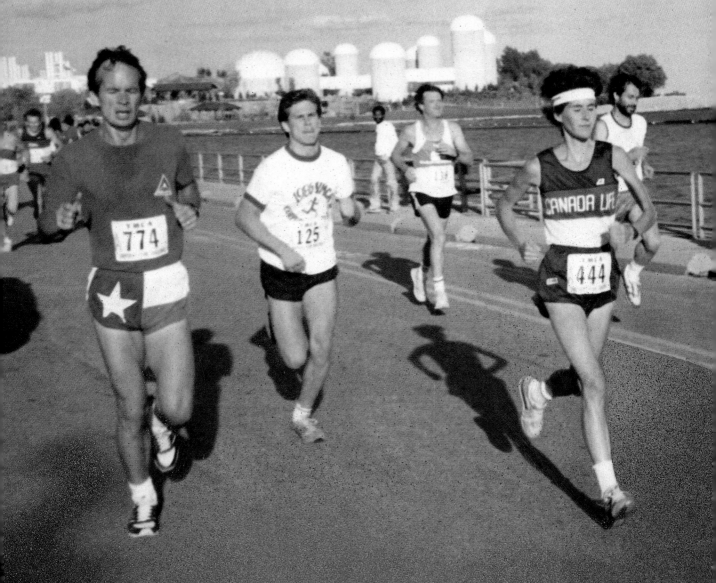

Running is one of the many activities companies
are sponsoring for improved employee health.

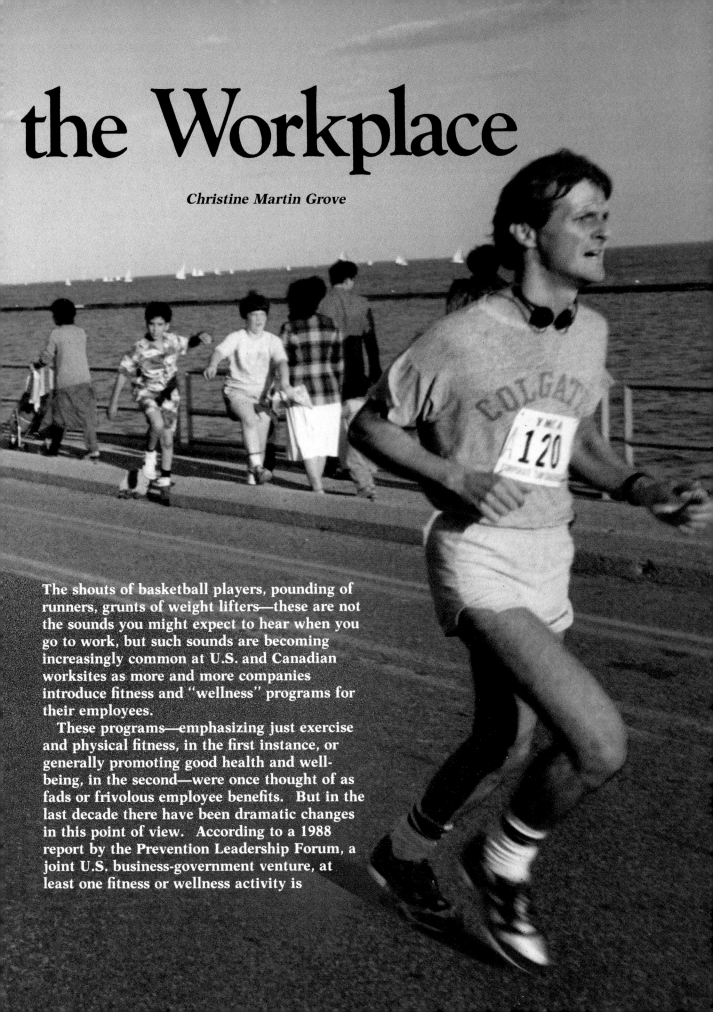

the Workplace

Christine Martin Grove

The shouts of basketball players, pounding of runners, grunts of weight lifters—these are not the sounds you might expect to hear when you go to work, but such sounds are becoming increasingly common at U.S. and Canadian worksites as more and more companies introduce fitness and "wellness" programs for their employees.

These programs—emphasizing just exercise and physical fitness, in the first instance, or generally promoting good health and well-being, in the second—were once thought of as fads or frivolous employee benefits. But in the last decade there have been dramatic changes in this point of view. According to a 1988 report by the Prevention Leadership Forum, a joint U.S. business-government venture, at least one fitness or wellness activity is

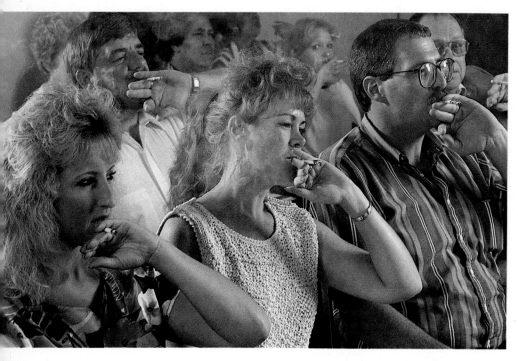

Kicking the Smoking Habit

Company support can range from stop-smoking seminars (left) to self-help kits (right), complete with cartoon-filled workbooks designed to make quitting seem like fun.

now found in almost two-thirds of U.S. worksites with 50 or more employees. (The group defines such activities as those dealing with smoking control, stress management, nutrition education, physical fitness, and so on.) The Canadian government agency Fitness Canada reports some form of program in almost 15 percent of Canadian companies with 100 or more employees.

Why the turnaround? A major cause is escalating health insurance costs, which according to a Stanford University economist now amount to more than 40 percent of U.S. business and industry's pretax profits. In addition, heart disease alone, the leading cause of death for Americans, is responsible every year for 29 million lost workdays. Estimates for lost productivity and earnings resulting from cigarette-related illnesses range from $27 billion to $61 billion per year. According to Blue Cross and Blue Shield, back ailments are the second leading cause of hospitalization (after pregnancy) and cost U.S. industry an estimated $14 billion annually. Add in the costs directly related to all other illnesses and injuries, plus the hidden costs of subpar job performance and personnel replacement or training expenses, and business is faced with staggering sums.

Protecting the Bottom Line

The business community's major strategy to contain its costs has been to cut back company health insurance programs, by making employees pay part (or a higher part) of their medical bills and absorb higher

Christine Martin Grove is a staff editor.

106

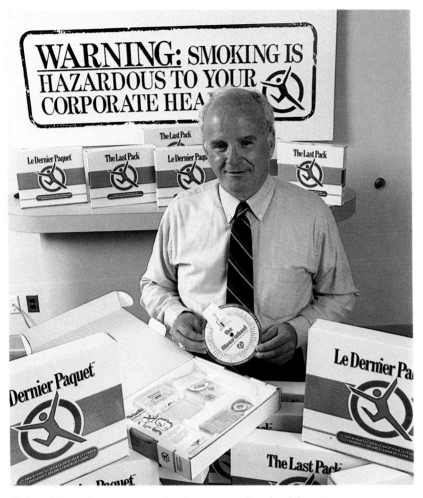

deductibles. Some companies have turned to health maintenance organizations, which aim to keep down costs by stressing prevention, or have joined business groups that are working to keep down hospital costs. But, according to some observers, it is the fitness/wellness programs that offer one of the best prospects for controlling costs.

A recent study by the Control Data Corporation of 15,000 of its employees showed that people with unhealthy life-styles use more medical care and generate higher total costs for health insurance claims than people with more healthful life-styles. Among the findings: one-pack-a-day smokers have health claim costs 18 percent higher than nonsmokers; people who wear safety belts less than 25 percent of the time have 54 percent more hospital inpatient days than those who use seat belts 75 percent of the time or more; and seriously overweight people are 48 percent more likely to have claims over $5,000 in a one-year period than people of normal weight.

According to the U.S. Centers for Disease Control, at least half of the chronic diseases in the United States can be prevented, or at least postponed, by "proper life-style behavior." Improve employee fitness and emphasize "proper life-style behavior," it is reasoned, and the health of both the employees and the company's finances will improve.

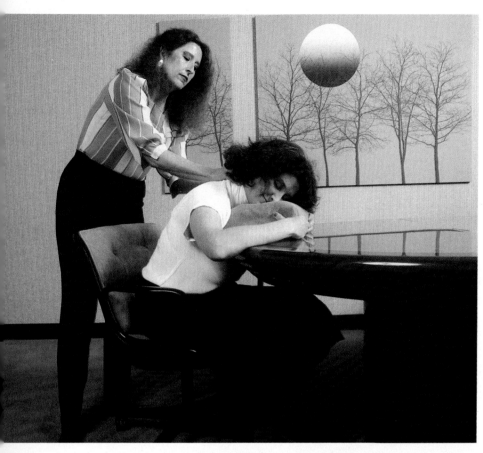

Working for Wellness

Although wellness programs include exercise activities (below and right), their focus is on modifying health-related behaviors. The woman at left is receiving a massage as part of a stress management program.

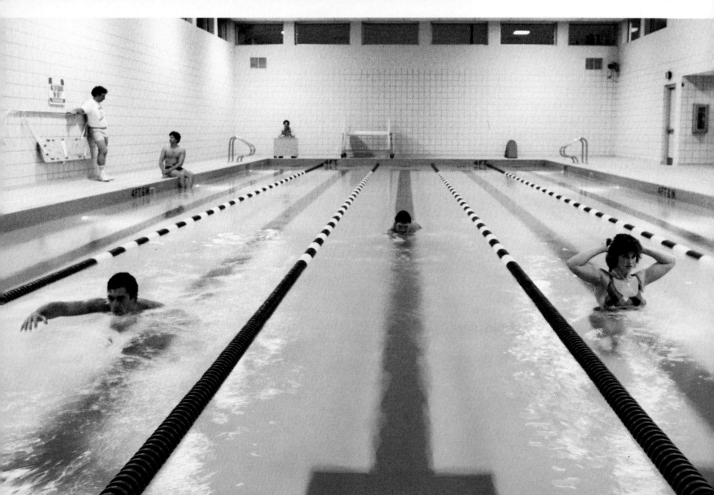

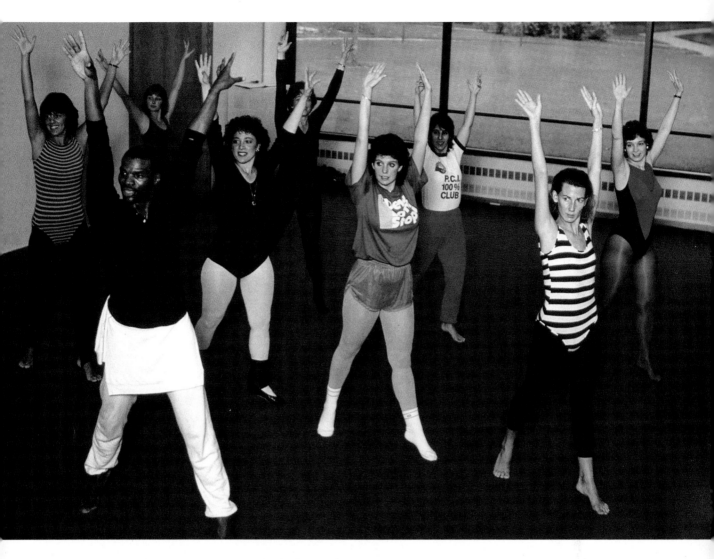

One approach is fitness programs, in which the emphasis is on exercise. A more comprehensive approach is wellness programs, which include exercise but go beyond it. In wellness programs (sometimes called health promotion programs), the emphasis is on modifying people's life-styles, which in this context means behavior specifically related to health, such as eating, drinking, exercise, and smoking habits, as well as attitudes toward family, work, recreation, and the world in general. Health promotion programs typically include components dealing with topics such as how to eat properly, control stress, and stop smoking.

The average participation rate in fitness/wellness programs is only 25 percent of eligible employees (such programs are, of course, voluntary). Nevertheless, the programs save companies a great deal of money. Although the earliest fitness/wellness programs were largely based on faith rather than actual evidence, there are now hard data to support the conclusion that they are good for both the employee and the employer.

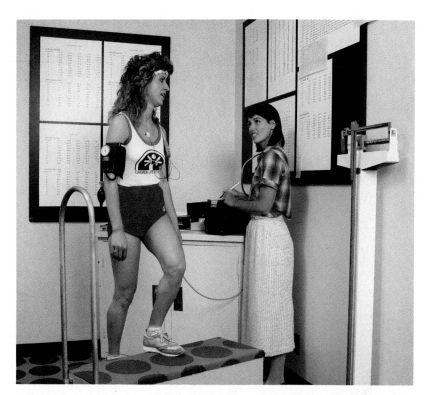

How Fit Are You?

Many programs help participants find out just how fit they are. At left, a staff member measures how efficiently a participant's heart and lungs work during exercise. Below, employees use computers to monitor their heart rates.

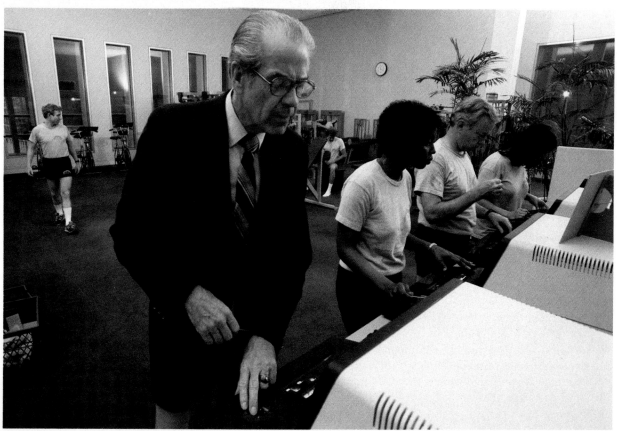

In Canada a government-sponsored study of Canada Life Assurance Company's pilot health program, Fit for Life, projected that if the program were offered to all employees, it would save the company up to Can$500,000 a year through reduced absenteeism and lower staff turnover. (Absenteeism of participants in the pilot was 22 percent lower than that of other employees; the turnover rate for participants was only 1.5 percent, compared with 15 percent for the company as a whole.) According to Canada Life, this projection turned out to be correct when Fit for Life was made available to all of the company's employees.

In the United States a study of Total Life Concept, a pilot employee health program at AT&T Communications, reported that if the trends shown in the pilot were to continue over the next ten years, AT&T would save $72 million because of fewer heart attacks and $15 million because of fewer cancer cases. A comparison over five years of medical costs for groups of Johnson & Johnson employees taking part in the company's health promotion program, Live for Life, and groups not taking part showed lower costs for the participants. A finding of particular interest was that hospital bills, which account for nearly two-thirds of the company's total health benefit costs, doubled for participants over the five-year period but increased four-fold for nonparticipants.

A five-year evaluation of Blue Cross and Blue Shield of Indiana's Stay Alive and Well program for its own employees showed that for each dollar the company invested in health promotion, it saved $1.45 in healthcare costs. And, finally, an investigation of teachers in the Dallas Independent School District found that teachers who participated in a fitness program took an average of three fewer sick days per year, at a savings of $452,000 in substitute pay alone.

What's in It for Me?

Hand in hand with the benefits to the company's bottom line go benefits to individual employees. The Canada Life study showed significant improvement in cardiorespiratory fitness and flexibility and a corresponding loss in body fat among those who worked out regularly. The general attitude of employees toward their jobs also improved.

A Control Data study of its StayWell program reported decreases in smoking rates, cholesterol levels, percentage of overweight employees, and percentage of sedentary employees at StayWell sites compared with other Control Data sites. In addition, 46 percent of employees not using seat belts began to use them after taking part in StayWell. The Johnson & Johnson study showed decreases in excess weight and blood pressure, leading to reduced heart attack risks, as well as reduced stress, improved morale, and improved job satisfaction.

At AT&T, workers' fitness levels improved, blood pressure decreased significantly, and cholesterol levels were lowered. Weight reduction averaged 10 pounds, and 60 percent of people with low back pain reported a decrease in the severity of the pain. And at a 12-month follow-up, 53 percent of participants in stop smoking programs were

BUILT-IN FACILITIES

An increasing number of developers of new office buildings and business parks are putting in fitness centers for tenant use, thus allowing companies to share the cost and benefits of an on-site facility that they couldn't afford on their own or that they don't want to be responsible for. Facilities range from small, unsupervised exercise rooms in office buildings to completely separate, 35,000-square-foot centers staffed by professionals, with swimming pools, jogging tracks, weight rooms, basketball courts, exercise rooms, and lecture rooms for wellness activities. Employers sometimes subsidize memberships and sometimes buy a block of memberships to provide to their employees at a discount. The larger centers are open to all building or business park employees. At others memberships are distributed to companies based on the percentage of eligible employees in each company.

A NEGATIVE SIDE OF FITNESS PROGRAMS?

The negative side of corporate health programs, according to a number of observers, is that some of them will keep workers from seeking needed outside medical care. Furthermore, critics argue, there is the danger that aggressive health promotion can change the perspective on illness and lead to a "blame the victim" syndrome. The 1988 proposal of the Circle K Corporation to cut off medical coverage to employees who became sick or injured as a result of what the company termed "personal life-style decisions" related to AIDS, alcohol, drug abuse, and self-inflicted wounds seemed to confirm some of the worst fears. Circle K, the second-largest chain of convenience stores in the United States, withdrew the proposal following a public outcry.

The issue of holding employees at least partly responsible for their health, however, has not gone away. Some insurance regulators, such as the insurance commissioner of Delaware, are considering forcing insurers to build into their programs economic incentives for healthful life-styles, believing that it is not fair for "clean livers" to subsidize people who choose to follow less healthful life-styles. If this idea takes hold, employers' costs could rise or fall 20 percent or more, depending on the health of their workers. In turn, workers might see their own health insurance contributions go up or down, depending on their life-styles. The issue is fraught with difficulties. Employer surveys of workers' habits might be regarded as invasions of privacy; verification of the healthfulness of someone's life-style away from the worksite would be virtually impossible; behaviors that impact on health claim costs affect different people differently; and forcing workers to pay more for health insurance based on conditions such as obesity could lead to questions of discrimination. Some employers are turning the question on its head. They are giving certain workers—those who can show they are healthy, or who are willing to take part in programs such as smoking clinics—discounts on their insurance costs, or paying a higher percentage of those workers' medical bills.

still not smoking. All of these factors translated into reduced health risks for program participants, including a decreased risk of dying in the next ten years and decreased risks of cancer and heart attack. Added to which, participants reported improved attitudes toward health and improved perceptions of AT&T. Interestingly, even workers at sites where the pilot program was being tried out who chose not to take part in it increased their positive perceptions of AT&T more than workers at nonpilot sites. This indicates that employees view corporate health promotion favorably even if they do not actually participate in corporate programs.

A Palette of Programs

Credit for the first true fitness program in an American company goes to John H. Patterson, president of the National Cash Register Company in Dayton, Ohio. In 1894 he authorized morning and afternoon exercise programs for employees, installed a gymnasium for their use, and built a 325-acre park for employees and their families.

Today's programs range from the very simple to the very elaborate. Many were initially set up with key executives in mind, but the trend now is toward making them available to employees at every level, from the executive suite to the factory floor.

A Comprehensive Program. HALO, the program offered by Steelcase, Inc., an office furniture manufacturing company in Grand Rapids, Mich., is fairly representative of a comprehensive wellness program. HALO—which stands for Health Awareness/Lifestyle Orientation—emphasizes a holistic approach to health. Participants (employees and their spouses) begin by filling out a health risk appraisal questionnaire with four categories of questions: environment, life-style, heredity, and personal health. They are also given a medical examination. After the results of the health risk appraisal and the medical exam have been analyzed, groups of employees meet with medical experts in follow-up workshops to discuss the results, ask questions, or seek advice.

Employees can then choose which of the programs and facilities offered by the company are of most interest to them. These include counseling services, stress management courses, nutrition instruction, aerobic exercise classes, and stop smoking programs. There is even a special menu in the employee cafeteria offering low-fat, low-sodium, low-cholesterol items at a 5 percent discount.

An integral part of HALO is the nearby fitness center, where employees can buy low-cost memberships for themselves and their families. (The center is also open to retirees.) The center has the latest in exercise equipment, including treadmills, exercise bikes, weight-training equipment, rowing machines, and heart monitors. The building also houses a swimming pool, whirlpool, half-court basketball gym, two racquetball courts, and steam room and sauna facilities.

The fitness center has a full-time manager and a staff of certified fitness instructors. An exercise physiologist counsels members about the best way to achieve their health goals. A fitness-screening test helps them determine their strength, flexibility, and cardiovascular conditioning levels. On the basis of the test data, a computer prints out exercise programs personalized to fit each member's particular needs. Monthly computer printouts help assess fitness, showing aerobic points accumulated and calories burned. (As is true of all HALO health data, this information remains confidential.)

A light workout on the job can perk up staff meetings.

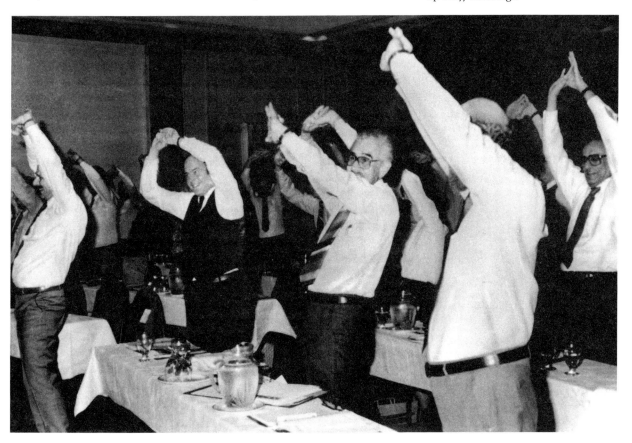

To help keep track of how HALO is affecting employee health, monthly health screenings are offered, such as cancer and blood pressure checks, cholesterol testing, and an examination of life-style habits. To make sure that the programs and activities zero in on employees' health needs, health risk appraisal data and insurance claims data are monitored to see what aspects of employee health require the most attention.

Variations on the Theme. There are, of course, many variations on the comprehensive program theme. SmithKline & French Laboratories' program, PATH (Programs to Achieve Total Health), does not have its own physical fitness center but has made arrangements for employees to use the athletic facilities of a nearby community college. On the health promotion side, PATH offers 25 or so wide-ranging activities, including a program on drinking and driving (offered around prom time) for the children of employees, a "wheezing and sneezing" workshop that teaches parents of new babies when a doctor's care is really needed, AIDS education, and help with caregiving for employees' elderly relatives and friends. An on-site dispensary, staffed by a physician and three nurses, is estimated to save the company well over $1 million in annual medical bills, because people are willing to come to work and use the dispensary rather than take a day off to visit a doctor. And a weekly Laugh Clinic offers a half-hour video of Bill Cosby or a live comic performance.

An important element in Control Data's StayWell program is fitness-related voluntary peer groups, which generate the peer support that is essential if there is to be long-term interest and participation in the program. These groups meet for any purpose, so long as it's consistent

Attending a Laugh Clinic can make employees feel better about life.

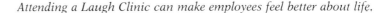

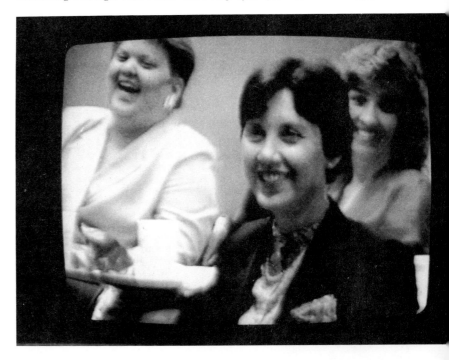

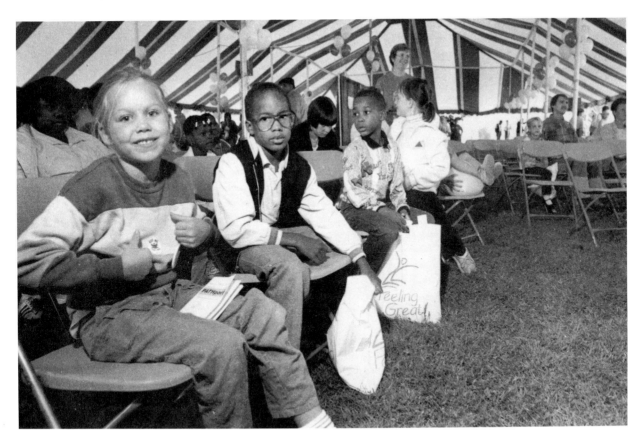

with StayWell program goals. There are groups of dieters, of runners and joggers, and of people who want to walk during their lunch hour, as well as groups that meet to help members quit smoking and groups that take canoe trips together. There has even been a square dancing group in the New York office.

Some companies regard Employee Assistance Programs as an integral part of their program. EAPs provide professional counseling to help employees and their families with personal and work-related problems such as those involving finances, mental and emotional disturbances, drugs, and alcohol. Some companies prefer to keep EAPs completely separate so the wellness program will not be thought of as dealing with "problem people."

Certain companies allow employees to exercise and attend class on company time, some make time available on a 50-50 basis at the beginning and end of the day or during an extended lunch hour, and some provide programs and facilities to be used on the employee's own time. In some programs employees at all levels work out together, while in others executives have separate facilities. Only employees are covered by certain programs, while in others family members can take part in at least certain activities. Membership fees may be charged to cover the cost of a fitness center, or use of the center may be free. Sometimes the cost is shared by the company and the employee because the company believes that payment of a nominal fee increases employee commitment.

Family members are sometimes encouraged to take part in company health promotion programs. Here, children at a company health fair listen to an explanation of the workings of the body.

115

Some companies have on-site programs run by a fitness/wellness director and support staff on the company payroll, while others bring in an outside organization to take charge. Groups such as the YMCA, the Association for Fitness in Business, and the American College of Sports Medicine, as well as consulting firms, may run corporate programs or can be used as a resource. Numbered among the consulting organizations are offshoots of Johnson & Johnson and Control Data, which had such success with the programs they developed for their own employees that they decided to market them.

On a Smaller Scale. Most companies cannot offer such full-service programs as Steelcase's HALO, Johnson & Johnson's Live for Life, or AT&T's Total Life Concept. They can, however, put something together for their employees. Companies can bring in medical and fitness personnel for health screenings. They can contact local heart, lung, and cancer associations, which often offer screening programs and give health courses, such as the American Heart Association's Heart at Work program. Local hospitals offer fitness classes, hypertension programs, quit smoking programs, and nutrition education. Companies using health maintenance organizations can bring to employees' attention any prevention packages that the HMO offers, such as hypertension, weight, and cholesterol control programs. Local health clubs and Ys offer exercise facilities and classes, and companies can share membership costs with employees who wish to take advantage of them. At a really basic level, companies can provide lockers, showers, and bicycle racks so that employees can use nearby park and community facilities, or they can offer "paper" programs consisting of bulletins, newsletters, and other fitness literature.

Even healthcare insurers can be a source of program help. The Blue Cross and Blue Shield Association has introduced a flexible, low-cost program called Your Healthy Best that a company can tailor to its needs. Components include a motivational video, personal health assessments (basically, questionnaires dealing with health history and life-style), newsletters, instructional books, and fitness diaries. Depending on the needs and interests of the company (and of the employees, who are surveyed), Blue Cross and Blue Shield may be able to add further elements to the program, depending on local resources. New York's Empire Blue Cross and Blue Shield, for example, can integrate into the basic program a worksite health fair to raise the level of employee interest and awareness, workshops on such topics as stress management and how to quit smoking, aerobics classes, screenings for problems like high blood pressure, and even drama workshops, in which professional actors perform a half-hour drama on an issue such as drug abuse, to be followed by group discussion.

The Ideal

According to the President's Council on Physical Fitness and Sports, the ideal fitness/wellness program in the workplace would have the following characteristics:

• Support from top company management and employee labor organizations.

FOOD FOR THOUGHT

As part of its attempt to give its employees an increased awareness of health, Steelcase, Inc., has built "food pavilions" in its plants that are designed to both soothe the spirit and provide healthful food for the body. On the principle that "the environment positions the palate," the food pavilions, which are actually restaurants in the middle of factory floors, have subdued lighting and are decorated with everything from murals on the walls to silk flowers on the tables.

Meals are planned and prepared by degreed chefs from a local junior college culinary program and served by experienced waiters and waitresses. A nutritionist is available to help employees with special needs, such as people with diabetes or weight problems, work out healthful diets. By all of the foods are signs stating the number of calories they contain. At each meal, at least one entrée and several à la carte items have a HALO sign beside them. This tells employees that they are low in calories, low in sodium, and low in cholesterol—and that they are available at a 5 percent discount. That doesn't mean everyone buys the most healthful dishes all the time, of course, but there are days when HALO entrées sell more than the others. Providing more healthful options in this fashion, Steelcase believes, is the best way to get people to alter their eating habits.

- Strong and effective program leadership.
- Easy and convenient access for employees to programs and facilities.
- Initial health and fitness assessments, periodic testing, and careful monitoring of fitness activities so that progress can be measured.
- Personalized programs.
- Diversity in the program.
- A professional environment in which the fitness/wellness program is taken as seriously and run as well as any other company office or department.
- Total programming—that is, programs with both fitness and health promotion components.
- An enjoyment factor.
- Skillful public relations. As any health program must be voluntary, it needs to be sold through skillful marketing and public relations, which will keep the program visible and stimulate interest and motivation. Among the public relations devices used are personal invitations to new employees to join a program; orientation sessions for new employees given by fitness staff; in-house newsletters; educational workshops; films; talks by guest speakers; displays in the company cafeteria; and bulletins posted strategically throughout the company. Sometimes activities are linked to special events in the community, as when Canada Life ran a special "Go for the Gold" week to tie in with the 1988 Winter Olympics in Calgary.
- Incentives. Closely linked with public relations efforts are incentive programs to keep employee motivation and participation high. Johnson & Johnson gives prizes such as sweatsuits and smoke alarms to boost participation. Employees of McKee Baking Company can earn "McKee dollars," to be cashed in for sports-related items ranging from headbands to baseball jackets. Berol USA credits each employee with $500 a year, minus whatever it has to pay out in insurance claims, and King Broadcasting splits its savings with its employees.

The Future

Professionals in the fitness/wellness field are convinced that corporate programs are here to stay. They envision some changes—more emphasis on modifying employee life-styles, more ways of providing programs, and a greater emphasis on management skills for corporate health directors—but the major theme is growth. Given the enormous stakes for American business, they are very probably right. □

SOURCES OF FURTHER INFORMATION

Blue Cross and Blue Shield Association, 676 N. St. Clair Street, Chicago, IL 60611.
President's Council on Physical Fitness and Sports, Washington, DC 20001.
Prevention Leadership Forum, 229½ Pennsylvania Avenue S.E., Washington, DC 20001.

How to Prevent Childhood Obesity

Myron Winick, M.D.

Obesity, and all its attendant problems, very often start in childhood. A startling fact is that in the United States almost one in four children of school age (between the ages of 6 and 17) can be considered obese—that is, 20 percent or more over ideal weight. Childhood obesity is increasingly being recognized as a medical problem—to be treated as such or, better yet, actively prevented.

Over 60 percent of obese children and adolescents remain significantly overweight as adults. Their excess weight increases their risk for heart disease, high blood pressure, diabetes, certain cancers, gall bladder disease, and complications from surgery. Some evidence also exists that bad eating habits that start in childhood, even if later corrected, can contribute to the development of serious conditions ranging from osteoporosis to atherosclerosis (hardening of the arteries).

Nor are the consequences of childhood obesity purely physical. Overweight children are often the butt of ridicule from their peers, who can be notably cruel. They may also be subjected to constant criticism from their parents. The consequent loss of self-esteem can lead children to seek consolation by eating even more.

There is evidence that the situation is getting worse instead of better. From 1963 to 1980, according to a recently published study, the prevalence of obesity among American children in the 6 to 11 age bracket increased by more than 50 percent and the prevalence of adolescent obesity increased by nearly 40 percent. If childhood obesity were an infectious disease, it would certainly be called an epidemic.

In the past, the major concern of health professionals caring for children was to ensure optimal growth and development and to prevent and/or treat childhood diseases. Today, pediatricians also concentrate on lowering the risk of eventual development of the degenerative diseases of mature years. An important part of this new effort is the prevention of childhood obesity or successful treatment of it. There are many practical steps that can be taken to keep children from becoming overweight.

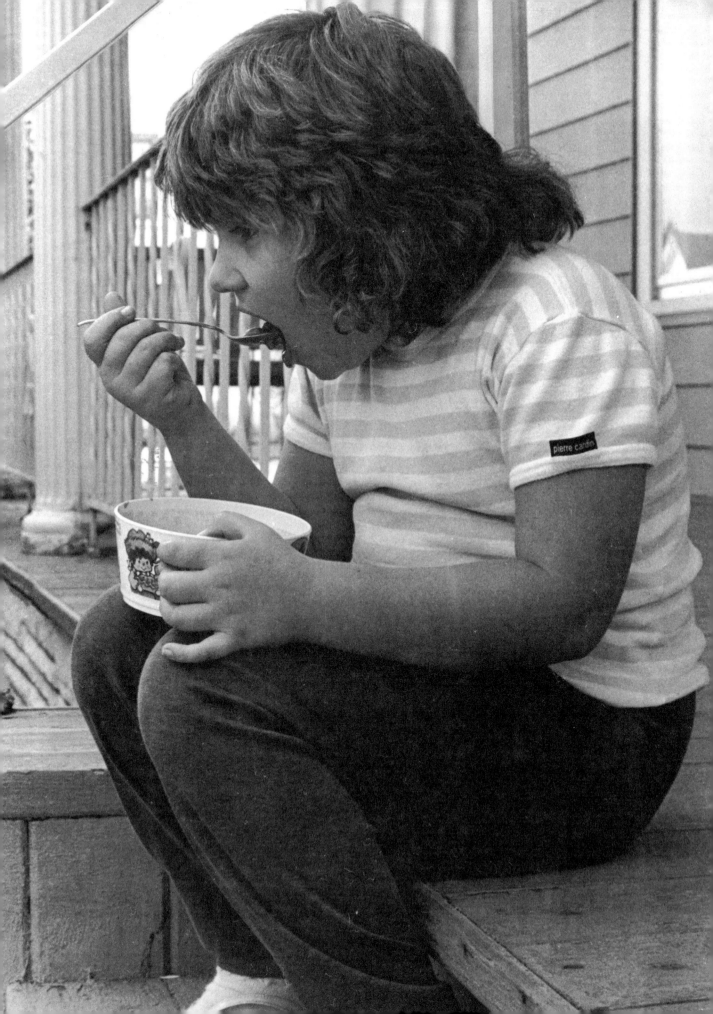

How the Body Stores Fat

Fat within the body can be packaged in different ways. All body fat is contained within cells known as adipocytes, each of which contains a single globule of fat. The size of each globule, and therefore of each cell, can vary enormously. In most people who become obese as adults, these fat cells are very large—sometimes five or six times normal size. However, people may be obese in another way. They may have too many fat cells, so that even if each cell contains a normal amount of fat, the total amount of body fat is too high.

The number of fat cells usually increases only from fetal life through adolescence. Thus, childhood and adolescent obesity tends to be due primarily to too many fat cells. Once a fat cell is formed, it remains throughout life. Weight reduction in adults reduces the size of fat cells

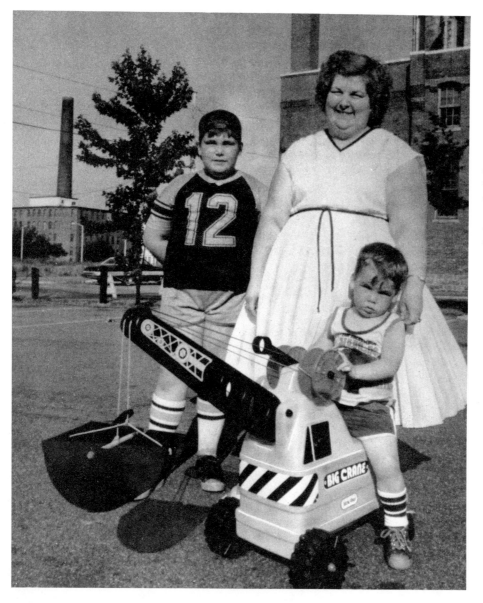

A child with one obese parent has about a 30 percent chance of becoming obese; if both parents are obese, the risk increases to 60 percent.

but does not affect their number. If obesity is caused by fat cells that are too large, then reducing their size returns tissue to normal. But if the problem is too many fat cells, then weight reduction will result in even more abnormal tissue: too many fat cells that are also too small. There is abundant evidence that obese people whose fat tissue contains this double abnormality almost always regain any weight they lose. This explains why obesity that begins in childhood often proves to be very difficult to treat once the person has become an adult.

The Genetic Factor

Scientists know that many chronic diseases are not caused by a single factor. Obesity, particularly childhood obesity, is no exception. Both genetic and environmental factors may increase the risk of any child's becoming obese.

The evidence that a genetic component often contributes to the development of obesity comes from several sources. First, studies have shown that if one parent is obese, the risk that a child will become obese is about 30 percent. If both parents are obese, the risk doubles to about 60 percent. Second, studies of identical twins have shown that even if they are reared in different environments (by different adoptive parents) they will be very similar in their body proportions: if one is lean, the other will be lean; if one is obese, the other will be obese. Almost invariably, both twins conform to the body types of their biological parents. Third, a number of strains of animal species are clearly genetically obese.

Most childhood obesity is caused primarily by the number of, rather than the size of, fat cells in the body.

In most people with a genetic propensity toward obesity, however, the genetic component increases the risk but does not absolutely determine that they will become obese. Since genetic makeup cannot be altered, people who are at risk must try to alter their environment, or behavior, in such a way as to lower that risk. Whatever form this environmental change may take, the person with a genetic tendency toward obesity will have to work harder than other people to avoid gaining weight.

Metabolic Differences

In the past few years, a number of important studies have begun to uncover the genetic defect that increases the risk of obesity, particularly childhood obesity. Health experts have long known that the difference between the number of calories a person takes in and the number that person burns up determines whether body fat increases or decreases. If people expend more calories than they consume, some of their body fat will be burned, and they will lose weight. By contrast, if they take in more calories than they expend, they will store the excess as fat. The implication, of course, is that fat people eat too much, exercise too

Myron Winick is R. R. Williams Professor of Nutrition and professor of pediatrics at the College of Physicians and Surgeons, Columbia University, New York City.

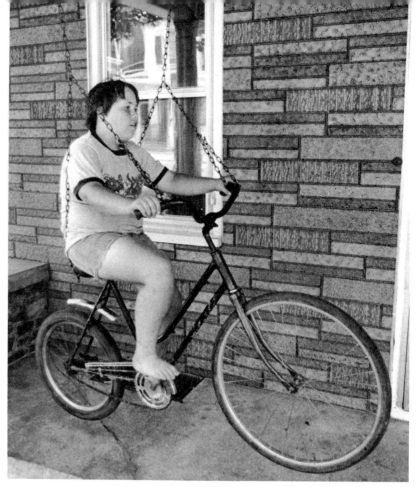

People at genetic risk for obesity must work harder to avoid it. For this Pennsylvania boy, an exercise bicycle replaces a porch swing.

little, or both. However, many obese people have noted that they did not eat more than their lean friends, nor did they exercise less. These observations were for many years dismissed as anecdotal and in violation of the laws of thermodynamics. Today, we know that they are probably correct.

It appears that many obese people handle calories within their bodies more efficiently than lean people. At any given caloric intake, obese people need fewer calories to maintain and operate the necessary functions of the body, and they have more calories left over to be stored as fat. For example, a lean woman who consumes 2,500 calories a day may use 1,500 to maintain body temperature, heart rate, respiration, digestion, and the like and to supply the energy required by all cells to function properly at rest; she expends 1,000 as a result of all the exercise she does during the day. She is in caloric balance and will neither gain nor lose weight. By contrast, an obese woman may also consume 2,500 calories a day but may need only 1,200 to run her body efficiently at rest. If she too expends 1,000 calories in exercise, but is left with a 300-calorie excess, or about 0.1 pounds of fat a day, 3 pounds a month, or 36 pounds a year. Thus, very small differences in the way the body handles calories can, over a long period of time, make a significant difference in one's weight.

This finding emerged only recently, as the technology became available to measure the small differences in the ways people use calories. Patients have been studied in chambers constructed to measure the amount of heat generated by the complex energy-consuming reactions in all of the body's cells. Such studies demonstrate that for any given calorie intake, many obese people will have a grater tendency than other people to accumulate fat.

This conclusion raises the question—answered even more recently—of whether the metabolic difference produces obesity or obesity produces the metabolic difference. Studies had indicated that obese people who lost weight and attained what is considered the ideal weight for their height and build would regain the lost weight even with the small caloric intake and the same energy expenditure as a normally lean

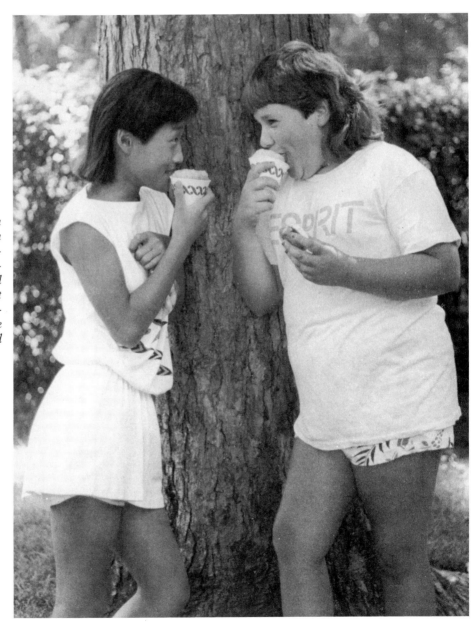

The same sweet treat can have different effects on different girls. Many children gain excess weight because their bodies need fewer calories to carry out necessary metabolic functions; thus, they have more calories left over to be stored as fat.

person of the same ideal weight. These studies suggested that metabolic differences could occur even if the patient was not obese at the time of measurement. But still to be determined was whether one needed to be obese first before the body became a more efficient calorie user or whether some people were *becoming* obese because their bodies used calories more efficiently.

Two studies released in 1988 suggest that the latter is true. One of them involved the Pima Indians of the American Southwest, who have an extremely high incidence of obesity. Although the obesity can begin at any age, it is usually manifest by the time a person reaches young adulthood. In studying young Pima adults who were not obese, researchers found two distinct groups: those who were very efficient in metabolizing calories and those who were not. Two years later the investigators found that a high percentage of those in the more efficient group had become obese. By contrast, few in the group that was metabolizing calories less efficiently had become obese. In this population, then, it was generally possible to predict who would become obese.

Is this difference in metabolism inherited from one's parents, and can it be demonstrated at a young age? To answer these questions, a group of investigators in Great Britain studied infants of obese and lean mothers. All of the infants were lean at the time the study began. A significant number of those whose mothers were obese metabolized calories more efficiently. One year after birth, those babies who had

Young people who are chronic television watchers are in more danger of gaining weight. Reason: lack of exercise and the temptation to snack.

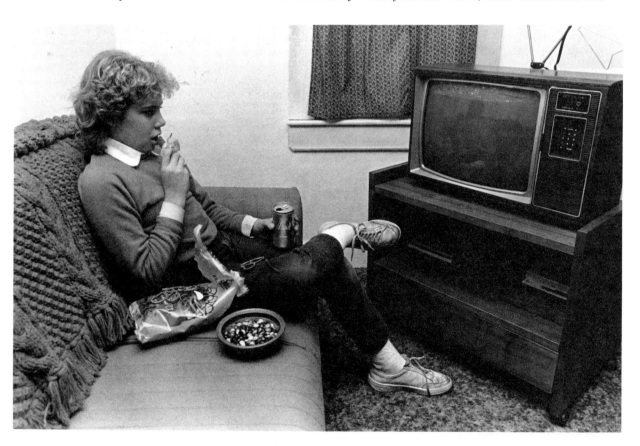

developed obesity were almost exclusively from the group of efficient calorie users. These two studies demonstrate that a portion of the population metabolizes calories in such a way as to be at higher risk for obesity. This type of metabolism is probably genetically determined and can be identified in children before they become obese.

The Effects of Environment

While genetics may determine who is at higher risk for obesity, environment appears to determine who actually becomes obese. Both the physical and the social environment play a role in the risk for obesity. There are a number of examples of the influence of physical surroundings: the chance of developing long-term obesity is 2½ times greater in the winter than in the summer, 3 times greater for those who live in the northeastern and midwestern United States than for those who live in the southern or western United States, and 1½ times greater for those who live in a large metropolitan area than for those who live in a small urban area. All of the factors associated with higher rates of obesity are probably related to life-style: they encourage an increased food intake and a more sedentary existence.

Obesity in children is more common among affluent families.

Perhaps even more important than physical environment are the social conditions that determine life-style. Obesity in adult women is more common among lower socioeconomic groups. By contrast, obesity in children is more common among higher socioeconomic groups, perhaps reflecting a tendency for affluent parents to overfeed their children. Larger families have less childhood obesity, and oldest or only children are at highest risk.

Probably the single most important social variable involved in producing obesity, however, is the amount of time a child spends watching television. There is a statistical relationship between television viewing and the incidence of childhood obesity, and the strength of that relationship suggests cause and effect. Besides discouraging children from physical activity, watching television encourages them to eat. This encouragement is not just indirect: during prime time, scenes with characters eating are shown an average of eight times an hour, and food, particularly high-calorie snack food, is advertised at almost every commercial break.

Guarding Against Childhood Obesity

Given these complex causes of obesity, which no doubt interact with one another, what can parents do to protect their children from obesity? First, they can try to determine if a child is at genetic risk for obesity. Is one or both parents obese? Is a sibling obese? Is there a history of obesity among close relatives? If the answer to any of these questions is yes, a child must be considered at high risk. If both parents are obese, the child is at very high risk.

Since parents cannot do anything about their child's genes, they must eliminate or reduce the environmental factors. The focus of prevention for a high-risk child is controlling caloric intake and encouraging caloric expenditure—allowing less high-calorie food and encouraging

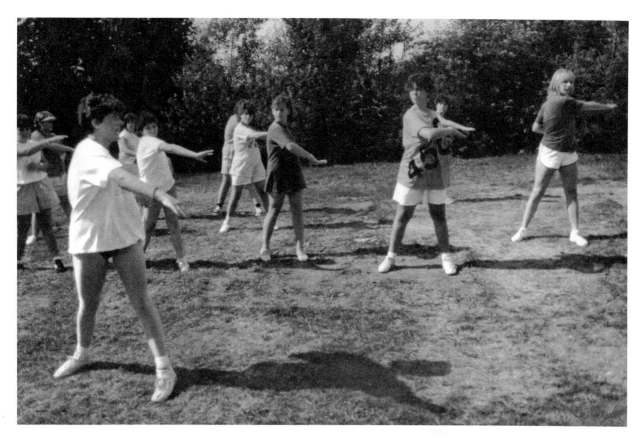

more exercise. To do this, parents must create an environment that fosters this kind of life-style, and they must understand that the restriction of calories may have to be greater than in a child whose risk for obesity is low. The child, of course, requires an adequate number of calories to grow and develop normally; caloric restriction cannot be too great, or the child's growth could be stunted.

For any child, the major principle in avoiding childhood obesity is to ensure that the child increases in height and weight proportionally. The child should be weighed regularly, and if weight is increasing at a greater rate than height, weight gain should be slowed or stopped temporarily (it is rarely necessary for a child to lose weight to prevent obesity). Because the child is growing, the diet must be balanced so that it contains adequate amounts of vitamins and minerals. Special high-protein or other unconventional types of diets have no place in preventing or treating childhood obesity.

Parents can do a number of things to ensure that their child does not gain weight at an inappropriate rate. Some of these are listed, and as noted above, such guidelines are especially important for children genetically at high risk. Perhaps most important, however, is setting a good example. Children have a better chance of avoiding obesity if the whole family eats and exercises sensibly.

Infancy. Infants should be breast-fed if possible. Breast-fed children tend to gain weight more slowly than children who are fed formula. Also, infants should not be given solid foods too early; when solids are

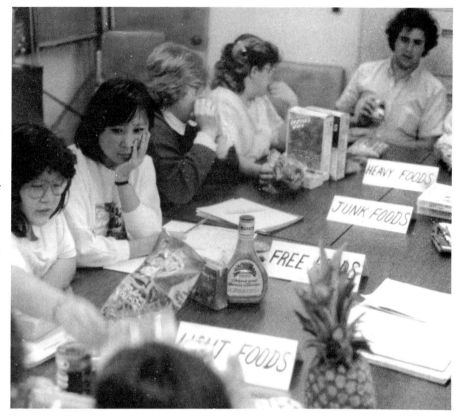

Treating childhood obesity is much more difficult than preventing it. Girls at a summer weight-loss camp near New York City (left) try to take off the pounds with aerobic dancing; at right, adolescents learn about nutrition in Shapedown, a nationwide program developed to treat obesity in children and adolescents.

introduced before four to six months, the child is likely to consume more calories than necessary.

Childhood. Discourage excessive consumption of foods that are high in fat. This may not be easy, since high-fat foods include such childhood delights as french fries, hot dogs, and hamburgers. The key to success may lie in encouraging moderation rather than total abstinence, which may be an unrealistic (and not absolutely necessary) goal. Dairy products, while they contain essential nutrients and are an important part of a child's diet, are also a source of fat. Children 2 to 5 years of age can be given low-fat (2 percent) milk and other dairy products, and children over 5 can use 1 percent or skim dairy products. (Children under 2 need a higher-fat diet and should not be given low-fat milk products.)

Minimize children's intake of foods high in refined sugar, such as cookies, candy, soda, and cake. (Again, limiting rather than trying to totally eliminate these foods may be the best way to go.) Refined sugar is not only bad for developing teeth but is also a source of calories unaccompanied by nutrients ("empty calories"). Encourage children to eat complex carbohydrates and foods high in fiber (fruits, vegetables, whole-grain breads and cereals). These foods are low in calories but high in vitamins and minerals.

Do not use food as either a reward or a punishment. Don't insist that children finish every morsel on their plate, and don't overindulge them with food—keep portion sizes and the number of "treats" moderate.

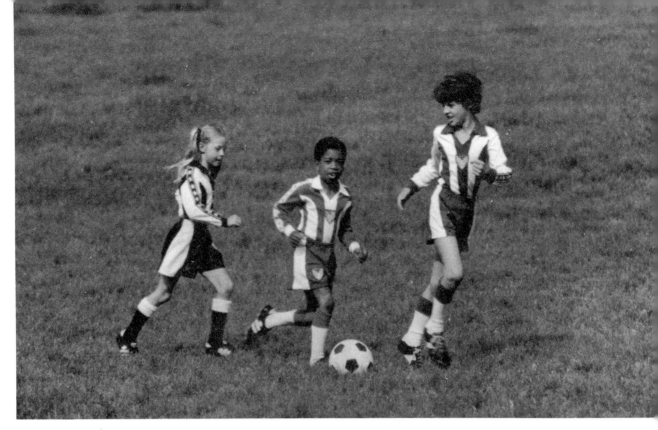

Physical activity and sports are key factors in keeping children trim.

Discourage excessive television viewing, and limit snacking during viewing periods. Some children sit in front of the television for as many as 25 hours a week. Reducing television time will reduce children's desire for high-calorie snacks and reduce the time they spend in sedentary activities. Instead, encourage physical activity and sports, which will increase caloric expenditure. Make a particular effort to encourage activities (indoor swimming, gymnastics and dance classes) that expend energy during winter months in cold climates.

Adolescence. Discourage adolescents from eating at fast-food restaurants, and encourage them to make proper choices when they do eat there. Fast foods are generally high in calories, fat, and sodium. However, more nutritious choices are often available, such as salad, juice, pizza, fruit, sherbet, and yogurt. Also, encourage teenagers to exercise restraint at parties. Those chips and dips can provide a lot of calories.

Discourage adolescents from snacking while watching television and while studying. Provide low-caloric snacks for these periods if they want something to munch on—carrots or raisins, for example, rather than cookies or ruffled potato chips.

Encourage physical activity and sports, which will increase caloric expenditure. Older teenagers might be reminded that they can walk rather than take the car if going only a short distance.

Stronger Measures

If the guidelines just outlined are followed and the child nevertheless starts gaining weight too rapidly, then more stringent action is called for to prevent obesity. A plan should be adopted, with the child's understanding, to limit calories while at the same time providing adequate amounts of all required nutrients. A multivitamin tablet containing the Recommended Daily Dietary Allowances (RDAs) for all of the vitamins and essential minerals can be taken for insurance. The diet should stress reducing fat, the most concentrated source of calories, and increasing intake of foods containing complex carbohydrates and fiber, which are lower in calories and high in nutrients. The trick is to make every calorie count. Foods of high nutrient density (a high content of vitamins and minerals per calorie) should be chosen. The child must be weighed frequently, and caloric intake adjusted as necessary. The child should not lose weight but rather should gain more slowly than height is increasing. The diet changes and monitoring of their effects should be supervised by a physician.

Correcting Obesity in Children

Treating childhood obesity is much more difficult than preventing it. The approach is the same, but the measures may have to be even more stringent and may take a considerable amount of time. A physician's supervision is advisable. Actual weight loss should still not be attempted unless the child is extremely obese. For the moderately or slightly obese child the goal is to choose a diet and exercise routine that will keep weight constant while allowing the child to grow normally. Literally, the child should grow out of the obesity. This may take months and sometimes years, but it is the safest course and the one most likely to succeed in the long run. The principles are the same as with preventive dieting; however, the goal is to prevent any weight gain rather than just to reduce the rate of gain. The number of calories permitted will again vary with the child; therefore, frequent weighing (once a week) is necessary, and the number of calories must be adjusted downward if any weight gain occurs.

Parents need to provide emotional support as well as nutritional guidance to obese children.

When this approach is used for treating childhood obesity, it is very important that calories not be restricted to any greater degree than necessary to stabilize weight. Crash diets or fad diets should never be used. They may reduce weight, but they may also stunt growth so that if the weight returns to its previous levels (which it often does), the child will have an even greater problem.

For children who are severely obese, the goal may have to be modified. Rather than ideal weight, which may be difficult to reach and almost impossible to maintain, a weight 10 or 15 percent above ideal weight may be used as a goal. Such a figure is enough to reduce significantly the risk for the complications of obesity that develop later in life.

While helping the child do the right thing nutritionally, parents should be emotionally supportive as well—praising progress and not being harshly critical either of occasional lapses or of the existence of a weight problem in the first place. (Criticism can be perceived not just from what is said but from facial expression or amount of affection displayed.) While many overweight children are undoubtedly happy and well-adjusted, others may suffer loneliness, isolation, and low self-esteem. In order to help their children achieve an ideal weight, parents need to be especially sensitive to these potential problems. □

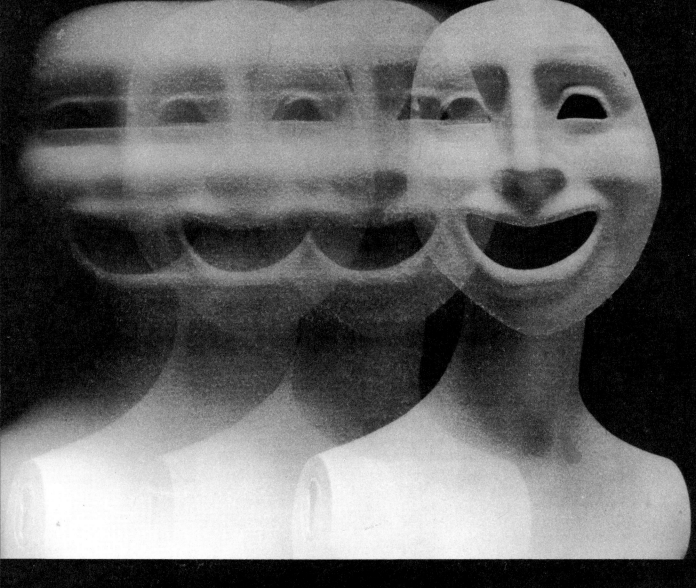

Mania and

Bruce Shapiro, M.D.

Ancient history is replete with stories of people afflicted with major depression and manic-depression. The Bible describes graphically the severe depression, self-destructive urges, and eventual suicide of King Saul and tells of others in states of pathological excitement that were probably manic in nature.

In the fifth century B.C., Hippocrates, the Greek physician celebrated as the father of medicine, was the first to use the

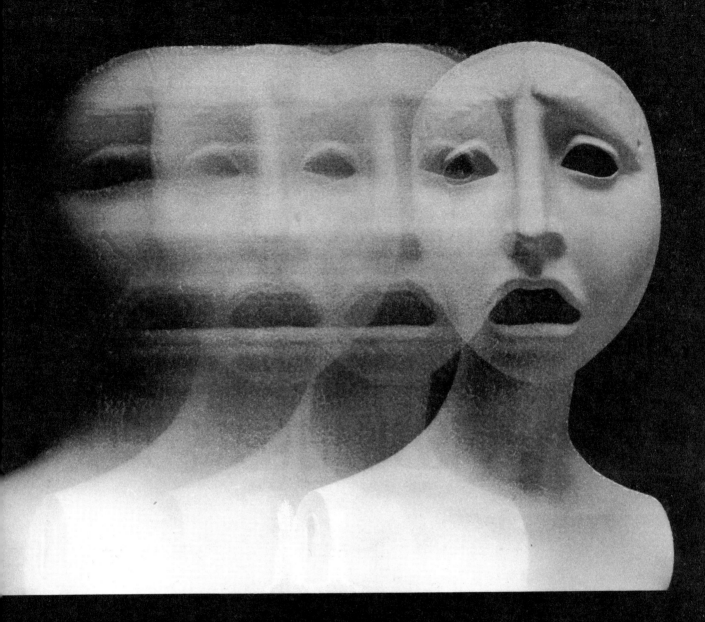

Depression

term "melancholia" to describe depression, which he attributed to an excess of black (*melan*) bile (*chol*). Hippocrates was also the first to note that mania (uncontrolled excitement) tended to occur episodically in individuals who also suffered from depression.

In the 1600s, English writer and clergyman Robert Burton said in *The Anatomy of Melancholy* that "other men get their knowledge from books, I get mine from melancholizing."

Burton detailed the sense of isolation, despair, anger, and pain that is so often felt in depression.

Individuals who suffered from depression or manic-depression have shaped the course of history. Some of the world's most famous leaders—including Winston Churchill and Abraham Lincoln—have had well-documented mood-swing disorders. Lincoln would at times be so deeply depressed that his aides would hide the guns in the White House to prevent his possible suicide. Churchill had periods of great energy and overactivity that alternated with severe depressions; he called the latter his "black dog."

Major depression, a disorder involving episodes of depression only, strikes approximately 15 percent of the U.S. population during the course of their lifetime and affects about 1 in 20 individuals at any given moment. Manic-depression, less common, involves both mania

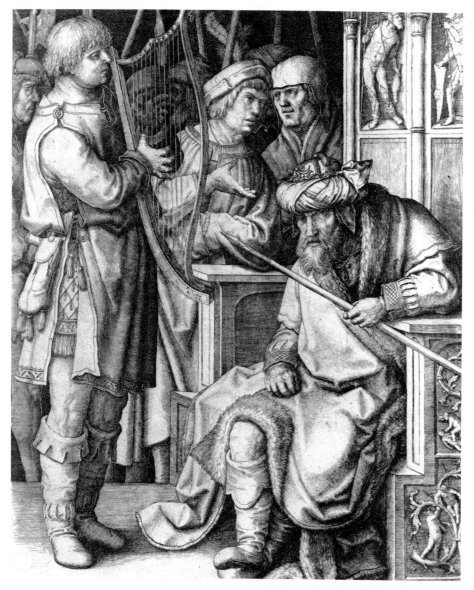

This 16th-century Dutch print shows David playing the harp before Saul, perhaps to ease the depression that was said to have afflicted the biblical king.

and depression and affects approximately 1 percent of the population. But these statistics apply to the more severe forms of depression and manic-depression; the prevalence of their less severe but still painful and disruptive forms is significantly greater. The episodes of depression that occur in both these disorders have similar characteristics, and their treatment, too, is essentially the same, although in the case of manic-depression, care is taken to avoid triggering a manic episode.

Major depression is more common in women (occurring in over 20 percent of American women) than in men (about 10 percent of whom are affected). Mania, on the other hand, occurs as often in men as in women. Although theories have been ventured of possible sex-linked inheritance of depression or cultural biases that allow it to be more acceptable in women, we still do not know why gender affects the prevalence of this illness.

Defining the Disorders

It was not until the turn of the century that German psychiatrist Emil Kraepelin established the modern view of manic-depressive illness and described its manifestations. He was the first to differentiate manic-depression from schizophrenia (or, as schizophrenia was known then, dementia praecox). Kraepelin described manic-depression as recurrent manic and depressive episodes without the disorganization of thinking and deterioration in personality and functioning found in schizophrenia, and he noted that it was marked by periods of illness and subsequent recovery.

The periods of illness in a person with manic-depression can vary in nature. An episode may consist of symptoms of both mania and depression or of only either one. (In rare cases, individuals experience episodes of mania without ever suffering any periods of depression.) Most people with manic-depression do recover rather fully between periods of illness. The modern psychiatric term for manic-depression is bipolar disorder.

Manic-depressive and depressive disorders occur in varying degrees of severity. An individual may suffer from *dysthymia*, a minor depression (what used to be called neurotic depression), or from *major depression*, in which depressive moods and psychological and biological changes significantly interfere with usual functioning. In *melancholia* as the term is now used in psychiatry, biological changes result in an even more severe form of depression, which brings on almost complete emotional paralysis. Similarly, the symptoms of mood expansion may be mild (hypomanic) or severe (manic). *Cyclothymia* is a term used to refer to a milder form of manic-depressive illness with shorter and less severe cycles of depression and hypomania. The milder forms of manic-depression often masquerade as—or are misdiagnosed as—other medical or psychological problems.

Major depression strikes about 15 percent of Americans at some point in their lives. Many more people suffer from less severe forms of depression.

Bruce Shapiro is psychiatrist-in-chief and chairman of the Department of Psychiatry, The Stamford Hospital, Stamford, Conn., and clinical associate professor of psychiatry at New York Medical College in Valhalla, N.Y.

Mania. An individual's first manic attack can occur at any time from the late childhood years through adulthood, but most commonly the attacks begin between the ages of 15 and 35. Affected individuals may be elated or irritable and are often overactive, physically restless, and talkative. Their speech seems pressured, as if they were trying to keep pace with racing thoughts, and they may have grandiose plans and expectations. They may also feel little need for sleep, be easily distracted, and have a decreased attention span. Not uncommonly they engage in activities that have a high potential for painful consequences. Examples include sexual indiscretions, buying sprees or foolish investments, and reckless driving. During bouts of mania, some individuals deplete their life savings or get into trouble with the law. In addition, a manic person may be paranoid or suffer from a mixture of grandiose, religious, and paranoid delusions. In its severe forms, mania may cause people to feel that they are at the center of a grand scheme and that, as a result, others (the police, the CIA) are in pursuit of them. Manic patients are often demanding and unreasonable and often seem to be at the center of confrontation and difficulties.

Untreated mania can have devastating consequences. It can lead to spouse and child abuse, family breakup, financial ruin, drug and alcohol abuse, other criminal behavior, even homicide. When the manic episode breaks, a depressive spiral ending in suicide is possible. In psychotic forms of mania, individuals may lose contact with reality and have hallucinations. Psychotic mania may represent a medical emergency.

Mild forms of mania (hypomania) may manifest themselves in overproductivity, heightened activity and energy, restlessness, and decreased susceptibility to fatigue. Often individuals with milder forms of mania become valued members of organizations and businesses. A certain percentage of workaholics and so-called Type A personalities (fiercely competitive, hard-driving people) are clearly hypomanic. Thus, society may seek out and reward those with milder forms of mania. In its severe forms, however, mania is clearly not adaptive—it is destructive.

Depression. The usual indication of major depression is a loss of ability to experience pleasure. This lack of enjoyment is often accompanied by sadness, worry, or irritability. Depressed individuals frequently suffer from decreased appetite, weight loss, insomnia, and loss of interest in sex (although occasionally, increased appetite, weight gain, and excessive sleepiness may occur). Depressed people often feel a sense of hopelessness, defeat, guilt, and worthlessness. They may be unable to concentrate or to remember things as well as before and may exhibit an indecisiveness that can impede daily functioning and be particularly painful to them. The depression usually brings a loss of energy, which may be compounded by painful anxiety—pacing, hand-wringing, and a furrowed brow are characteristic physical symptoms.

Suicidal thoughts are not uncommon during depression; the rate of suicide is much higher among manic-depressives and people suffering from major depression than among the general U.S. population. Suicide is the cause of death in 15 to 20 percent of those who have been diagnosed with these disorders, accounting for at least one-third of

A severe bout of mania may give rise to grandiose delusions.

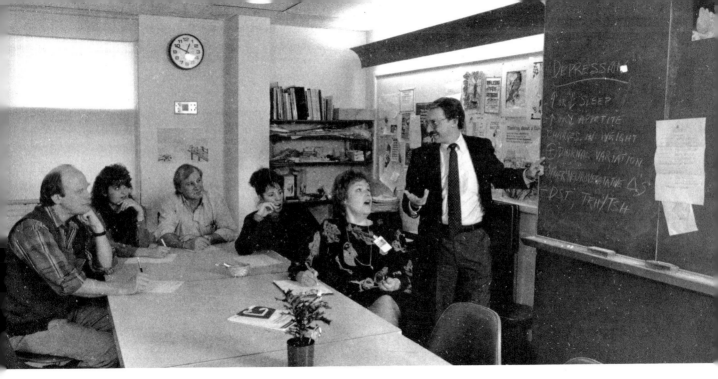

The author, Dr. Bruce Shapiro, reviews some common symptoms of depression with his staff.

completed suicides in the general population. The risk of suicide may be high early in the course of illness, with the turmoil and confusion of the first episode. Suicide attempts also tend to occur when the individual is just beginning to recover. Thus, the period following discharge from treatment in a hospital is one of increased suicide risk because at that time individuals may not be free of hopeless thoughts but may have more energy and therefore be more capable of completing a suicidal act. The risk of suicide increases with the length of illness and is particularly high in depressed elderly men.

The Course of Illness

The course of manic-depression or major depression can vary greatly. Between 20 and 30 percent of patients will have either rapid recurrences of episodes of illness or persistent disabling symptoms. A similar percentage will have just one episode. Most commonly, however, individuals will experience a number of episodes, separated by months or even years. Between episodes most individuals will have normal moods and mood shifts. They may hold responsible jobs and be very involved with family life.

In manic-depression the manic episodes can last for a few days or a few months, but they tend to be briefer than depressive episodes and to begin and end more abruptly. Depressive episodes are generally more frequent, and if untreated, they typically last six months or longer.

At times a manic or depressive episode may come on without any obvious cause. At other times a clear psychological or physical stressor leads to the episode. The rejection by or loss of a loved one, a recent failure, the loss of a job, or, interestingly, the stresses of success can precipitate both manic and depressive episodes. Sometimes these episodes are preceded by viral or other physical illnesses.

A relatively small psychological stressor may seem to initiate a major manic or depressive episode. It is often unclear, however, whether the

135

stressor truly precipitated the episode or whether the episode had already begun and the stressor was later perceived as its cause. The following case history illustrates this phenomenon:

> Mr. L., a successful professional, went through a period of feeling "wonderful" during which he took on multiple projects, overextended himself, began to invest impulsively, and felt "tireless." Mr. L. did not feel that he was experiencing a mood disorder—just an enjoyable sense of energy and involvement. He felt this way despite a history of two manic and three depressive episodes for which he needed brief hospitalizations, electroconvulsive (formerly called electroshock) therapy, and stabilization with the drug lithium. But as he planned to move to a new home, he began to feel tired, anxious, sad, and unable to concentrate. Although his finances were secure, he began to worry about his ability to pay his new mortgage, and he soon felt preoccupied, and then overwhelmed, by financial concerns. He came to believe that his planned move was the cause of his anxious depression, and feeling severely depressed and unable to cope, he requested treatment.

A simulated session in which a patient in a depressed state meets with his psychotherapist.

In examining this man's history, one should ask: Which came first, the chicken or the egg? Did this man's change of residence and new mortgage affect his ability to cope and precipitate a depression? Or did he have a major depressive mood shift that coincided with the timing of his planned move and that led him to erroneously identify the

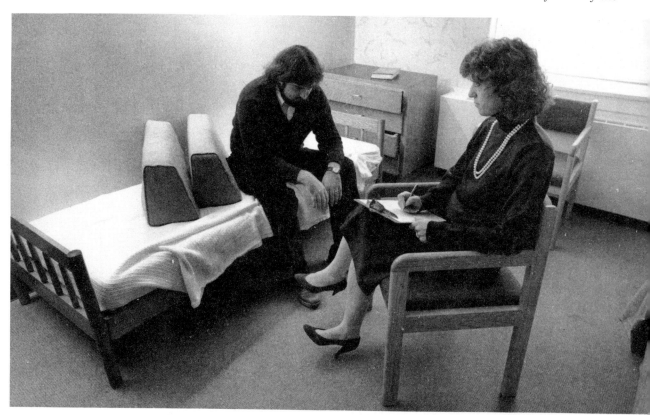

move as the cause of the depression? There is one further possibility—one that is actually more likely than either of the two above. Like other individuals with manic-depressive illness, Mr. L. may have been vulnerable to specific stressors—in this instance, having to deal with a major change in daily living habits. When he experienced such a stressor, he began to have changes in body chemistry (alterations in the quantities of certain brain chemicals, which lead to hormonal changes) that developed into a full-blown depressive episode.

The focus of medical attention is generally on major episodes of illness. But between episodes, individuals with manic-depression or major depression may display subtle psychological symptoms related to their disorder. These include a tendency to break down under stress, a lowered energy level, feelings of insecurity, a tendency to worry, a lack of assertiveness, and dependent and obsessional traits.

Mr. L., in the example above, clearly illustrates another hallmark of manic-depressive illness. During the manic (or hypomanic) phase, individuals feel that they are fine and often see no need for consultation or treatment. They deny their pathologically elevated mood and ignore the consequences of their behavior. In contrast, when they become depressed, they generally know that they are ill and are more likely to seek assistance. Nevertheless, at least two-thirds of those who suffer bouts of depression do not seek treatment. When the pain of depression is combined with a lack of treatment, suicide becomes a strong risk.

When the pain of severe depression is not treated, it may lead to suicidal impulses.

The Search for Causes

The question of what causes manic-depression or major depression has been with us for about as long as the illnesses themselves. Unfortunately, psychiatrists still do not have definitive answers, although they are now closer to being able to identify some probable causes. Starting with the black bile theory of Hippocrates, one can find almost as many swings in the theories of what causes mood disorders as in the moods of the sufferers themselves. The Middle Ages brought theories of demonic possession and witchcraft. Erasmus Darwin, the English physician and grandfather of Charles Darwin, thought that major mental disorders were the result of congealed blood in the brain. Psychiatrists of the mid-1800s classified psychotic states together with mental retardation.

The two major types of theories of causation over the past century have been the biological and the psychological. The psychological theories have focused on disturbing early childhood experiences—emotional loss, separation and its insecurities, and a sense of early emotional abandonment that prevented the development of a strong, stable sense of self able to withstand the pressures of life. Advocates of a biological cause of illness find support in the evidence that mood-swing disorders run in families and are responsive to medication and electroconvulsive therapy.

What is emerging today is an integrative approach. Current evidence indicates that there are significant differences among individuals who suffer from manic-depression or major depression and that many

Drugs for Depression and Mania

Commonly Used Drugs[1]	Advantages	Possible Side Effects
DEPRESSION		
Tricyclic antidepressants: imipramine (Tofranil), amitriptyline (Elavil), doxepin (Sinequan)	Generally effective; work in 1–4 weeks; used for over 30 years	Weight gain; dry mouth; constipation; blurred vision; light-headedness
MAO inhibitors: phenelzine (Nardil), tranylcypromine (Parnate), isocarboxazid (Marplan)	Very effective in atypical depressions that involve anxiety or panic	Insomnia; may interact with certain foods or other drugs to produce severe hypertension[2]
Other: maprotiline (Ludiomil)	Some side effects occur less frequently than with tricyclics	Dry mouth; constipation; blurred vision; light-headedness
fluoxetine (Prozac)	Side effects even less likely to be a problem than with maprotiline	Anxiety; insomnia
ANXIETY ASSOCIATED WITH DEPRESSION		
Minor tranquilizers: alprazolam (Xanax), lorazepam (Ativan), chlordiazepoxide (Librium)	Relieve anxiety	Sedation; tolerance; withdrawal symptoms when drug discontinued
MANIA		
lithium carbonate, lithium citrate (Eskalith, Lithobid)	Most effective antimanic agents; work in 10–14 days	Weight gain; increased thirst and urination[3]
carbamazepine (Tegretol)	Helps patients who do not respond to lithium or who have rapidly recurring bouts of mania or depression (more than four a year)	Decreased white blood cell count[3]
PSYCHOSIS ASSOCIATED WITH MANIA		
haloperidol (Haldol), thioridazine (Mellaril), trifluoperazine (Stelazine)	Rapidly controls psychotic symptoms such as hallucinations	Dry mouth; sedation; stiffness

[1]Common brand names in parentheses   [2]Patients need to be on special diet   [3]Blood level of drug must be monitored

factors come together to cause mood-swing disorders. Thus, it is likely that genetic vulnerability, physical illness, personality, and specific life events all play a role—to different degrees in different individuals.

Investigating a Genetic Link

Studies of the incidence of illness within families do indeed suggest inheritance as a significant factor in the development of manic-depression, and some interesting recent research has focused on genetic vulnerability. Although clusters of cases within families have been recognized for some time, it has not, until recently, been clear whether it was the psychological problems of a troubled family that were transmitted or a "manic-depressive gene" itself. As noted earlier, manic-depressive illness has a prevalence rate of approximately 1 percent in the general population. Yet the incidence of bipolar disorder in sisters, brothers, and parents of patients with the illness is five to ten times higher. Studies of twins support the theory of genetic transmission of vulnerability to illness, since identical twins have a

138

much higher rate of bipolar disorder or depression than do fraternal twins. (These studies do not separate cases of manic-depression from cases of major depression.) In one study of 12 pairs of identical twins who were brought up living apart, 67 percent of those individuals who had a twin suffering from either mania or depression were stricken with a mood-swing disorder, even though the twins grew up in different households. Furthermore, studies of individuals adopted early in life who later developed manic-depression indicate a higher rate of illness in their biological parents than in their adoptive parents—strong evidence for a genetic factor in the illness.

More recent research has focused on the nature of the genetic transmission of vulnerability to illness. The evidence suggests that genetic transmission takes different forms. Early reports suggested transmission via one of the sex chromosomes, specifically the X chromosome, which might have helped explain the greater prevalence of major depression in females (females have two X chromosomes, while males have only one). It now seems likely, however, that most cases of genetic transmission are not sex-linked. A study published in 1987 identified a region of chromosome 11 that seemed to contain a gene involved in causing manic-depression in a group of Amish people in Lancaster County, Pa. Soon after the report's publication, researchers in France and at the U.S. National Institute of Mental Health were unable to replicate its findings in small numbers of individuals coming from families with a high incidence of manic-depressive illness. This failure is consistent, however, with the belief that there are probably a number of chromosomal sites involved in genetic inheritance of manic-depression and that chromosome 11 represents just one site. It is also important to observe that only 60 to 70 percent of those Amish who inherited the apparent gene on

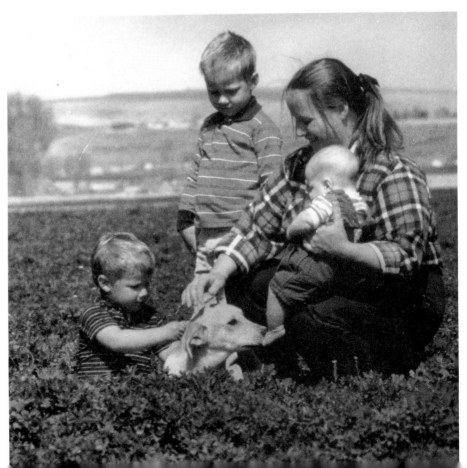

Manic-depression has appeared in at least four generations of this young woman's family. She and one of her sons (standing) have both been diagnosed with the disease.

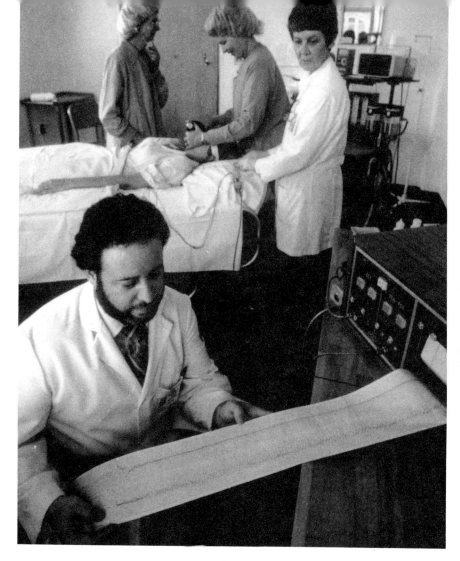

As electroconvulsive therapy is being administered, a doctor checks the patient's EEG (or electroencephalograph). "Shock" treatment has proven to be very effective for severely depressed patients.

chromosome 11 came down with the illness. This fact is consistent with the evidence that what is inherited is vulnerability to a mood-swing disorder, not the illness itself. Lastly, scientists know that this specific region of chromosome 11 is responsible for producing an important enzyme (tyrosine hydroxylase) which is known to be involved in the metabolism of dopamine, a chemical messenger in the brain involved in major mental disorders. Although a linkage between this enzyme and manic-depression has not been established, it is clear that researchers are moving closer to the day when a truer understanding of the genetics and chemistry of manic-depression will be available—and thus perhaps more specific means of prevention or cure.

Methods of Treatment

Many of the effective treatments for manic-depression and major depression are of relatively recent origin. Lithium, one of the most widely used drugs for manic-depression, was first found to be effective in treating mania in 1949. Antidepressant medications have become available only over the past 30 years, and even electroconvulsive therapy has been available only since 1938. Before modern treatments were introduced, individuals with severe mood-swing disorders suffered painfully and were often hospitalized for years, not uncommonly dying by suicide. Today, however, from 70 to 90 percent of sufferers can get relief through treatment.

The first step in effective treatment is accurate diagnosis. Treatment should be undertaken only after a thorough evaluation of the patient by a skilled psychiatrist, who can determine whether the individual is suffering from manic-depression or major depression or from one of a number of other psychiatric illnesses showing symptoms of mood disturbance. There is also the possibility that the mood swings are the result of an underlying physical illness or a reaction to a drug. (Symptoms of mania or depression can be produced by a number of illnesses, among them multiple sclerosis, diseases of the thyroid gland, seizure disorders, and tumors, as well as by such drugs as steroids, alcohol, cocaine, amphetamines, and barbiturates.)

Many people have misconceptions and unwarranted fears about psychiatric consultation. It should be realized that the modern psychiatrist talks with those coming for consultation much as an internist or family physician would. Most individuals who consult a psychiatrist feel relieved after the meeting.

Psychotherapy. Modern psychiatrists, once they have determined that an individual does indeed have a mood-swing disorder and evaluated its severity, have a wide range of treatments available. During depressive episodes, psychotherapy can be extremely helpful, particularly in educating patients about the nature of the disorder. In milder cases, it can have a beneficial effect on the depression itself. Some studies have found psychotherapy as effective as medication for milder depressions. The medication option should not, however, be abandoned. Even mild depressions, although not completely disabling, rob the individual of a good quality of life, and a significant number of such cases respond to antidepressant medications.

Psychotherapy is not the treatment of choice for more severe depressions and, if not used in conjunction with medications, may at times delay more effective treatment. Depressions that involve bodily changes (such as weight loss and severe insomnia with early morning awakening), significant deterioration in daily functioning, or suicidal thoughts often warrant medication or electroconvulsive therapy.

Medications. There are numerous effective medications for the treatment of depression. Antidepressants, first discovered in the late 1950s, are effective in over 70 percent of patients suffering from major depression. These medications may take from one to four weeks to achieve their effect, and their full effectiveness depends upon an adequate dosage. New laboratory techniques allow doctors to monitor blood levels of the drug in patients taking some antidepressant medications and may be important to utilize for patients who are slow to respond or seem to respond incompletely.

There are a number of classes of antidepressant medications (see the table on page 138, Drugs for Depression and Mania). Each has its own side effects—such as dry mouth, constipation, or light-headedness—although all are generally well tolerated and very effective. Newer antidepressants have fewer side effects and may be particularly effective for certain subgroups of patients. One recently introduced

Psychotherapy can be helpful in coping with episodes of depression.

141

medication, fluoxetine (sold under the brand name Prozac) affects the production of serotonin, one of the brain chemicals thought to be involved in certain forms of depression. Since antidepressant medications can actually induce mania in susceptible manic-depressive patients, it is important for patients to remain under the care of the psychiatrist while taking these drugs. Most individuals on antidepressants function normally and are not bothered at all by the medication. For depressed patients who also suffer from anxiety, several drugs are available to treat that condition.

The drugs used to treat mania are as effective as, if not more effective than, those used for depression. Lithium (lithium carbonate tablets or lithium citrate liquid) is the most commonly used antimanic agent. It is successful 80 percent of the time in treating mania, and it prevents most recurrences of both mania and depression in manic-depressives. Remarkably, lithium generally works within just 10 to 14 days. When the manic episode is severe, with paranoid and psychotic symptoms, other drugs (antipsychotic medications) are also needed in the beginning of treatment.

> **The drug lithium is successful 80 percent of the time in treating mania.**

Before lithium treatment is begun, blood and urine tests are done to make sure the patient can tolerate the drug and to get baseline information (for comparison purposes) on such things as blood count and hormone levels. After recovering from the episode of mania, most patients continue to take the drug at least for a while. The period of maintenance on lithium varies from six months to a lifetime and is determined by the number and severity of previous episodes. Patients taking lithium should be aware that there is a narrow margin between the blood level of the drug that is helpful and the level that can cause toxic side effects. Blood levels must be monitored once or twice a week at first, then every month or two later in the course of treatment.

Lithium does not leave people feeling sedated or "zombie-like" and is generally well tolerated. The vast majority of those taking the drug have few or no side effects and, like many people on antidepressants, are not bothered by the medication. However, it is important for patients taking lithium to maintain a normal salt and fluid intake and to be aware that such side effects as weight gain and increased urination may occur. The experienced psychiatrist knows the methods available to counteract unpleasant side effects.

In the past few years, other medications have been used to treat those manic episodes that are not responsive to lithium. The most effective has been carbamazepine (brand name, Tegretol), which is thought to work by reducing the sensitivity of nerve cells to abnormal electrical and chemical discharges that may be involved in mania. Patients taking carbamazepine should also have blood levels monitored, and the drug should be administered by a physician skilled in its use.

Electroconvulsive Therapy. Often referred to as shock treatment and shrouded in myth, fear, and misconception, electroconvulsive therapy (ECT) is an extremely effective—in fact, the most effective—treatment both for very severe depression and for mania that cannot be controlled by drugs. ECT is successful over 90 percent of the time in relieving severe depression within the first week or two (as noted earlier,

142

antidepressant drugs may take up to four weeks) and has undoubtedly saved many lives by preventing suicides. It is the only treatment left for the severely depressed who cannot take or fail to respond to medications.

The modern administration of ECT in no way resembles the horror film depictions of painful shocks given in a "snake-pit" setting. While the patient is asleep under anesthesia, two electrodes are placed on the patient's head through which an electric current flows to the brain—typically for one to four seconds. This produces a small seizure. For reasons still unknown, a series of such controlled and monitored seizures rapidly reverses severe depression. Generally, 6 to 12 ECT treatments are given over a period of two to three weeks. (As a follow-up, antidepressant drugs are often prescribed.) Because ECT is administered under anesthesia, it involves no pain, and medications which relax muscles minimize the less-controlled seizures that used to occur in the past. Although there have been reports of memory loss following ECT, especially concerning the weeks or months around the treatment period, there is no documented evidence of significant long-term memory disturbance in the vast majority of those who have received this therapy. And newer treatment techniques, involving improved placement of the electrodes and better regulation of the electric current, have reduced the number of complaints of memory loss. Professionals familiar with the treatment can cite many cases of patients who were tormented by depression and deeply suicidal and who, after receiving ECT, went on to lead normal and productive lives. The focus upon past abuses with ECT has at times obscured the relief and life-saving benefits that it can offer. (*See also the Spotlight on Health article* UPDATE ON "SHOCK" THERAPY.)

SOURCES OF FURTHER INFORMATION

American Psychiatric Association, 1400 K Street, N.W., Washington, DC 20005.

Canadian Mental Health Association, 2160 Yonge Street, Toronto, Ontario M4S 2Z3.

National Depressive and Manic-Depressive Association, Merchandise Mart, Box 3395, Chicago, IL 60654.

National Institute of Mental Health, 5600 Fishers Lane, Rockville, MD 20857.

SUGGESTIONS FOR FURTHER READING

FIEVE, RONALD. *Moodswing: The Third Revolution in Psychiatry.* New York, Bantam Books, 1976.

GREIST, JOHN H., AND JAMES W. JEFFERSON. *Depression and Its Treatment.* New York, Warner Books, 1985.

PAPOLOS, D. F. *Overcoming Depression.* New York, Harper & Row, 1987.

WENDER, PAUL H., AND DONALD F. KLEIN. *Mind, Mood, and Medicine: A Guide to the New Biopsychiatry.* New York, Farrar, Straus & Giroux, 1981.

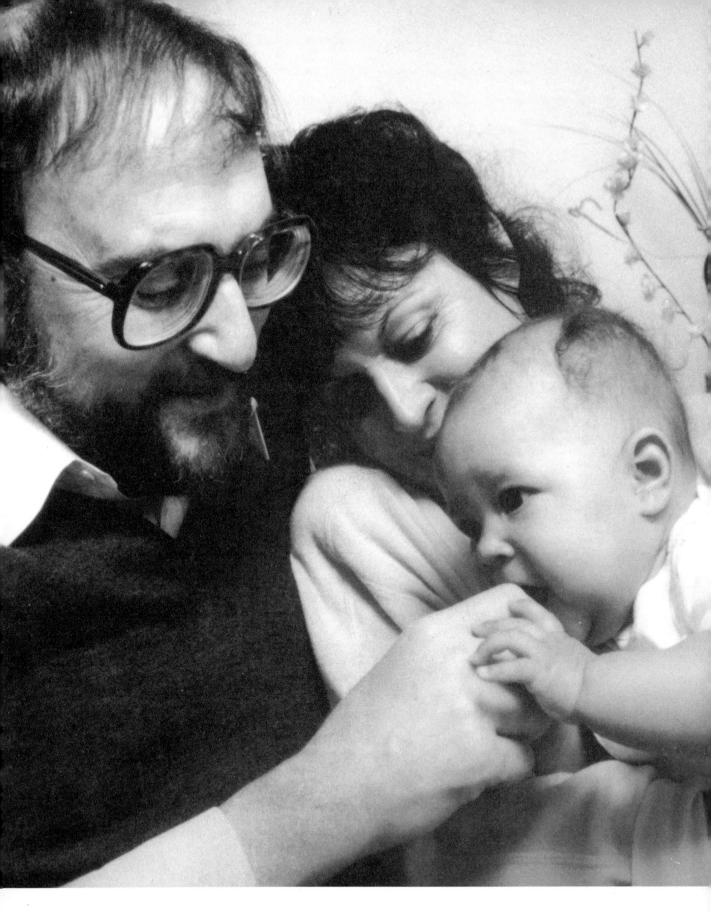

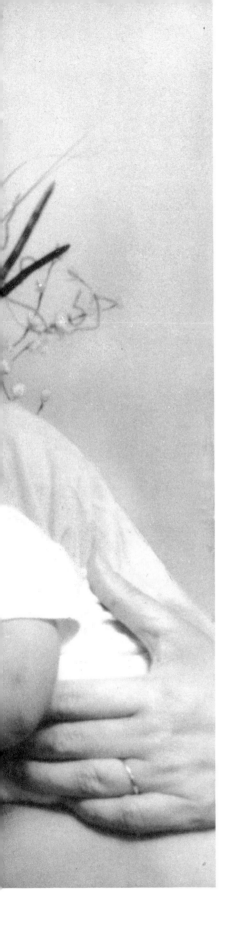

Having a First Child After 35

Johanna F. Perlmutter, M.D.

The belief that childbearing should occur at an early age has long been entrenched in American thinking, both in medical circles and among the general public. In recent years, however, a growing number of women—especially those at the higher end of the socioeconomic scale—are delaying childbearing into their late 30s and early 40s. (In the context of childbearing, they are often referred to as "older women.") This trend has a number of important implications for mother, father, and child. There is much concern about medical implications—specifically, whether older women face special problems in becoming pregnant and in delivering healthy babies.

Johanna F. Perlmutter is an assistant professor in the Department of Obstetrics and Gynecology at Harvard Medical School.

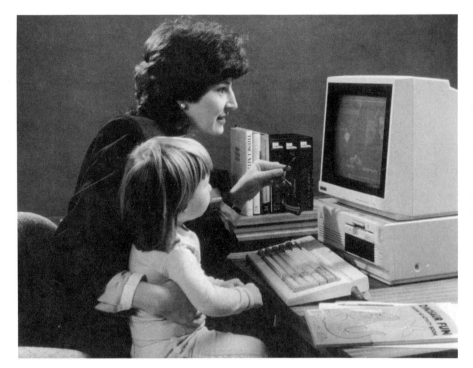

An increasing number of women are delaying childbearing until their careers are well under way. At left, a working mother introduces her child to the facts of office life. Right, recognizing the trend, specialty shops are catering to career mothers.

A Growing Trend

Women who delay a first pregnancy are still very much in the minority, but their numbers are increasing. Between 1970 and 1979, the percentage of 30-year-old American women who had had children dropped from 86 percent to 72 percent. Although this does not appear to be a drastic change, these same figures, looked at another way, show that there was a doubling in the percentage of 30-year-old women who were childless—a much more impressive statistic. In addition, between 1972 and 1982, first births per 1,000 women, aged 30 to 34, doubled; in women aged 35 to 39, there was an 83 percent increase. (Second pregnancy rates have not risen in the same fashion and are consistent with the fact that more than 60 percent of women over 30 who become pregnant for the first time plan to have only one child.)

The trend toward delaying childbearing is likely to continue, and at the same time, the total number of women aged 35 to 49 is expected to increase. It has been estimated that by 2010, the proportion of births to women over 35 will have risen to 9 percent of total births—nearly double the 1982 figure of 5 percent. (The large majority of births, as these statistics show, will still occur in younger women.)

Why Do Women Delay Childbearing?

There are many reasons why women delay pregnancy. Overall, women are marrying later; the number of unmarried women between the ages of 25 and 34 is increasing. Unstable relationships and divorce—both now common—also tend to delay childbearing. Furthermore, a growing number of women are entering the job market for professional

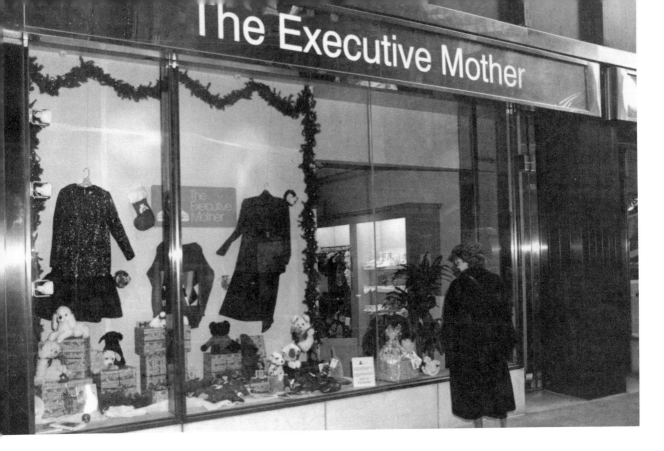

as well as financial reasons; such women may be reluctant to interrupt their careers (even for a three-month or six-month pregnancy leave) until becoming established in their profession to the greatest possible extent. Other reasons for delayed childbearing include a woman's need for personal growth, desire to complete her education, and pursuit of other interests, as well as a couple's need to ensure financial security.

Impact on Parents and Child

Having a first child means bringing a third person into a partnership, which places strain on that relationship. In addition, it means appending another full-time job to a couple's busy daily affairs. Old life-styles must be altered. Because older parents are more certain of their decision to have a baby, they tend to accomplish the transition with less difficulty than do younger parents. They are better equipped to handle their new life-style and are able to adjust more comfortably.

If parenthood is considered a crisis state, then the older parent, generally speaking, is more equipped to handle it. The maturity that ordinarily accompanies the additional years usually means better coping mechanisms and more wisdom in handling family relationships. The older mother and father's concept of what is needed to be a good parent is more realistic and less romantic—they are more flexible and more aware of the complexity of child care. Older parents are also generally better off financially, which takes some of the emotional stress out of raising young children.

There is a down side to being an older parent. Lack of sleep, trying to keep up with the many needs of an active toddler, and running after a young child can be physically exhausting. The problem is compounded if increasing age has decreased one's energy level and physical vigor. There also may be a sense of isolation because one's peers—from whom most information, communication, and support usually comes—may not have dealt with similar problems for ten years or more. Assistance and advice from the baby's grandparents may not be available. In fact, if grandparents have reached an age where chronic illness and infirmity are a reality, they too may need constant care and attention. It may be a struggle for new mothers and fathers in their late 30s or 40s to juggle the everyday demands of a baby with the problems associated with their own aging parents.

For the new mother, attempting to reenter the work force may not be as easy emotionally as anticipated—she may discover that she would like to stay home with her baby. It is not uncommon for new mothers to be torn between their reluctance to leave the infant with a baby-sitter or other caretaker all day and their need for the intellectual stimulation, social contact, and sense of accomplishment that can come from working. Some women compromise by seeking part-time employment, others do return to work full-time, and a few choose to stay at home.

As the child grows, each age range brings its own set of problems. Among the most trying times for any parent are the teenage years. One needs extra patience and tolerance at this time, but parents in their late 40s and 50s may be more short-tempered than they were when they were younger and not as permissive or understanding. As the years

Once a baby joins the household, candlelit dinners and leisurely brunches give way to more down-to-earth mealtimes.

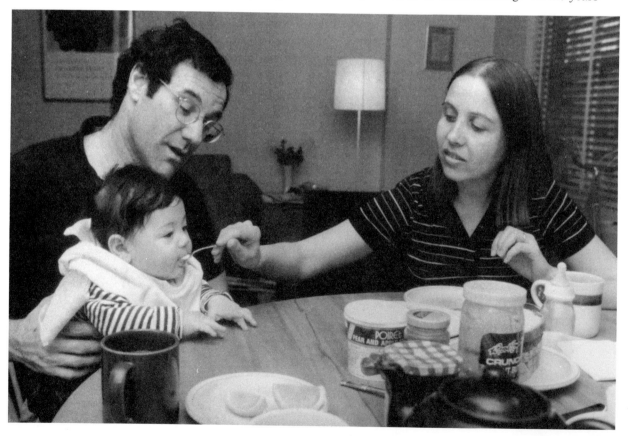

148

continue to pass, college and graduate school tuition payments may come just about the time parents are considering retirement—possibly making it impossible.

Finally, this discussion cannot be considered complete without taking into account the impact of delayed childbearing on the child. The children of older parents are very much wanted and very special. They are doted on and are given lots of love and affection. Typically, they do not have any siblings, and they are frequently spoiled and self-centered. Like most only children, they tend to be achievers, to have greater earning potential, and to hold more prestigious jobs as adults than do other people. But they too may have special problems to deal with. They grow up with parents who are older than and thereby different from the parents of many of their peers. They may lose one or both of their parents while they are still quite young. They may be deprived of the love and attention of grandparents. Moreover, they may become responsible for the care of their aging and ill parents while they are still in their 20s.

Fertility and Infertility

Are Infertility Rates Higher? As a childless woman enters her 30s, pressure is put on her to consider becoming pregnant soon, "before it's too late." There is concern about how much longer her "biological time clock" will run. This is not an unreasonable concern, as one-third to one-half of women who marry over 30 remain involuntarily childless.

Increasing age brings with it an increasing decline in a woman's fertility. A woman is at her most fertile right after puberty. Her ability to reproduce remains high when she is in her 20s; when she reaches her 30s, it decreases at an accelerated pace until menopause. This is part of the normal aging process. It does not mean that women in their 30s and 40s cannot become pregnant. If they are still menstruating, many women will be able to bear children, although a higher proportion of them will not.

A first look at statistics dealing with fertility might give the mistaken impression that it is almost impossible for an older woman to have a baby. The statistics show, for example, that while 25 percent of teenage girls who have unprotected intercourse become pregnant each month they are exposed, less than 8 percent of women over 40 do. The fertility rate (the number of live births per year per 1,000 women 15-49 years of age) shows the same kind of drop. As of 1986 (the most recent figures available), the fertility rate for women in their early 30s was just under 70. For women between 40 and 44, it was just over 4.

But statistics like this, often widely publicized by the media, can be misleading, and close scrutiny and analysis are needed to understand fully their significance. In the first instance given above (pregnancies after unprotected intercourse), the rate given is a monthly one. It does not tell how many women conceive after six months or a year of attempting to do so. The fertility rate statistics are just as problematic, covering as they do *all* women between the ages of 15 and 49, even those who are sterile, have already gone through menopause, or are using contraceptives to prevent conception.

Childless women in their 30s are concerned with the biological time clock.

149

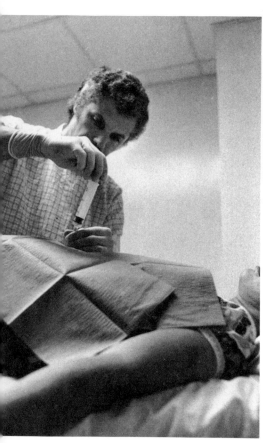

Amniocentesis is a test commonly recommended for pregnant women over 35, to discover birth defects.

Traditional teaching has been that as a woman approaches menopause, she does not ovulate, or release an egg, as often. Thus, the chance of becoming pregnant is reduced because fewer eggs are available. There is some evidence to support this.

A very large and rigorous study, done by French researchers several years ago of women undergoing artificial insemination because their husbands were sterile, indicated that it does take *longer* for older women to become pregnant. Three-quarters of women in the study between the ages of 20 and 30 became pregnant within 12 months, as compared to just over 60 percent of participants between 31 and 35 and just over half of those over 35. Once again, the statistics—which were disseminated to the general public through front-page newspaper articles—are difficult to interpret.

Most such data are generated in and gathered from infertility clinics, whose clients are a self-selected group with fertility problems. Are the older women in this group currently in the "older" category because of long-standing difficulties with conception that began when they were younger? This is unknown. Does the older woman in general really have as much difficulty as these statistics suggest? This is another unknown. There is little statistical data available on women who never needed or sought the services of a fertility specialist.

Are Some Causes of Infertility More Common to Older Women?
Specific medical or physical conditions, which can affect women of all age groups, can contribute to infertility. A condition as common as emotional stress can shut down the pituitary gland—which controls many of the hormones crucial to fertility—resulting in the loss of the menstrual cycle and an end to ovulation. Eating disorders like anorexia nervosa, a condition called polycystic ovarian disease, and extremely vigorous exercise such as that undertaken by ballet dancers and marathon runners can also interfere with ovulation.

Damage to the fallopian tubes is frequently associated with decreased fertility. Such damage may result from use of the older intrauterine devices (those currently on the market are not believed to produce this problem) or from pelvic inflammatory disease (PID, an infection that is usually transmitted venereally). There are other causes as well. Endometriosis, in which the kind of tissue that lines the uterus grows on the outside of the uterus or elsewhere in the pelvic cavity, sometimes leads to scarring of the fallopian tubes. Even when the tubes are not directly affected, endometriosis may interfere with conception, in a way that is not precisely understood. Even minor flaws and difficulties in seemingly normal menstrual periods can prevent a pregnancy; for example, there may be problems when the time interval between ovulation and menstruation is too short or too long.

The statistics seem to suggest that some of these causes of infertility are more prevalent in older women. But again, the information is gathered mostly from the records of infertility clinics. It is impossible to know exactly what relevance they have for the general population of older women. What can be said is that the older woman has had more time in which to develop conditions such as pelvic inflammatory disease that interfere with pregnancy and that she has fewer childbearing years ahead in which to have them treated.

The aging process itself does leave women at risk for serious illnesses that can impact on the decision to have children and interfere with the ability to become pregnant. As women get older, they are more apt to develop cancer of the endometrium (the lining of the uterus) or the ovaries. Treatment of these cancers frequently leaves a woman sterile. Today, however, another reproductive tract malignancy, cancer of the cervix, can be treated without hampering a patient's reproductive capabilities unless the cancer has already begun to spread.

Nongynecologic cancers, also more likely to occur in older women, do not usually directly affect fertility. Nevertheless, certain cancer drugs can lead to premature menopause. In general, when a woman has a type of cancer that depends on hormones for its growth, like breast cancer, pregnancy is not recommended because the hormones involved in pregnancy might cause the cancer to recur. Although this is still the current philosophy, the rules have become less rigid, and some women who have had breast cancer have become pregnant, delivered healthy babies, and remained in good health themselves.

The aging process does put women at risk for illnesses that can interfere with the ability to become pregnant.

A discussion of fertility problems cannot be complete without considering the role of the male. Approximately 30 percent of infertility problems relate to the male, and it has been estimated that there is a 10 percent decrease in male fertility per decade—which is significant for those older women whose husbands are about the same age. Low or absent sperm counts, infections of the reproductive tract, and testicular varicose veins are factors that can contribute to male infertility. If a couple first discovers while in their mid-30s that the husband has a fertility problem, they may be close to 40 by the time it can be cured.

Pregnancy Difficulties and Outcomes

Most frightening to the older expectant mother are the reports of increases in pregnancy complications and adverse outcomes in older women. The literature of the 1950s and 1960s, in particular, suggested that pregnancy in women over 35 was hazardous to both mother and infant. Most of these data, however, are not applicable to the modern-day woman who has chosen to delay childbearing. Many of the surveys from which they were drawn included women who had had numerous children and unplanned, closely spaced pregnancies, as well as couples with long-standing histories of infertility who were now over 35 and had finally achieved pregnancy—all high risk groups.

It is widely believed that older mothers are more likely to suffer from complications such as placenta previa—abnormal placement of the placenta, which can be dangerous for both mother and child. It is also thought by many that older women are more likely to give birth to small babies. The reality is that age is not really a factor. The greater the number of full-term pregnancies a woman has had, the greater the chance of placenta previa. By the same token, infants of low birth-weight are seen commonly in women with large families, particularly when the pregnancies were closely spaced. Small babies can also result from inadequate nutrition or high blood pressure, which are not necessarily connected with age.

Birth Defects. Although many of the medical difficulties associated with having a baby after 35 are overstated, there definitely are certain problems that occur with increasing frequency with advancing age. An example is the higher proportion of babies with chromosomal and congenital abnormalities born to older mothers. The most common condition caused by a chromosomal abnormality is Down's syndrome, which occurs when there is an extra copy of a specific chromosome.

Most women in their 20s do not worry about birth defects because they occur so infrequently in young women. The risk of such abnormalities increases with every year, so that as a woman enters her 30s, concern about having a child with a birth defect rises dramatically. Of the babies born to women under 35, the proportion having a major birth defect is 15 per 1,000 live births; the figure rises to 17 out of 1,000 live births for women between the ages of 35 and 39. The numbers escalate as women get older, reaching 31 out of every 1,000 live births for women 40 to 44, and 76 out of 1,000 for those who are 45 or older. Even though these figures appear astronomical, it should be remembered that over 90 percent of 45-year-old women will still have a normal infant. Also, most of the abnormalities can be found relatively early in pregnancy if blood tests and other diagnostic tests— amniocentesis or a newer technique, chorionic villus sampling—are done.

Amniocentesis is usually recommended for all women who will be 35 or over at the time of delivery. Age 35 was chosen when the test initially became available because that was the age at which the risk of having a baby with Down's syndrome exceeded the hazard posed by amniocentesis itself (possible miscarriage). Newer technology and the use of ultrasound while the procedure is being performed have made the test quite safe. As a result, a higher proportion of younger women are also opting for such screening.

Miscarriages. The risk of having a miscarriage increases as a woman gets older. For a pregnant woman in her 20s, the chance of a miscarriage is 11 percent. This percentage doubles for women in their 30s. By age 40, there is a twofold to fourfold increase over women in their 20s. An interesting observation from studies of women undergoing artificial insemination is that the older women who miscarried generally took longer to become pregnant than the older participants whose pregnancies ended in live births. This suggests that older women who miscarry have more difficulty in getting pregnant in the first place, although data derived from participants in artificial insemination studies may not accurately reflect the degree of risk for those who have voluntarily postponed pregnancy.

It has long been recognized that most miscarried embryos and fetuses have abnormal chromosome numbers. This could explain the increase in early pregnancy losses that older women experience.

Role of Maternal Health. Numerous studies show that adverse pregnancy outcome is often a direct result of a health problem suffered by the mother. Some of the maternal health problems that can affect the fetus do increase in frequency with age, although they by no means affect all women who become pregnant in their late 30s or beyond.

Hypertension, or high blood pressure, is the most common disorder

Miscarriages occur more frequently in older women.

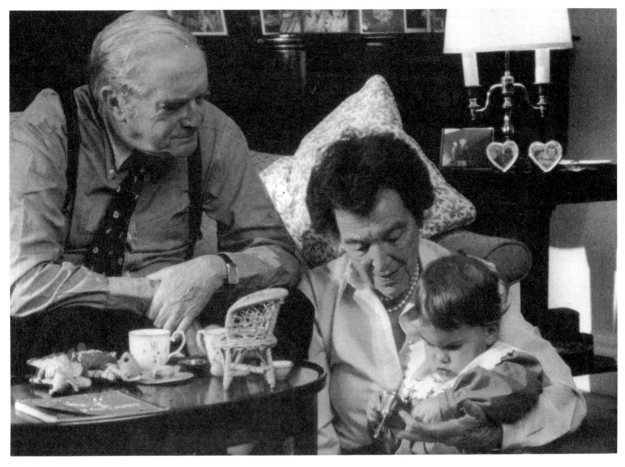

that affects pregnancies, afflicting approximately 35 percent of pregnant women. It is more than twice as common in older pregnant women. Hypertension proves to be more of a determinant of whether a pregnancy will end in a stillbirth than maternal age alone. Women who have hypertension are at increased risk for the disorders called toxemia (preeclampsia, in its less severe form, and eclampsia, in its more severe form). In its severest form, this condition involves a drastic increase in blood pressure and the risk of convulsions in the mother, and it can endanger the lives of both mother and baby.

Low-birth-weight infants, late fetal deaths, stillbirths, and an increase in deaths among newborns are all associated with high blood pressure problems. In fact, although the hypertensive disorders are seen in one-third of pregnancies, they are responsible for two-thirds of perinatal deaths (fetal and infant deaths occurring in the period shortly before and after birth). Hypertension has also been found in the majority of women who have abruptio placentae, in which the placenta separates before delivery and hemorrhage occurs in the uterine cavity.

Diabetes, a disorder that is seen more frequently in people over the age of 40, is associated with an increase in miscarriages and in fetal morbidity (sickness rate) and death. Although only 7 percent of pregnant women have this disorder, it is responsible for 22 percent of perinatal mortality. Older pregnant women are more likely than

Children of older parents are fortunate if they have grandparents who are fit and well enough to love and cherish them.

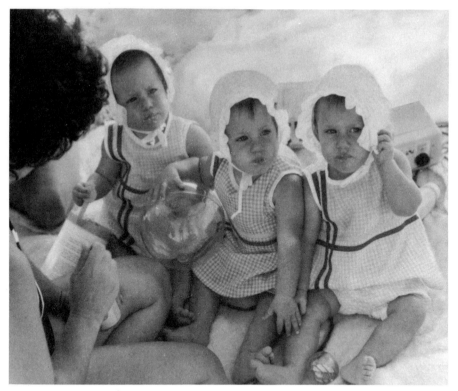

The use of fertility drugs often leads to multiple births, as the mother of these triplets can attest.

younger pregnant women to develop gestational diabetes—the type of diabetes that occurs with pregnancy.

Another condition that becomes more common with age is obesity. Being significantly overweight at the start of a pregnancy is associated with both hypertension and diabetes. Thus, overweight women are at greater risk for the complications associated with those conditions.

Fibroids—usually benign growths of uterine muscle that tend to enlarge and distort the uterus—can affect a pregnancy negatively. Only about 5 percent of women in general have them, but 20 percent of women over 40 do. Fibroids are associated with miscarriages, premature deliveries, and fetal malposition; when the baby is positioned incorrectly in the uterus, vaginal birth becomes more difficult. Fibroids can also impede labor, and because they may prevent the uterus from contracting properly after delivery, they are associated with postpartum hemorrhage.

Prolonged Labor and Cesareans. Prolonged labor and an increase in cesarean rates have been reported for older pregnant women. Older women tend to be given more painkillers than younger women during labor, which appears to account for their prolonged labor. Once cases involving significant medication have been removed from the statistics, the total length of labor does not seem to be any different than in younger women.

There is, however, a higher rate of cesarean deliveries in older women—even when researchers take into account the size of the infants born to older mothers and complications of pregnancy. Perhaps both mothers and doctors are more anxious during these deliveries—and therefore quicker to opt for a cesarean—especially if it is a first birth and the woman may not have many more years to become pregnant again. Whatever the reason, the cesarean rate tends to be two to three times higher than in younger women. Since cesareans are major operations, they do entail some risk to the mother, as well as considerable pain and a slow convalescence.

Mortality Rates. Although women who become pregnant over 35 are at higher risk of maternal death than younger women, in recent years that risk has dropped by almost 50 percent, from an average of 47.5 maternal deaths per 100,000 live births during the years 1974-1978 to 24.2 by 1982. (The mortality rates include deaths from abortions.) The decline has been attributed to the higher socioeconomic status of older women having babies in recent years, since such women are more likely to be in good health and to receive good medical care during pregnancy and delivery.

Multiple Births. Multiple births are more common in older women. The incidence of identical twins is about the same as that found in teenagers, but the incidence of fraternal twins quadruples, possibly because as a woman ages, she is more likely to release more than one egg during ovulation. Overall, twins are found in just under 2 percent of pregnancies in the over 35 age group. The use of fertility drugs and to a lesser extent of in vitro fertilization, in which several fertilized eggs are implanted in the uterus, also increase the chances of having a pregnancy with two, three, four, or more fetuses.

Older women who have good prenatal care and who deliver in a modern facility are probably at no greater risk for an adverse outcome than younger women.

Older Mothers and Healthy Babies

How likely is it, then, that a late first pregnancy will end successfully for mother and child? The answer to this question is somewhat complex but encouraging. First, a *healthy* woman who elects to delay childbearing has a good chance of having an uncomplicated pregnancy and a healthy baby. For such a woman there does not appear to be an increased risk of most major complications associated with childbirth.

Age does bring with it, however, a greater incidence of some chronic illnesses and other conditions that can adversely affect pregnancy and its outcome. But medical knowledge and prenatal care have changed dramatically in the past 25 years. There is better understanding of medical problems, a host of new treatments, and improved technology. As a result, even in complicated pregnancies, outcomes have improved. On the whole, women over 35 today who have good prenatal care and who deliver in a modern facility are probably at no greater risk for an adverse outcome than younger women. □

SUGGESTIONS FOR FURTHER READING

"Delayed Pregnancy: How Safe Is it?" *Mayo Clinic Health Letter*, November 1988, pp. 3-4.

MENKEN, JANE, JAMES TRUSSELL, AND ULLA LARSEN. "Age and Infertility." *Science*, September 26, 1986, pp. 1389-1394.

"Pregnancy: Age and Outcome." *Harvard Medical School Health Letter*, October 1985, pp. 1-3.

What Killed Napoleon?

William B. Ober, M.D.

Was Mozart poisoned by a rival composer? Would Marfan's syndrome have killed Lincoln if an assassin's bullet didn't? Did Henry VIII really have syphilis? Did Napoleon die of natural causes?

For biographers and historians the answers to questions about the health, illness, or cause of death of their subjects can be of some importance. In the case of 20th century figures, the answers are generally to be found in medical records. For important figures of earlier times, however, some medical detective work is called for. The nature and cause of disease has to be reconstructed from whatever evidence is available, usually written materials based on the observations of nonprofessionals. Present-day diagnoses for historical figures are, in fact, retrospective inferences made by applying modern medical knowledge to historical data, and the inferences should not be made when the data are insufficient or contradictory. Medical detective work has been called armchair diagnosis, but it is best done by using many armchairs in many libraries or manuscript collections.

Analyzing the Clues

In history books of bygone eras the reader is often informed that a given king or nobleman "died of a surfeit." To a modern physician this usually suggests that the victim in fact died of a heart attack after overindulgence in food and drink. (Sudden heart attacks often masquerade as "acute indigestion.") In some cases, however, death

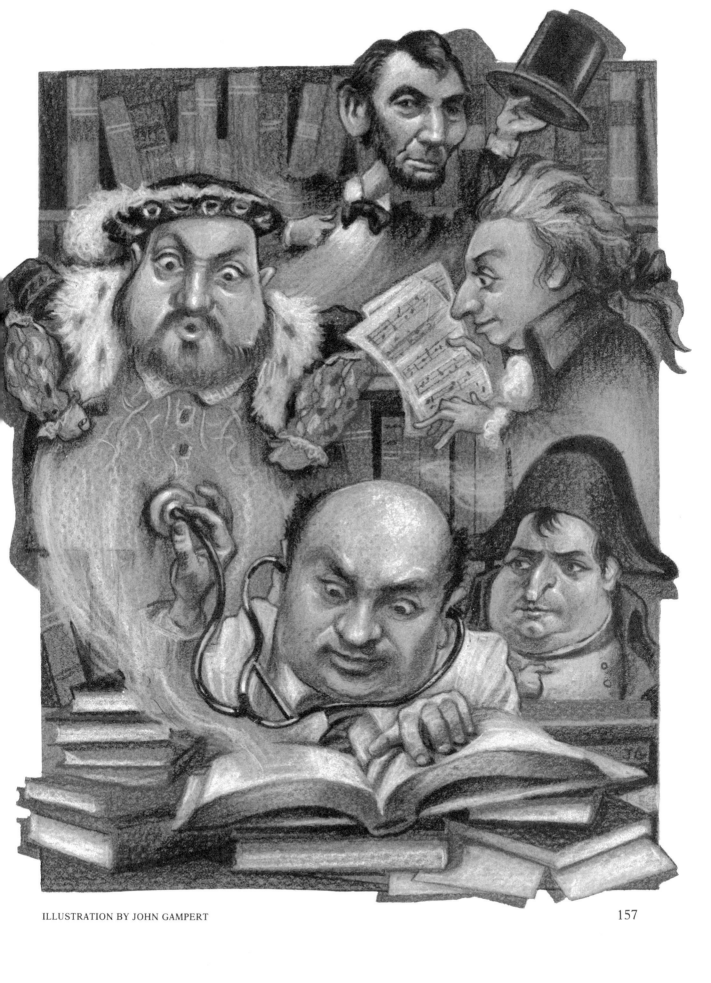

ILLUSTRATION BY JOHN GAMPERT

157

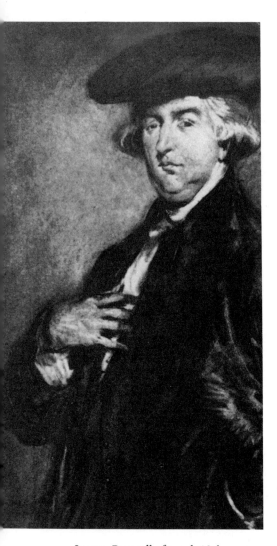

James Boswell, famed 18th-century biographer, provided the clues to the eventual cause of his death in the racy details of his journal.

may have been due to acute hemorrhagic pancreatitis (inflammation of the pancreas accompanied by bleeding). In one such celebrated case reported by Hermann Boerhaave, the great Dutch physician of the late 17th and early 18th centuries, an autopsy revealed that the victim, Admiral de Wassenaar, had died of a rupture of the lower part of the esophagus and stomach, the result of violent vomiting caused by the disease. In most instances, autopsy findings provide conclusive evidence of a diagnosis. (Autopsies have been performed for hundreds of years, dating back to when people first took a rational interest in disease. The first forensic autopsy is said to have been ordered at the beginning of the 14th century.)

Sometimes a diagnosis is clear but incomplete. James Boswell, best known for his biography of Samuel Johnson, had no qualms about recording in his journals the frequent attacks of gonorrhea incurred by his visits to prostitutes. Since the publication of the journals in the 20th century, one can document 19 such attacks. But the clue to the immediate cause of Boswell's death in 1795 lies in a cryptic diary entry for January 31, 1790: "Earle's; was sounded; almost fainted." An interpretation of this notation is as follows: Boswell had developed a urethral stricture (scarring and narrowing of the urethra), which prevented him from urinating normally. One of the causes of this disorder is gonorrhea. Boswell consulted James Earle, a surgeon who pioneered in treating diseases of the genitourinary tract, and had his urethra dilated, or stretched, by an instrument called a sound. Five years later, in April 1795, he collapsed at a meeting of London's Literary Club, overcome by chills, fever, a violent headache, nausea, and vomiting. This constellation of symptoms, taken in conjunction with Boswell's reference (in a letter) to "mortification of the bladder," leads to the diagnosis of an infection that had moved all the way up the urinary tract to the kidneys—and proved fatal a month later. Urinary tract infections are common when there is urethral stricture.

Other victims of urethral stricture following gonorrhea included the philosopher Jean-Jacques Rousseau and the composer Gioacchino Rossini. In Boswell's case, more interesting than the diagnosis is the psychology underlying his almost compulsive exposure to the risk of gonorrhea, behavior one would not expect from a happily married man of good family, considerable education, and prominent social connections.

Until recent years medical records for most patients were not preserved, and much retrospective diagnosis must rest on the observations of nonprofessionals found in memoirs, correspondence, or diaries. But the medical records of royalty and other exalted personages are sometimes preserved, and it was by examining notes

William B. Ober, presently assistant medical examiner in Bergen County, N.J., is a former clinical professor of pathology at New Jersey College of Medicine and Mount Sinai School of Medicine in New York City. His books include Boswell's Clap and Other Essays: Medical Analyses of Literary Men's Afflictions *and* Bottoms Up! A Pathologist's Essays on Medicine and the Humanities.

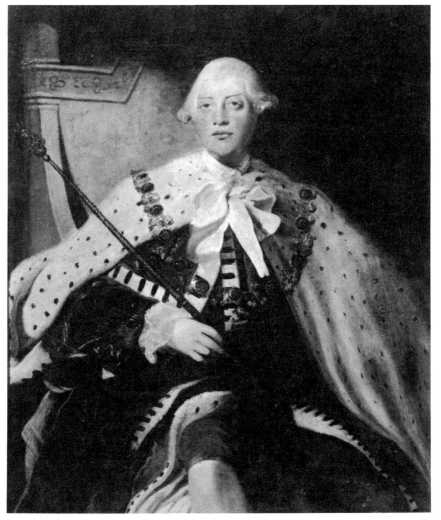

The cause of George III's recurring attacks of insanity, a mystery to his physicians, was uncovered by modern medical detective work.

made by the physicians who attended George III that two British psychiatrists were able to diagnose porphyria, an abnormality in body chemistry, as the cause of the monarch's recurring attacks of insanity. The pivotal observation was that his urine turned wine-colored when left to stand.

Disorders Rare and Common

A good general rule in the diagnosis of afflictions of historical figures is that if the disease is a common one and follows a typical course, there is little reason to question what seems an obvious diagnosis. In 1818 the poet John Keats, who had studied medicine, nursed his younger brother Tom, who was ill with tuberculosis. Tom died in December of that year. A few months later Keats developed progressive malaise, a low-grade intermittent fever, and tightness in the chest, and on February 3, 1820, he suddenly started spitting up blood. This persisted, accompanied by a cough. Keats died 13 months later in Rome. Although his death came more than half a century before the discovery of X rays and of the bacterium that causes tuberculosis, no one can reasonably doubt that Keats died of tuberculosis. The case of the composer Frederic Chopin also seems beyond dispute. One of Chopin's sisters died of tuberculosis when he was still an adolescent, and he himself developed symptoms of the disease in his mid-20s. Unlike Keats, in whom the disease spread rapidly, Chopin had a slowly progressing form and survived for 13 years. For the writer F. Scott Fitzgerald the diagnosis of tuberculosis remained unsupported until over 30 years after his death. Fitzgerald often told his friends that he had tuberculosis, but he rarely had any symptoms of respiratory disease. His alcoholism, on the other hand, was an obvious problem, which may explain why his friends and his early biographers tended to dismiss the possibility of tuberculosis and put down his claims as romantic braggadocio. It was only when his most recent biographer took the trouble to consult Fitzgerald's medical records that he was able to find chest X-ray reports and a bacteriology report that supported Fitzgerald's claim. Fitzgerald survived for at least 15 years—and perhaps longer, since the date he contracted tuberculosis is not clear—only to die of a heart attack in 1940. No autopsy was performed; therefore one cannot assess the extent of his lung disease nor determine whether the heart attack was due to hardening of the coronary arteries or to alcoholic cardiomyopathy—heart disease brought on by alcoholism.

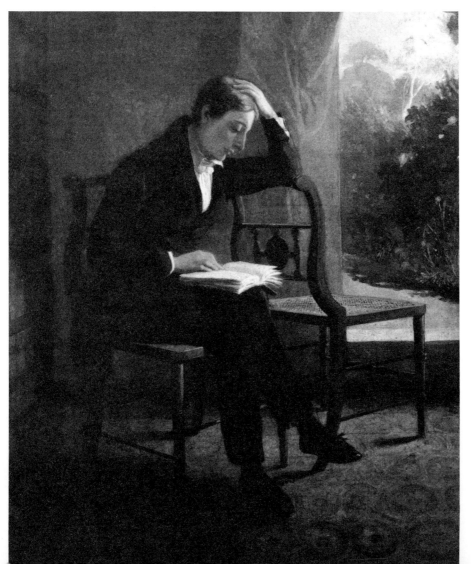

The Romantic poet John Keats was known to suffer from tuberculosis, although the diagnostic methods of his time were primitive.

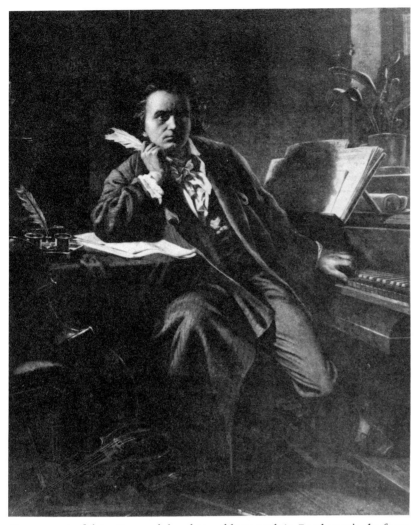

No amount of detective work has been able to explain Beethoven's deafness.

Syphilis has been imputed to many historical figures, sometimes on flimsy evidence. In the case of Henry VIII of England, the supposed syphilitic tumor of his knee may equally well have been chronic osteomyelitis—long-term infection of the bone accompanied by leaking pus from an ulcer—caused by frequent falls from horseback while hunting or jousting. Henry's death at the age of 56, accompanied by symptoms of progressive swelling of the legs and shortness of breath, seems more likely to have been the result of congestive heart failure (probably from hardening of the coronary arteries) than of the heart problems caused by syphilis, though the latter cannot be absolutely excluded.

Modern tests for the diagnosis of syphilis were not available until after 1900. However, a diagnosis of syphilis can be made with some assurance in the cases of the composers Donizetti, Smetana, and Hugo Wolf, the writers Guy de Maupassant, Flaubert, and Jules de Goncourt, and the poet Baudelaire, because they all developed dementia of

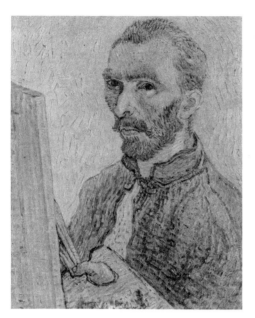

Vincent Van Gogh's mental instability was undoubtedly heightened by heavy drinking of absinthe, now known to produce hallucinations.

general paresis, a form of insanity characteristic of the final stage of syphilis. The poet Alfred de Musset developed an aneurysm, or bulging weak spot, on his aorta, the large blood vessel leading from the heart, because of syphilis. Controversy has raged over whether composer Franz Schubert died of a form of neurosyphilis (syphilis affecting the nervous system) or of typhus fever; the weight of the evidence favors the former. It is highly unlikely that Beethoven had syphilis, though the claim has been made. The composer Robert Schumann likewise did not have syphilis; his insanity was manic-depressive psychosis.

Much ink has been spilled on the subject of Mozart's last illness. The persistent gossip that Antonio Salieri, a rival composer, poisoned him is an absurdity. Various diagnoses have been proposed—tuberculosis, typhus fever, septicemia (blood poisoning), acute rheumatic fever—but none can be supported. From the age of 6 to his mid-20s, Mozart had many upper respiratory infections caused by streptococcus bacteria. The first of these was followed by erythema nodosum, an inflammation of the skin that is a rather unusual complication of some infections. His terminal illness at the age of 35 was heralded by the onset of fever, generalized edema (swelling due to fluid retention), recurrent attacks of vomiting, and, later, diarrhea. All of these symptoms are consistent with uremia, a condition in which impurities build up in the blood because of kidney failure. In Mozart's case the kidney failure was probably caused by the chronic inflammation of the kidneys that sometimes follows streptococcal infections. About two hours before he died, he had a convulsion and became comatose, possibly as the result of a stroke. Patients with kidney failure usually have hypertension (high blood pressure) and often die from a stroke.

The music of Bach and Handel is inevitably compared and contrasted. But physicians, at least, can agree that the cause of death was the same in both cases. Bach, probably hypertensive, died of a massive stroke following inept treatment of his cataracts by the quack "ophthalmiater" John Taylor. Handel died of a stroke nine years later, following a series of small strokes that first caused blindness, then incapacity. These diagnoses can be made with assurance because the illness followed a typical course. But when the composer Vincenzo Bellini died in Paris in his 34th year after a short illness, it took an autopsy to show that he died of a large liver abscess, or pus-filled sac, most likely caused by a parasite. Brahms died at the age of 63 in Vienna; his biographers agree that liver cancer was the cause of death, and his rapid weight loss and jaundice certainly suggest a malignant process involving the liver. Primary liver cancer is, however, quite rare in Europe, whereas cancer of the head of the pancreas, which has similar symptoms, is not uncommon. In Brahms's case, an autopsy would have provided conclusive evidence.

An autopsy was performed on Beethoven, but unfortunately it gave no clue to the cause of his deafness. The autopsy did show that the cause of death was advanced cirrhosis of the liver. It could not have been alcoholic cirrhosis because Beethoven drank only wine and that in moderation. Presumably it was the cirrhosis that sometimes follows hepatitis—Beethoven had been ill six years earlier with what was described as jaundice. Beethoven suffered from many ailments during his life, notably recurrent digestive disorders; although a variety of diagnoses for these ailments have been proposed, they rest on tenuous evidence.

When present-day physicians attempt to diagnose an uncommon or rare disease in a historical figure, the retrospectoscope is often difficult to focus. It has been suggested that Abraham Lincoln suffered from Marfan's syndrome, an inheritable disorder of connective tissue in which the prominent features are excessive height, unusually flexible joints, a hollowed sunken chest, and a tendency to develop aneurysms of the aorta. To be sure, Lincoln was tall, but there is little firm evidence of the other features of the syndrome. An assassin's bullet killed him before he showed any signs of aortic disease. He does not seem to have passed the disease to any of his sons.

Poisoning and Addiction

Retrospective diagnoses of poisoning (intentional or accidental) are difficult to support in the absence of toxicological evidence. In 1793, Francisco Goya, then 47 and well established as a painter, came down with a serious illness characterized by abdominal pain, dizziness, buzzing in the ears, partial loss of sight, severe headaches, and partial paralysis of the right side. It took him several months to recover, and when he did so, he was irremediably deaf. The illness marked a turning point in his work; from a painter of predominantly happy, colorful scenes, he became a painter of the darker, crueler side of life. Many conjectures have been made about the cause of his illness, but the leading hypothesis is that he developed lead poisoning from contact with his paints. When he died in 1828, no autopsy was performed. The symptoms of Goya's 1793 illness do not suggest an infectious disease. Lead intoxication has been known to produce similar symptoms—acute illness which leaves behind some permanent damage. A definitive answer could be found if Goya's skeleton were exhumed and a small piece of bone analyzed for lead content.

Poisoning has been suggested as the cause of Napoleon's death. The autopsy showed that he had cancer of the stomach, a condition consistent with the symptoms and downhill course of his last illness. But recent analysis of a lock of his hair showed a high content of arsenic, resurrecting the charge made by Bonapartists that the British had poisoned their former enemy during the years that he spent as their prisoner. Arsenic can be given in small, unnoticed doses until enough accumulates in the body to be fatal. Parenthetically, it has been suggested that Napoleon's failure to follow up his initial advantage at the battle of Waterloo, the scene of his final defeat in 1815, was due to a sudden attack of hemorrhoids.

History shows us that even nonfatal toxins can have dramatic effects. Vincent Van Gogh was introduced to the liqueur absinthe by fellow painter Paul Gauguin, and as Van Gogh's emotional instability gradually worsened, he drank more and more. Absinthe, now illegal in the United States and many other countries, was flavored with oil of wormwood, which contains a neurotoxin that produces hallucinations. There is adequate evidence that on several occasions, Van Gogh had

Playwright Eugene O'Neill was one of many literary figures who abused alcohol.

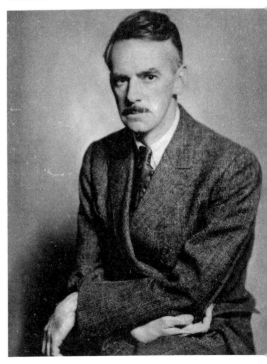

163

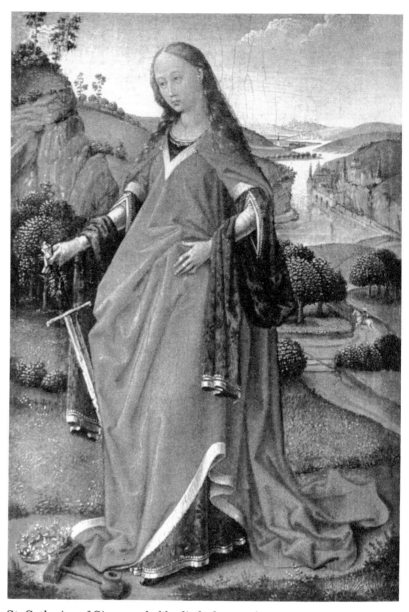

St. Catherine of Siena probably died of anorexia nervosa.

agitated hallucinatory fits following drinking bouts. However, he was mentally and emotionally unstable before he met Gauguin and began drinking absinthe, and this may have made him more susceptible to the toxin.

The poet Arthur Rimbaud also drank considerable amounts of absinthe when he was living with Paul Verlaine; the hallucinatory quality of Rimbaud's poems can partly be attributed to the effects of the liqueur, which he drank in a deliberate attempt to derange his senses and become a prophetic poet. That experiment ended in emotional and poetic burnout; Rimbaud wrote no poems after the age of 21. Instead he became a drifter, went into the gunrunning trade in

Africa, and died at the age of 37 of a cancerous tumor near his right knee.

Alcohol is another familiar toxin, and any number of well-known figures have been alcoholics. Although it is sometimes difficult to draw the line between heavy drinking and alcoholism, alcohol abuse clearly figured prominently in the lives of several leading American novelists, including the Nobel laureates Sinclair Lewis, Ernest Hemingway, William Faulkner, and John Steinbeck, and at one stage in his life, the playwright Eugene O'Neill. A notorious political figure, U.S. Senator Joseph McCarthy, who gained worldwide attention in the 1950s with his charges that communists had infiltrated the U.S. government, died of acute alcoholic hepatitis, a diagnosis confirmed by an autopsy.

The list of famous drug abusers is also long, and again includes a number of literary figures. Samuel Taylor Coleridge, the poet and critic, was addicted to laudanum, which is nothing more than a tincture (or solution) of opium. Other opium addicts were Thomas De Quincey, author of *Confessions of an English Opium-Eater*, and the poets George Crabbe and Francis Thompson. And, in his *Ode to a Nightingale* Keats betrays evidence of having experimented with small doses of opium. Aldous Huxley has left a brilliant account of his experiences in using the hallucinatory drug mescaline.

The experiences of drug use have been portrayed by such writers as Thomas De Quincey and Aldous Huxley.

Medieval Mystics

Religious beliefs can be an indirect cause of death; history is filled with stories of those who died a martyr's death for beliefs others considered heretical. But one does not usually count piety as a disease. Nonetheless, there are instances in which a medically definable disease can be diagnosed in an intensely religious person. In her *Book*, taken down from her own dictation, the 15th-century English mystic Margery Kempe provides evidence that she suffered from hysteria as well as from a postpartum depression, both most likely the result of a sense of guilt for premarital sexual relations. Kempe, whose *Book* remained in manuscript until the mid-1930s, also had occasional hallucinatory experiences.

St. Catherine of Siena, a 14th century devout, was declared Italy's patron saint in 1939 and in 1970 she was made a doctor of the Church, a title honoring her greatness as a teacher of Roman Catholic doctrine. At the age of 7 she vowed her virginity to God, and at 16 she entered the Dominican order. Catherine spent much of her time living in solitude and silence in her cell and became renowned for her holiness; at 21 she had a "mystical espousal" to Christ. A woman of great strength of mind and unusual charm, she attracted a following of important men and women, and was able to play the role of peacemaker in the long-running feud between the city-states of Italy and the papacy. Catherine had always eaten sparingly and fasted with devotion, but at the age of 33, when she was separated from her confessor, Raymond de Capua, who had been sent off on a papal mission, she no longer ate and merely swallowed small amounts of water. She lost weight, became weak, and wasted away after four months of this regimen. It is difficult to escape a diagnosis of anorexia nervosa. ☐

Premature Babies

Sanjivan V. Patel, M.D., and Aruna J. Parekh, M.D.

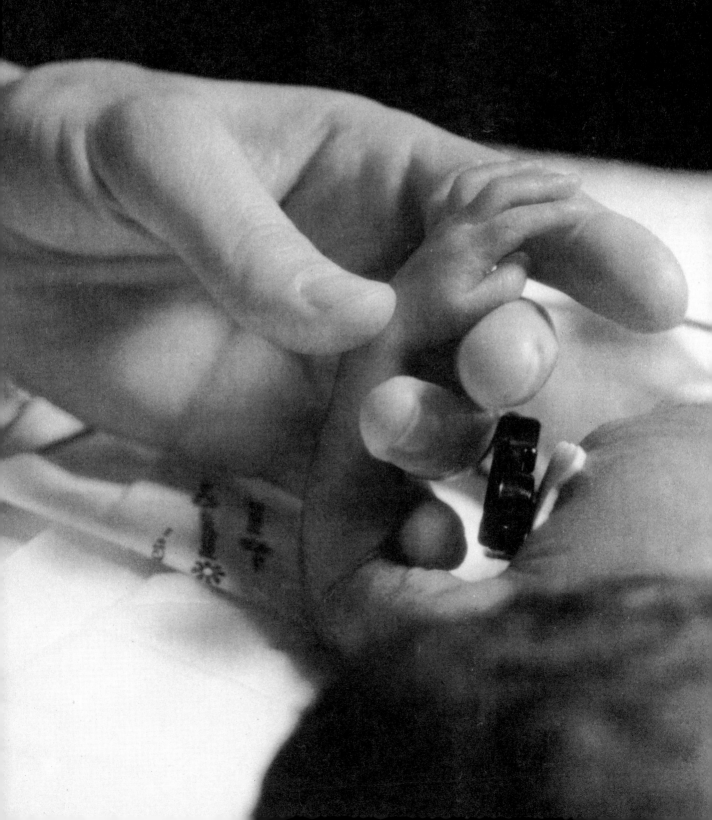

Premature babies are babies born earlier than the 38th week of pregnancy. Over the past five to six decades, and particularly in the past 20 years, the care of such babies has changed dramatically. Technological advances, better understanding of prematurity, and more aggressive treatment have led to a whole new era of neonatal (newborn) care. Ten or even five years ago, there was virtually no chance of survival for a baby born after only 24 weeks in the uterus and weighing little more than a pound. Now there is up to a 20 percent chance that doctors can save such a baby. For babies born between 24 and 28 weeks, the chances of survival rise steadily. Those born at 28 weeks and weighing between 2 and 3 pounds—more than half of whom would have died a quarter of a century ago—now have a survival rate of 90 to 95 percent.

Most premature babies, or preemies, go through a period of adjustment during which their not fully developed organs gradually take over body functions. Today, doctors can provide special medications, constant monitoring, and mechanical intervention if necessary until the baby's body has sufficiently matured. Still, the switch from total dependency on the mother before birth to independent existence is often fraught with difficulties and is not always successful. Babies born close to term may have few problems and may be sent home after only a short stay in the hospital. In contrast, the earliest and tiniest babies, who are least developed at birth, suffer many problems. Although the vast majority of premature babies will go on to live normal or near-normal lives, others will die after days or weeks in the neonatal intensive care unit. Still others will survive, but with disabilities so severe that normal life is impossible. According to one study that followed premature babies until they reached school age, a third were leading normal lives, half had relatively minor problems, and the rest were moderately to severely disabled. No one is sure how these proportions will change now that greater numbers of 24-week babies are surviving.

Neonatal Intensive Care

Intensive care for newborns was first brought to the United States in 1902, by the French physician Martin Couney. Dr. Couney showed that if premature babies were kept warm in incubators and fed via tubes through the nose, more of them survived. Subsequently, many hospitals across the country opened neonatal intensive care units (ICUs), beginning with Sarah Morris Hospital in Chicago in 1923. Neonatal intensive care has come a long way since then, with major milestones being the understanding and control of infections, the ability to help premature infants breathe using mechanical respirators, the understanding of the need to maintain the baby's glucose level and other chemical balances, and the understanding of nutritional needs.

The modern neonatal intensive care unit is a bewildering place—a brightly lit, high-tech setting in which the noise of the equipment is constant. The main purpose of all the equipment is to mimic the functions normally carried out in the womb and keep a careful watch

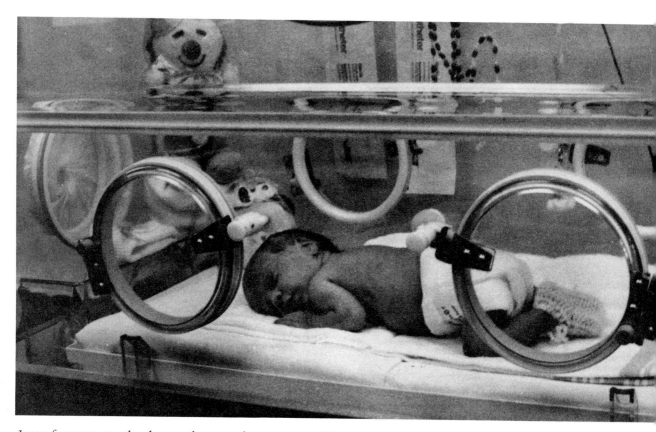

Just a few years ago the chances that severely premature babies would survive were slim. But because of technological advances and aggressive treatment, more of these infants can be helped until their bodies have sufficiently matured. Here a premature baby is kept warm in an incubator.

on each baby's condition. Respirators help babies breathe, warmers prevent them from becoming cold, and pumps ensure that an accurate flow of fluids and nutrients enter the body through tubes or intravenous needles. Cardiac monitors keep track of the babies' vital signs. An electronic thermometer is taped to the skin, while oxymeters and other monitoring devices help keep the baby's body chemistry as close to normal as possible. Teams of specially trained nurses and physicians are on the alert, 24 hours a day, for the problems that may well occur.

Sanjivan V. Patel is attending physician in neonatology at Long Island College Hospital and clinical instructor at the State University of New York's Downstate Medical Center, both in Brooklyn, N.Y. Aruna J. Parekh is chief of neonatology at Long Island College Hospital and assistant professor of pediatrics at the SUNY Health Science Center in Brooklyn.

What Causes Prematurity?

There are many reasons why a baby is born prematurely. Among the most important are the mother's low socioeconomic status and the inadequate prenatal care that often accompanies it. The mother's age is also a factor, with women under 18 and over 35 having the highest rates of prematurity. Habits such as smoking, drinking, and using drugs are contributing factors, as are severe emotional stress and poor nutrition. Various medical conditions and illnesses during pregnancy increase the risk of premature delivery, including high blood pressure, diabetes, urinary tract infections, and rubella (German measles). Women are also at risk of having a premature baby if they have a history of premature births, are carrying twins, have had many abortions, and/or have abnormalities of the cervix and uterus.

In many cases, premature births are avoidable if preventive measures are taken. Adequate prenatal care can increase dramatically a woman's chances of carrying a child to term. This includes treatment of known medical conditions where possible, sound nutrition, avoidance of risk factors like smoking and drinking, bed rest where appropriate, and careful monitoring of women for whom premature labor seems a risk. Women can also be taught to recognize the signs of premature labor. If contractions are caught early, they can sometimes be stopped by a combination of bed rest and drugs, allowing the pregnancy to continue.

Common Problems

The problems that can befall premature babies are many, and the most sickly preemies commonly develop not just one problem, but several. Fortunately, medical advances—many made only in the past five years—have led to better treatments for these problems.

Breathing Difficulties. Two major kinds of breathing difficulties can affect premature babies. The first is respiratory distress syndrome, formerly known as hyaline membrane disease; it remains the number one cause of death among premature infants. Normally, the lining of the lungs is coated with a chemical substance known as surfactant. In premature babies the lungs are underdeveloped and the surfactant may be missing or insufficient. Without surfactant, the lungs cannot inflate—instead, the air sacs in the lungs stay collapsed and stick together. As babies mature, the surfactant appears naturally and respiratory distress subsides. In the meantime, many infants need both supplemental oxygen to inflate the lungs and mechanical help with breathing. Respirators expand and contract the babies' lungs for them, which can be life-saving but carries the risk of long-term lung damage or of the child's becoming dependent on the respirator. However, recent technical advances have made it possible for the respirators to deliver oxygen in such a way that minimal damage is done to the baby's fragile lungs.

Sometimes, when there is high risk of a premature birth or a woman is having early contractions, a sample of the amniotic fluid is tested to determine whether the unborn baby's lungs have enough surfactant. If they don't, the mother can be given steroid drugs, which help the baby's lungs mature faster. If a child is born with insufficient surfactant, a promising new approach to respiratory distress syndrome involves "blowing" into the infant's lungs (via a tube inserted into the windpipe) surfactant extracted from the lungs of calves or from amniotic fluid donated by women undergoing cesareans. This treatment is still experimental.

Another type of respiratory difficulty—frequently faced by infants born before 34 weeks—is apnea, in which the baby "forgets" to breathe for a short time. Apnea generally occurs because the respiratory center in the brain, which is responsible for controlling breathing, is underdeveloped. In most cases, apnea is temporary and self-limiting. Until it does resolve, though, some babies need to be given drugs to stimulate respiration. At times, stimulation provided by an oscillating water bed seems to help. Occasionally, the baby has to be put on a respirator until a regular breathing pattern is established.

Keeping Warm. Stress from being cold is detrimental to most newborn infants and particularly to premature infants. Lacking an insulating layer of fat, having a smaller muscle mass and decreased muscle activity, and perhaps unable to feed and digest milk, many preemies cannot generate enough heat to maintain their body temperature. They must be kept warm in incubators or under special warmers until they get older and stronger and are able to maintain an adequate body temperature themselves. By the time they are ready to be sent home from the hospital, the majority of these infants can be kept warm with just a blanket and a head cover.

Nutritional Problems. Premature babies need more calories than other newborns; they also need higher levels of protein, calcium, phosphorus, salt, specially composed fats, vitamins, and trace minerals. But babies born before the 34th week of pregnancy are often too weak to suck or to swallow without choking, and they may lack the necessary swallowing/sucking reflexes. In such cases they are fed either formula or breast milk (expressed by the mother) through a tube that goes through the nose and down the throat into the stomach. If they can't take in enough milk this way, or have problems dealing with milk because of an underdeveloped digestive system, essential nutrients can be given intravenously. Before discharge most infants are able to breast-feed and/or bottle-feed normally.

Jaundice. Jaundice—yellowish discoloration of the skin, eyes, and, at times, body fluids—is perhaps the most common disorder afflicting newborns. Almost 50 percent of all healthy newborn infants and up to 70 percent of premature infants have jaundice in their first week of life. It is caused by accumulation in the blood of a yellow pigment known as bilirubin, which is produced by the breakdown of red blood cells. All of us throughout life produce this pigment, which is normally cleared from the bloodstream by the liver. However, the liver in newborn infants, particularly premature infants, can't always cope with bilirubin, and it accumulates in body fluids. A high enough level of bilirubin can harm the developing nervous system.

In the majority of cases, light treatment, or phototherapy, is enough to lower the bilirubin level. The baby is placed in a special chamber bathed in ultraviolet light, which helps the liver make the chemicals needed to get rid of the bilirubin. The baby's eyes are shielded from the light during phototherapy to prevent damage. In some instances, when bilirubin levels are increasing faster than can be countered by phototherapy, babies are given an exchange transfusion, in which their blood is completely replaced. Doctors are now actively looking at a promising new treatment for jaundice called Sn-protoporphyrin therapy, which would replace exchange transfusions. It utilizes a synthetic blood protein that acts to block the production of bilirubin.

Infections. Most premature infants have underdeveloped immune systems and also lack certain maternal antibodies against disease that ordinarily cross the placenta in the late stages of pregnancy. Thus, infection, a hazard for all newborns, is particularly dangerous for preemies. Premature infants are exposed to infection in many ways—while still in the uterus, during birth, and even in the ICU, where all the tubes they are connected to offer pathways for bacterial and viral invasion. Infections may cause pneumonia and meningitis. A baby showing evidence of infection must be treated at once, often with antibiotics, intravenous fluids, and sometimes infusion of blood products.

To add to the premature baby's problems, in recent years a serious and steady rise in the incidence of sexually transmitted diseases has increased the likelihood that a baby will pick up an infection during its passage through the birth canal at the time of delivery. There has been a steady rise in the number of babies born with congenital syphilis, streptococcal diseases, gonococcal conjunctivitis (inflammation of the eye), and AIDS.

Except for AIDS, most of these infections are treatable, but occasional serious complications cause lifelong disability. As with all infections, premature babies are more vulnerable to these problems than are full-term babies.

Brain Damage. The premature infant's brain, not fully developed at birth, is extremely vulnerable to infection, changes in blood pressure, lack of oxygen, and accumulation of unusually high levels of carbon dioxide in the blood. When premature infants fall victim to any of these conditions, they are likely to suffer hemorrhaging in the brain. As many as 40 percent of premature infants have "brain bleeds"; the most immature show the highest incidence.

The damage or disability caused by brain hemorrhages differs markedly from one baby to another and depends on the degree and the site of the bleeding. In smaller hemorrhages, the blood is absorbed spontaneously without any consequences, while larger hemorrhages can have serious effects such as seizures, hydrocephalus (excessive water inside the brain), paralysis, and mental retardation.

Ultrasound and sophisticated CT scans allow physicians to diagnose and follow the course of a hemorrhage, although there is little they can do to treat it. However, steps can be taken to treat hydrocephalus. If it does not go away spontaneously, it can often be dealt with by the insertion of a tube through which excess fluid can drain.

Although brain bleeds are the major neurological problem facing premature infants, some of them may suffer from other nervous system disorders. Lack of oxygen, and at times decreased blood supply, can lead to the death of brain cells, which may cause paralysis or mental retardation. In some instances, infections such as meningitis cause neurological problems.

Intestinal Disorder. Anywhere from 2 to 15 percent of premature infants develop an intestinal disorder called necrotizing enterocolitis (NEC), in which the lining of the large intestine breaks down, leaving babies vulnerable to infections from bacteria that normally live in the intestine. All sick premature infants are at risk for NEC, especially those who did not breathe on their own at birth, those who may have suffered from shock, lack of oxygen, or infections, and those who required exchange transfusions. Initially, the baby develops abdominal distension, followed by passage of blood in the stool—signs doctors and nurses look for in order to treat NEC promptly. For the most part, careful monitoring, intravenous fluids, the withholding of oral feedings so the intestine can rest, and antibiotic therapy are enough to cure the condition. Sometimes, however, the intestine ruptures and spills its contents into the abdomen. When this happens, the damaged part of the intestine must be surgically removed. Surgery may not cure the baby of NEC, but removal of the damaged part of the intestine promotes the healing process. Occasionally, a temporary colostomy (a hole in the abdomen with a bag attached to collect the baby's stool) is necessary.

Vision Problems. Retinopathy of prematurity (ROP) is a vision disorder caused by injury to the retina, the light-sensitive tissue that lines the eyeball. The immature retina is extremely sensitive to the amount of oxygen and carbon dioxide in the blood, as well as to changes in the volume of blood flow. The retina sometimes reacts by suddenly producing new blood vessels. After a few weeks, these vessels result in scar tissue, which contracts, pulling on the retina. Eventually, if the process continues, the result may be blindness. Approximately 20 percent of premature infants—and as many as 50 percent of those weighing less than 2.2 pounds—show evidence of injury to the retina. A small percentage of infants with ROP become blind. Where the disorder does not cause blindness, it either disappears completely or results in a reduction in the child's vision.

Until recently, retinopathy of prematurity was untreatable. All that doctors could do was monitor oxygen levels in the baby's blood—too much oxygen being a known risk factor for the disease—and if necessary adjust the amount of oxygen in the air the baby was breathing. In 1988, however, the U.S. National Eye Institute recommended that a new treatment, called cryotherapy, be used in all severe cases. In cryotherapy, part of the retina is frozen and destroyed, thus stopping the spread of the new blood vessels. Cryotherapy can reduce by half an affected infant's chances of becoming blind or losing some vision. It must be recognized, however, that ROP is not always preventable and that some children will suffer vision problems in spite of appropriate care.

Heart Defect. Normally, the heart pumps oxygen-rich blood to the body via a blood vessel called the aorta, and oxygen-poor blood to the lungs for reoxygenation via the pulmonary artery. Before birth, however, fetuses receive oxygen from the

mother through the placenta. The lungs are inactive, and blood bypasses them by means of a temporary channel called the patent ductus arteriosus, which connects the pulmonary artery to the aorta.

In a normal, full-term baby, the lungs take over the job of providing oxygen right after delivery, and the now-unnecessary ductus closes 10 to 15 hours

An infant may be hooked up to machinery with a tangle of wires, but loving human contact is important too.

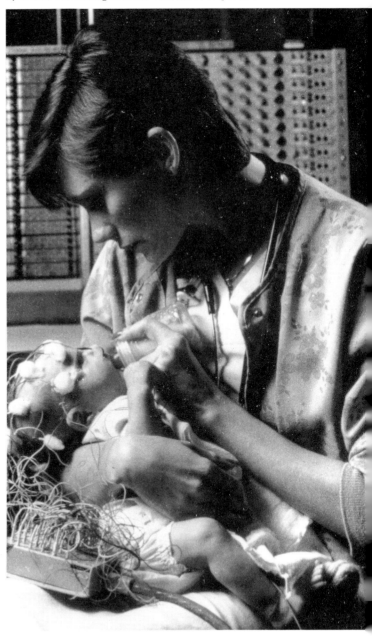

later. In premature infants the closing takes longer, perhaps as long as two to three weeks; a closed ductus may even reopen. In either case the baby can go into heart failure or develop breathing difficulties as the heart and lungs try to deal with the abnormal circulatory pathway.

The drug indomethacin (Indocin IV), which stimulates closure of the ductus, may be given. Often, though, surgery is needed. Surgical closure of the ductus has become a very common procedure, performed at bedside in most neonatal ICUs.

Anemia. At some point in their first three months of life, almost all premature infants develop anemia, which can slow their weight gain or even send them into heart failure. Anemia means that the body has fewer red blood cells than it needs to carry oxygen to body cells. In premature infants it can be caused by many factors—decreased blood volume, inadequate formation of blood cells by bone marrow, insufficient iron and protein stores in the body, a shorter than usual life span for red blood cells, infections, and the frequent drawing of blood for tests. Anemia of prematurity can easily be corrected by proper nutrition, iron and vitamin E supplements, and at times blood transfusions.

The Parents

As the smallest and most fragile premature babies confront one problem after another in the fight to survive, their parents try to cope with a situation full of seemingly never-ending stress. As with most critical patients, anything can go wrong with such an infant. A baby that is doing just fine one day

In a neonatal intensive care unit, a baby who was born prematurely is being helped to breathe with a mechanical ventilator.

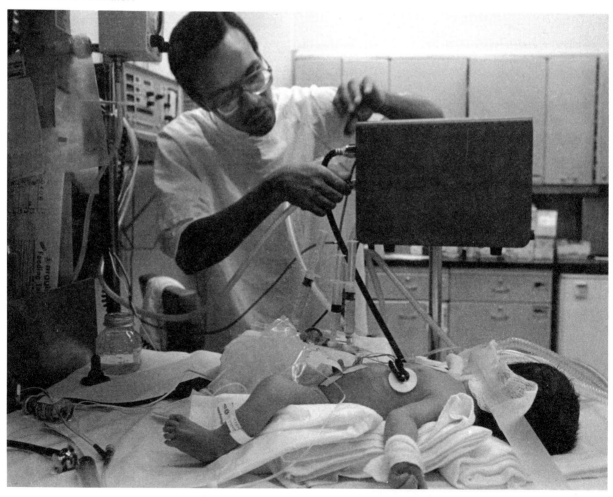

may be near death the next. Thus, a premature baby's course in the ICU can best be described as a roller coaster of unexpected events. The parents' emotions follow the same course.

From the minute a premature child is born, the fact that the baby is not perfect weighs heavily on most parents, who typically experience guilt and fear. Did they do something to bring on the early birth of their child? Are they responsible for its condition? While the infant's state is critical, anxiety virtually paralyzes the parents. Most soon learn not to take anything about their child's progress for granted and become very dependent on nursery personnel for reassurance.

The parents of a healthy full-term baby get to hold and caress it immediately after birth and to take it home only a few days later. This is usually denied the parents of a premature baby. The physical separation imposes fear and frustration. An important factor in how comfortable and secure the parents come to feel with their baby is how much time they spend with the child while it is in the hospital. Parents are encouraged to visit their babies in the neonatal ICU as often as possible and to interact with them, however sick or small the babies may be. If the baby is in an incubator, parents can reach in and touch it through glovelike openings. When the child is stronger, parents can hold, rock, and bathe the baby. This contact is also important for the babies. They seem to thrive more readily and are more active and responsive when they are touched, held, rocked, and talked to.

Throughout an infant's stay in the neonatal ICU, support and counseling by physicians and nurses are extremely important for the parents' well-being. A hospital social worker is also often involved, forming a vital link between parents and the medical staff. If a baby dies, it may be helpful for the parents to meet with the doctors and a social worker to have all their questions answered and allay inappropriate guilt feelings. Some parents require long-term counseling.

Lasting Effects of Prematurity

As might be expected, infants who undergo and survive what is essentially an artificial existence in a neonatal ICU do tend to have special problems in the long run. Some of them are relatively minor ailments, including recurrent colds, pneumonia, bronchiolitis (a lower respiratory tract infection),

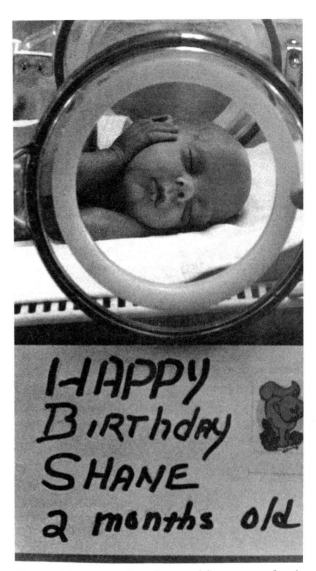

The road home can be a long and bumpy one for the smallest and most fragile premature babies.

middle ear infections, and anemia. These illnesses are easily treatable and usually do not have serious consequences. Inguinal hernias, in which there is a protruding bulge of tissue near the groin, are very common among premature infants; they can be corrected surgically once the baby weighs about 5 pounds. Many premature infants show delayed physical growth during their first year. This usually gives way to accelerated growth by the middle of their second year, allowing them to catch up to full-term children. Some premature infants tend to spit up and vomit frequently. This may be due in part to parental anxiety, which can communicate itself to

173

the child, but at times it is due to gastroesophageal reflux, caused by looseness of the valve that stops food from coming back out of the stomach. This condition disappears without treatment.

Some of the problems facing survivors of the neonatal ICU are, however, more serious. From 15 to 30 percent of infants who were on respirators develop disabilities that require special attention later in life. Among them is a chronic lung disorder called bronchopulmonary dysplasia—a condition in which fibrous tissue develops in the lungs. Children suffering from bronchopulmonary dysplasia have frequent wheezing episodes and occasional respiratory failure requiring hospitalization. Sudden infant death syndrome (crib death) is three to four times more common among survivors of neonatal ICUs than among babies generally. Some of the infants who have had surgery for NEC cannot absorb fat or glucose well and have to be fed special formulas; their growth may never catch up to that of their peers.

Children with impaired vision as a result of retinopathy of prematurity are more likely to have developmental disabilities and require special education. Premature children also may suffer minor neurological disabilities, which may be late in appearing. These include speech and language disorders, hearing problems, and problems with cognitive abilities such as analytical thinking. Fortunately, major neurological disabilities, including seizures, mental retardation, and motor retardation, are seen less frequently.

Lastly, the aftereffects of prematurity can go beyond physical and mental disabilities. When they come home from the hospital, many premature infants require much more care from their parents than ordinary babies. At the same time, they may not be as responsive as bigger babies. Long-term medical or developmental problems may be a constant source of parental stress. All of these factors are reflected in higher rates of child abuse or neglect and failure to thrive than is found among full-term children. Support groups have been established to help parents deal with the problems that stem from having a premature baby.

Ethical Issues

We have come a long way since the first premature baby was treated in a neonatal ICU. Modern technology has made it possible to save the lives of many babies who only a few years ago would have died at birth or soon after. In most cases the value of this capability is beyond question. But not always. With the new ability to help premature babies survive have come new, seemingly unanswerable questions that go beyond issues of sustaining life to issues of the quality of the lives being sustained. Should doctors treat with aggressive means those premature babies who will inevitably be so severely damaged by their medical problems that any semblance of a normal life is impossible? Who should decide what quality of life is acceptable? Who should make the decisions about starting treatment, continuing it, or stopping it? Should society be spending up to $500,000 each for the very sickest babies who require months of intensive care? Should more than half of all the money that goes to newborn care in the United States be spent on premature babies—who represent only about 10 percent of infants born every year? Would it make more sense to spend the money on prenatal care, so that many premature births could be avoided?

These are questions that affect everyone to a greater or lesser extent. Most immediately involved are the parents of a premature infant, the intern who stays up all night providing care for the child, and the nurse who knows that a baby is not going to make it and sees a team of physicians trying to save the baby anyway, even if their efforts involve pain without benefit. There are neonatologists and neurologists who know that a baby's brain will be severely damaged by treatment, yet feel they have to go along with the heroics of modern medicine. And there are the citizens whose hard-earned dollars are being spent on neonatal care.

These issues are a constant challenge to society and the medical profession. Doctors involved in the care of premature infants know their duty is to provide the best care so as to ensure the best possible outcome, which occasionally may mean letting a child go. Although most of these issues have remained unaddressed for a long time, over the past five years or so, medical societies, the courts, and individual institutions have begun to offer choices whereby such infants are allowed to die in a dignified manner.

We cannot lose sight of the fact that these extreme cases represent a minority. For most premature babies, modern medicine promises a chance to live and to thrive. □

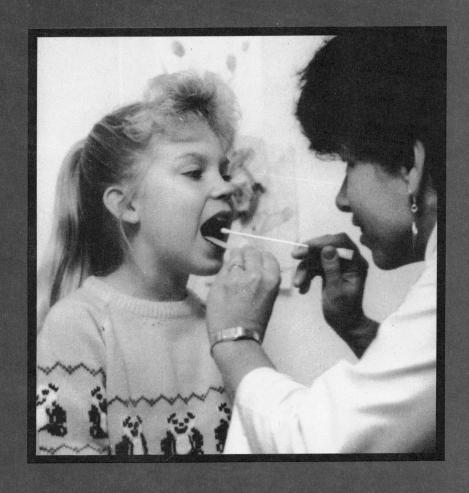

SPOTLIGHT ON HEALTH

Facts About OAT BRAN

Eleanor R. Williams, Ph.D.

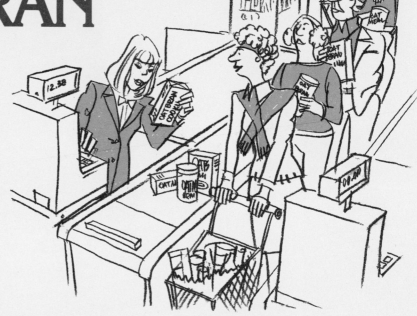

One of the biggest health food fads to hit the United States in recent years has been the public's passion for oat bran. At some health food stores, sales of oat bran products tripled in 1988. One company estimated that sales of its oat bran cereal increased 600 percent, and the Quaker Oats plant in Cedar Rapids, Iowa, had three shifts working daily to try to keep up with demand. Oatmeal sales were up 20 percent overall, and manufacturers put out dozens of new products—from cold oat bran cereals to oat bran animal cookies.

Fiber and Cholesterol

What is oat bran, and why the sudden interest in it? Oat bran is the outer layer of the whole oat grain, after the husk has been removed. It is a source of soluble dietary fiber and is capable of lowering blood cholesterol—a potentially significant benefit, since high cholesterol levels have been linked to heart disease (and a benefit widely publicized in a recent bestseller). Rolled oats and steel-cut oats are made from the whole oat grain and therefore also furnish oat bran, although they contain only about half the soluble fiber in an equal measure of pure oat bran.

Fiber, the indigestible organic material found in plant foods, comes in two types, called soluble and insoluble (depending on whether they dissolve in water). Both types may help prevent or alleviate constipation, hemorrhoids, and intestinal disorders like diverticulosis. Insoluble fiber, the kind found in wheat and many other grains, may help prevent colon cancer but has no effect on cholesterol. Soluble fiber is found in peas, beans, and many fruits and vegetables, as well as in oat bran.

Several types of soluble fiber have been shown to lower blood cholesterol levels (all types have not yet been tested, so scientists do not know if they all have this effect). Researchers are not quite sure why soluble fiber does this. In the case of oat bran, it may be because the fiber absorbs bile acids, which are chemical derivatives of cholesterol, from the gastrointestinal tract and carries them out of the body. The liver then must break down more cholesterol to form new bile acids, which results in lower total cholesterol in the blood.

Effects of Oat Bran

The fact that rolled oats lower blood cholesterol was first observed in the early 1960s, long before the current interest arose in dietary fiber and its possible relationship to disease. Later research confirmed the original findings, but because it was unclear whether some component of oats other than bran might be the effective agent, investigators began studying the effects of pure oat bran. These studies concluded that oat bran did lower blood cholesterol, generally to a greater extent in people who have high as opposed to normal cholesterol counts.

Recent studies have shown that blood cholesterol could be lowered as much as 19 percent in people with cholesterol levels above 260 milligrams per 100 milliliters of blood. (A normal level would be between 180 and

200.) But to achieve this degree of lowering, study participants consumed 100 grams of oat bran daily, in the form of one bowl of hot cereal plus five oat bran muffins. Research shows that people with normal blood cholesterol levels can achieve a 3 percent lowering by consuming 35 grams of oat bran a day (about 1.2 ounces). A 3 percent lowering is considered to be significant, since each 1 percent drop in blood cholesterol level results in a 2 percent drop in the risk of heart disease.

The type of blood cholesterol lowered by oats or oat bran is called LDL (low-density lipoprotein), sometimes referred to as the "bad" cholesterol, which forms fatty deposits in artery walls. It should be noted that oat bran does not affect blood levels of HDL (high-density lipoprotein), the "good" cholesterol that actually helps remove excess cholesterol from the blood.

Proper Diet

A practical and effective way to reduce blood cholesterol levels is to combine moderate amounts of oatmeal daily with the American Heart Association diet, which calls for individuals to take in no more than 30 percent of their daily calories as fat, including no more than 10 percent as saturated fat. A recent study demonstrated that subjects with normal cholesterol levels at the beginning of the study achieved a 9 percent reduction in blood cholesterol as a result of this combination. About one-third of the reduction was attributed to the added oatmeal they consumed.

One of the dangers of the oat bran craze is that people will think that they only need to consume some product containing oat bran to lower blood cholesterol levels, regardless of the quality of their usual diet. It is now clearly established that eating a low-fat, low-saturated fat, low-cholesterol diet is the best way to bring down blood cholesterol levels. Such a diet should contain larger amounts of vegetables, fruits, and whole grain products than many Americans usually eat. Adding oat bran to such a diet will likely result in additional benefit, but oat bran is not a panacea—it should not be *substituted* for a healthful diet.

Checking Oat Products

How do consumers find their way in a marketplace that is adding oat bran (often in minuscule amounts) to cold cereals, graham crackers, animal crackers, muffins, cookies, and breads? First, one should keep in mind that about 35 grams of oat bran is required to lower blood cholesterol by 3 percent. Check each product's package to see how much oat bran is in one serving (and note the serving size to be sure it is not unreasonably large). Cold oat bran cereals generally contain relatively small amounts of oat bran. Some manufacturers do not specify how much is in each serving, in which case it can probably be assumed that the amount is low.

In many cases it will turn out that 10 to 15 servings of a product would have to be eaten each day to yield the desired 35 grams of oat bran. In fact, one investigator noted that a person would have to eat 90 cookies marketed by one manufacturer to take in the desired 35 grams.

Once you have found a product that does contain 35 grams of oat bran in one or two servings, check the label to be sure the product does not also contain coconut oil, palm oil, beef tallow, butter, eggs, or cream, all of which can raise blood cholesterol levels. Oat bran muffins and cookies, which are currently very popular sources of bran, often are made with large amounts of butter, eggs, and cream to make them moist enough to be palatable, since oat bran makes the product dry. Any cholesterol-lowering effects from the bran in the muffin will likely be offset by the fat.

Finally, remember that rolled oats themselves can be quite effective in lowering blood cholesterol. A recent study showed that eating 35 grams of oatmeal (a little less than half a cup, dry) every day also lowered blood cholesterol by 3 percent, even though oatmeal has only half the soluble fiber of pure oat bran. If rolled oats are used in packaged baked products, again, be sure that large amounts

Oat bran is a valuable dietary source of soluble fiber, which can significantly lower blood cholesterol levels and thus reduce the risk of heart disease.

of butter, eggs, or cream are not in the product as well.

Oats can easily be incorporated into home recipes. For example, oat bran can be added to meat loaf, pancakes, and baked goods. Oatmeal can also be ground in a blender or food processor to make oat flour, which can be used like wheat flour for breading and thickening sauces. It cannot be substituted entirely for wheat flour in making bread because it lacks gluten, but oat flour can be mixed, half and half, with wheat flour in bread recipes.

Peas and Beans

Other sources of soluble fiber have been shown to be as effective as oat bran in lowering blood cholesterol, although these have yet to catch the fancy of consumers and advertisers. Dried beans and peas—such as chick-peas, split peas, lentils, and pinto, kidney, navy, and black beans—are excellent sources of soluble fiber. About half a cup of cooked beans or peas is as effective as a bowl of hot oat bran cereal in lowering blood cholesterol levels. □

How Drugs Are Approved

Virginia Cowart

In the United States, about 1.6 billion drug prescriptions are filled every year. There are also billions of purchases of over-the-counter drugs. The government agency charged with approving new drugs for use by the general public is the Food and Drug Administration (FDA). The process by which drugs are approved is often long and complicated—to ensure that the medications on the market are as safe as possible and will do the job they claim to.

Such stringent government oversight is actually fairly new. It was not until 1906 that any federal regulation of medications began, with a law requiring only that drugs meet official standards of purity and strength. Over 30 years later, the Federal Food, Drug, and Cosmetic Act of 1938 required drugs to be proven safe; a 1962 amendment added a requirement for proven effectiveness.

Every new prescription drug must obtain FDA approval of safety and effectiveness before it can be sold to the public. Most new over-the-counter drugs do not need specific FDA approval as long as they meet the agency's standards for the category of drug they belong to (laxatives, for example, or antacids). If a proposed over-the-counter drug is one of a class of medications that was not generally recognized as safe and effective before 1938, it must go through the same stringent review procedures that prescription drugs face.

The Role of the FDA

The FDA seeks to ensure that drugs are safe and effective not by testing drugs itself but by carefully reviewing the evidence about a drug submitted to the agency by its manufacturer. The agency is often criticized for being overcautious, for taking an average of 24 months to review a new drug application (in agency jargon, an NDA). Critics point out that new drugs come on the market much faster elsewhere. This is not true of all countries, however. In Canada, for example, the federal government's Drugs Directorate usually takes as long as the FDA to approve a new drug.

The FDA is sensitive to the time its reviews take. Dr. Stuart L. Nightingale, the FDA's associate commissioner for health affairs, has said, "Obviously, we are trying to speed up the approval process and make it as efficient as possible." The agency is working on a system that would allow companies to submit new drug applications in electronic form (for example, on computer disk). Since a new drug application can amount to 150,000 pages or more, electronic submission would eliminate mounds of paperwork and therefore should allow for faster FDA review. Electronic submission has already begun on a limited basis, but no standards have yet been set as to the exact form it should take.

Beginning the Process

Following a drug from its conception to market may make the approval process clearer. First, though, it must be noted that despite frequent headlines about "major scientific breakthroughs" or "miracle drugs," the reality is seldom so simple. Most of the media reports are premature, exaggerated, or inaccurate. The truth is that really significant advances in drug treatment are rare. Aside from anti-infective agents, drugs that make a disease disappear are almost unknown.

The research process at U.S. pharmaceutical companies is costly, sophisticated, and time-consuming—an average of $6\frac{1}{2}$ years is spent on initial synthesis and testing of a drug, most of it on testing alone. Sometimes a company sets out to develop a drug for a particular disease; sometimes a new drug results from research into something else.

The FDA first becomes involved in the process when a company files what is called an investigational new drug application, or IND. At this point, the manufacturer has already done tests, using animals, of the drug's safety and effectiveness. The IND includes information on the drug's chemical structure, the results of the animal tests, manufacturing details, and the complete plan for testing on people. All this material is reviewed by the FDA before approval is granted for human testing. Within 30 days after receiving the IND, the FDA lets the company know if human tests can begin or if the agency has questions about the application.

The human tests—or clinical trials, as they are called—are carried out by physicians and hospitals and usually have three phases. Phase 1 tests mainly the drug's safety, on small numbers of healthy volunteers; phase 2 involves several hundred patients and tests mainly the drug's effectiveness; phase 3 involves up to several thousand patients and consists of extensive tests for safety, effectiveness, and optimal dosage levels. The FDA receives regular progress reports throughout the testing process.

New Drug Applications

When the human tests are satisfactory, the company files its new drug application (NDA). The day the FDA receives it, a "review clock" is started, and the agency has 180 days to review the application and either approve or reject it. This 180-day period, however, tends to get stretched into about two years because the review clock may be stopped for several reasons. The most common is that the FDA requests more information from the company.

The length of the review process also depends on the priority as-signed to the drug. The FDA assigns priority based on a drug's potential benefit and chemical type. From a clinical standpoint, a drug may effectively treat a disease for which there is no adequate treatment, or it may offer just a modest advantage over other products already on the market. In a chemical sense, a new drug may be a new molecular entity, meaning that it has an active ingredient that has never been marketed in the United States. It could be a new derivative—that is, a chemical derived from an active ingredient that is already on the market. It could be a new formulation or a new combination of marketed drugs or a drug that duplicates an already marketed drug. Top priority currently goes to AIDS drugs, followed by drugs that combine a new molecular entity with an important therapeutic gain.

The actual process of review begins with the assembling of an FDA team to study the NDA from several viewpoints. (The NDA contains the same information as the IND, plus the results of the human trials and the proposed wording of all printed material to accompany the drug, including the so-called package insert distributed to doctors and pharmacists.) A chemist examines how the drug is put together and whether the manufacturing controls and packaging are sufficient to keep the drug stable. A pharmacologist looks at the short-term and long-term effects of the drug. A physician examines the results of the tests on humans, including both good and bad effects. A statistician looks at the designs of the

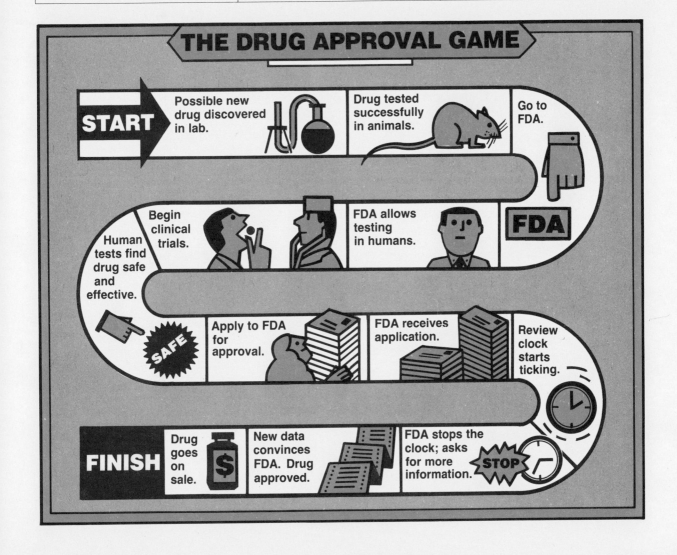

studies to see if the statistical analyses are valid. Other members of the team evaluate the way the drug is distributed in, metabolized by, and eliminated from the body. If the drug is an anti-infective (an antibacterial, antiviral, or antifungal agent), a microbiologist reviews the data.

In the end, the decision on whether to approve comes down to two basic questions:

- Is there substantial evidence that the drug is effective for the condition it is intended to treat?
- Is the product safe under the conditions of use in the proposed labeling?

After the agency review team has made its recommendation that a drug is "approvable," the FDA's upper management may concur or disagree. If this review is favorable, a drug can be on the market as soon as the manufacturer gets approval of its final labeling (all of the printed material distributed with the drug) and its production and distribution systems are set up. About 75 percent of NDAs are approved. If the drug is not approved, the company can amend the NDA by supplying new evidence, can withdraw the NDA, or can ask for a hearing.

Experimental Drugs

Suppose a drug is developed that appears to have promise in treating desperately ill people. Can the approval process be speeded up or the drug made available prior to approval, at least on a limited basis? The answer is a qualified yes. The FDA has for years permitted the use of experimental drugs in certain circumstances. A recent example is zidovudine (formerly known as AZT) for AIDS patients. The FDA allowed limited use of the drug while it was still experimental after early very promising results, and this enabled more than 4,000 desperate patients to be treated pending full FDA approval. The drug, marketed as Retrovir, was fully approved in March 1987, after only a four-month process.

In May 1987 the agency issued a new regulation, effective the following month, to make some experimental drugs available to more people at earlier stages in the testing process if no other effective treatment for a serious or life-threatening condition existed and early results were promising. The regulation recognized that patients for whom such experimental drugs are prescribed accept a greater risk of adverse effects.

In early 1988 trimetrexate, used to treat the pneumonia that often afflicts AIDS patients, became the first medication for an AIDS-associated disorder allowed to be used under the 1987 rule. However, the new regulation did not silence the controversy over the availability of AIDS drugs—a controversy that was a major reason for the rule's promulgation. The FDA contended that it could not approve drugs that did not exist; critics complained that there were drugs in the pipeline but that the FDA was too rigid in applying the new standards.

In October 1988 the FDA announced new procedures for the approval of drugs to treat life-threatening illnesses. Under the new system, the second phase of clinical trials for such drugs would involve more people and last longer, thus providing more information on the drug. Phase 3 of the trials—generally the longest phase—would be eliminated. The FDA could then approve the drug after phase 2, in some cases making that approval conditional on the manufacturer's agreeing to do follow-up studies of the drug while it is on the market.

Monitoring the Market

Once most drugs are on the market, both the manufacturer and the FDA collect reports of adverse reactions from physicians, pharmacists, and so on. If these reactions are serious—causing hospitalization, disability, or death—the manufacturer must report them immediately to the FDA. Data on less serious reactions may

be sent in quarterly or annually. These reports are put into a computer that searches for significant patterns. If a new drug proves to be toxic, changing the dosage or directions for use may be all that is necessary. In some cases, though, the product may be voluntarily withdrawn from the market by the manufacturer, or the FDA may order it withdrawn.

Following drugs on the market can uncover long-term effects not detected during the testing stages. An example is the drug diethylstilbestrol (DES), which was frequently prescribed in the 1940s, 1950s, and 1960s to prevent miscarriage. In the early 1970s, vaginal tumors caused by this drug began to be seen in the daughters of women who had taken DES.

Sometimes drugs with serious side effects are kept on the market because their benefit is deemed greater than the risk involved in taking them. In that case, the package insert should alert the doctor, pharmacist, and patient to potential adverse reactions. A recent example is isotretinoin—sold under the brand name Accutane— a vitamin A derivative that is used to treat severe, intractable cystic acne. Accutane has long been known to cause serious birth defects and was so labeled at the time of its approval. Despite the warning, however, many women taking the drug were still becoming pregnant. In May 1988 the FDA decided not to withdraw Accutane from the U.S. market, as some experts had urged. Instead, the agency required the drug's manufacturer to provide new labeling, including a picture of a deformed infant and a black-bordered warning statement to alert potential users of the dangers. In addition, women using Accutane are urged to have a monthly pregnancy test and to discontinue use if they plan to become pregnant. Patients taking the drug must sign detailed forms stating that they are aware of the risks; doctors must sign forms stating that patients have been fully informed. □

ANEMIA

Ernest Beutler, M.D.

Taken literally, "anemia" means "no blood." Of course we could not survive for even a minute without blood; the word actually refers to a deficiency of one component of blood, namely the red blood cell. When there is such a red blood cell deficiency, body tissues do not get enough oxygen, resulting in weakness, fatigue, pallor, headache, palpitations, and shortness of breath. In severe cases heart failure or shock can occur.

Like fever or a toothache, anemia is a symptom that can have many causes, and treatment must be directed at the underlying cause. The common type known as anemia of chronic disease, ordinarily quite mild, disappears when the disorder producing it is cured.

Blood tests help determine whether a person has anemia—and if so, what kind. Other tests may sometimes be needed, such as analysis of a sample of bone marrow.

Red Cells in Action

To better understand how anemia comes about, we need to look at the red blood cell. It is a small, highly specialized disk-shaped cell that carries oxygen from the lungs to body tissues by means of a red protein known as hemoglobin. This protein has the unique property of combining with oxygen in the lungs, where that substance is relatively abundant, and then releasing oxygen quickly when its concentration falls, as in the oxygen-consuming tissues of the body. Everything about the red blood cell is designed to maintain its hemoglobin in top working order. The cell contains dozens of

---

Fatigue, headache, shortness of breath—any or all of these symptoms can make life a struggle for people with anemia.

---

enzymes that help to maintain the integrity of the cell membrane and the hemoglobin.

In humans, red blood cells normally live approximately 120 days. There are 25 trillion of them in the average normal body. More than 200 billion are destroyed each day, mostly in the spleen, liver, and bone marrow, and are replaced by new ones manufactured in the bone marrow. The bone marrow seems to know how many red cells are required, obtaining its information through a sensor in the kidney that makes a hormone called erythropoietin (EPO) that stimulates red cell formation. Anemia results when the balance between red cell production and red cell destruction is disturbed.

Blood-Loss Anemia

One way the balance can be upset is if red cells are lost from the body. A bleeding stomach ulcer, a knife or bullet wound, can cause blood to be lost much more rapidly than the bone marrow is able to replace red cells. Anemia develops as the blood is lost. When the blood loss stops, the body quickly corrects the anemia, as long as it has sufficient building

blocks with which to make more red cells. The building block that is most likely to be in short supply is iron, an essential component of the hemoglobin molecule.

Hemolytic Anemia

Anemia can also occur if the red cell life span is shortened to substantially less than the normal 120 days. This is called hemolytic anemia. The bone marrow can compensate for moderate degrees of shortening of the red cell life span, but when the average red cell survives less than 20 or 30 days, the marrow cannot produce enough new cells. Red blood

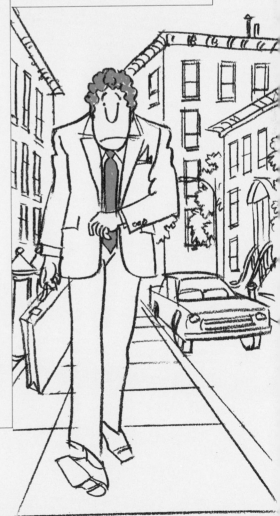

cells may be destroyed at an increased rate because they are defective (usually for genetic reasons) or because there are abnormal components in the bloodstream—the red cell's environment. Sometimes both factors play a role.

Sickle Cells. One of the more common red cell defects causes sickle-cell disease, which affects mainly blacks—about 3 out of every 1,000 in the United States. This disorder is due to the genetically determined presence of an abnormal kind of hemoglobin. In parts of the body where the oxygen supply is low, this hemoglobin forms rods that distort the red cells into a sickle shape. The red cells also become quite rigid, so that they are no longer able to pass

has, unfortunately, not yet been translated into a cure, although there is treatment for symptoms.

Enzymes and Membranes. Abnormalities of red cell enzymes or the cell membrane can also decrease the cell's life span. Two of the more common enzyme defects are deficiencies of pyruvate kinase and of glucose-6-phosphate dehydrogenase. The latter abnormality causes shortening of red cell life span, particularly when the red cells are subjected to an additional stress such as that imposed by infection or taking certain medications, such as some antimalarial drugs and the antibacterial drug nitrofurantoin (Furadantin).

The most common inherited membrane defect is hereditary spherocytosis. In this disorder the

occur as a complication of chronic lymphocytic leukemia or in subacute lupus erythematosus, diseases involving disturbances of the immune system. The anemia that results, called autoimmune

> **In sickle-cell anemia red cells become too distorted and rigid to pass through small blood vessels, thus interrupting the supply of blood to body tissues.**

hemolytic anemia, is diagnosed by demonstrating the presence of a coating of antibodies on red cells in a blood sample. Production of the antibodies can sometimes be stopped by treatment with such drugs as prednisone and cyclophosphamide. Sometimes destruction of cells can be greatly reduced by removal of the spleen.

Various drugs and poisons can shorten the red cell life span. Examples are toxins produced by spiders and bacteria and metals like copper or arsenic. Some drugs, such as the antibacterial medication dapsone, act directly on the red cell, producing damage that decreases its life span. Other drugs, such as L-dopa, may act less directly, stimulating the formation of antibodies that then damage the red cell. Treatment consists of stopping use of the drug.

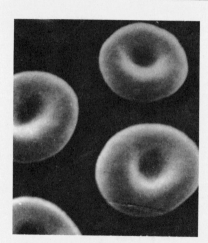

NORMAL CELLS

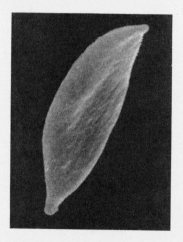

A SICKLE CELL

through small blood vessels. The resulting interruptions in the blood supply to tissues are responsible for the attacks of pain—in the abdomen, bones, and joints—and many other problems that occur in sickle cell anemia.

Sickle-cell hemoglobin is only one of many abnormal hemoglobins that may result in hemolytic anemia. Although medical scientists have accumulated a wealth of information about how these disorders come about, this knowledge

shape of red cells approaches that of a sphere rather than a disk, making them much less flexible. They become trapped in the tiny blood vessels of the spleen and are destroyed. Surgical removal of the spleen cures the anemia.

Bloodstream Problems. The life span of normal red cells can be greatly shortened if there are antibodies in the blood that attack components of the cell membrane. Such antibodies sometimes appear for no known reason, or they may

Low Red Cell Production
Another major cause of anemia is failure of the bone marrow to deliver normal numbers of red cells to the bloodstream. There are many possible reasons why this might happen. Simply administering EPO seems to help when kidney disease is the underlying

cause. Although the substance has been difficult to obtain in purified form, a genetically engineered version of the hormone was expected to gain approval from the U.S. Food and Drug Administration in 1989.

Iron Deficiency Anemia. Often the bone marrow's failure to produce the necessary red blood cells is due to a shortage of building blocks for red cells, notably iron. Iron deficiency is probably the most common cause of anemia. The amount of iron normally stored in the body is relatively meager, and the body's capacity to absorb it from food is limited.

Ordinarily, when red cells reach the end of their life span and are destroyed in the liver, spleen, or bone marrow, the iron in the hemoglobin is recycled. Losses of iron from the body are normally very small and are replaced by iron from the diet. There is usually little need for a healthy individual to take extra iron, except perhaps for rapidly growing infants and children and, to some extent, pregnant women.

But when a person bleeds, the red cell iron is lost to the body. Blood loss is, in fact, the most important cause of iron deficiency. The iron deficiency itself can usually be treated with iron tablets, but it is of vital importance that the cause of the iron deficiency be identified, so that it can be treated if necessary. Most commonly the cause is merely heavy menstrual bleeding or chronic bleeding hemorrhoids, but it can also be an ulcer or a cancer of the digestive tract.

Pernicious Anemia. The bone marrow requires a supply of two B vitamins—B_{12} and folic acid—to make red blood cells. When not enough of these vitamins is available, greatly reduced numbers of red cells, each larger than normal, are produced. Since most people's diets have enough B_{12}, a deficiency of the vitamin is usually due to an inability to absorb it. This disorder, pernicious anemia, most often has a hereditary basis

and usually occurs in middle or old age. The problem is readily corrected through lifelong injections of the vitamin.

Folic acid deficiency is most common in alcoholics, since alcohol interferes with the body's ability to process the vitamin, and since alcoholics' diet is often lacking in it. Some people may develop the deficiency because of inability to absorb folic acid. This problem may occur not only in individuals with gastrointestinal disease but also in women in whom birth control pills interfere with the processing of dietary folic acid. Treatment may include folic acid tablets.

Thalassemia. One of the more common causes of anemia is a group of disorders called the thalassemias. These affect the genes that direct hemoglobin production.

Alcoholics may become anemic because alcohol prevents proper processing of folic acid, needed to make red cells.

Unlike the hereditary disorders that cause sickle cells and other cell abnormalities that result in hemolytic anemia, these genetic disorders influence chiefly the rate at which hemoglobin is made. The hemoglobin that is manufactured by the bone marrow is usually quite normal; there is simply not enough of it.

The vast majority of people with thalassemia have very mild forms, called thalassemia minor. Such thalassemias are most common in persons of Mediterranean, Oriental, or African ancestry but occur in all races. Characteristically, the red cells are smaller than normal and poorly filled with hemoglobin. The number of red cells may be quite normal, but the

Anemia can be mild enough to go almost unnoticed or severe enough to require repeated blood transfusions.

amount of hemoglobin in the blood is low. Thalassemia minor does not cause any symptoms, because the anemia is so mild that the body can compensate for it.

Severe forms of thalassemia—thalassemia major—are devastating diseases. They occur when an individual receives genes for thalassemia from both parents. The disorder may cause the death of a fetus before birth or produce severe anemia requiring repeated blood transfusions.

Radiation, Cancer Drugs, Leukemia. The continuous production of red cells by the bone marrow depends on primitive "precursor" cells dividing repeatedly to create new cells that will mature into red blood cells. When these so-called stem cells are destroyed or become abnormal, severe anemia is the result. Stem cells can be destroyed by radiation or by anticancer drugs. This is largely why people who are exposed to radiation in nuclear accidents or who undergo chemotherapy become anemic. In leukemia normal stem cells are crowded from the marrow by leukemic cells, causing anemia.

In some instances a deficiency of stem cells can be corrected by transplanting bone marrow from a closely related person. Unless the donor is an identical twin, it is necessary to destroy the recipient's own immune system and replace it with that of the marrow donor. Otherwise, the new marrow will be rejected. Marrow transplantation is a hazardous procedure, but nowadays about three-quarters of marrow recipients survive the procedure. □

Dealing With a Colicky Baby

Raymond Karasic, M.D.

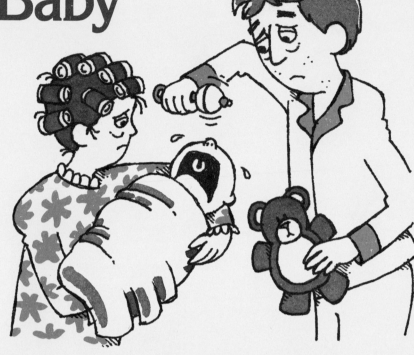

Next to adolescence, colic might be the meanest trick Mother Nature ever played on parents. After all, what else besides colic can instantly transform a placid young baby into a screaming demon and reduce the most even-tempered parent to a raw bundle of nerves? Although much has been written about this age-old condition, to this day no one knows for sure what causes colic or how to treat it effectively. The only consolation is that most colicky infants are otherwise healthy and all babies with colic eventually grow out of it.

What Is Colic?

Colic is an affliction of young infants that is characterized by frequent and intense bouts of crying, fussiness, and, often, abdominal pain and gas. It is extremely common, affecting about one out of every ten newborns. The disorder usually begins without warning during a baby's first month of life, wreaks havoc on the family for several weeks, then disappears by the third or fourth month just as mysteriously as it arose. During episodes of colic, babies typically clench their fists, tense their abdomens, and draw up their knees, often giving the impression that they are suffering severe stomach cramps. Some babies' attacks come at the same time every day. And although attacks vary in duration, they generally last for three or more hours. In between crying jags, babies with colic often seem to be fine.

Obviously, colic is not the only reason why babies cry. As any parent knows, infants get cranky when they are hungry, wet, cold, tired, bored, or sick—and sometimes for no good reason at all. The question is, how can a parent tell if a baby has colic? For the most part, infants who are fussy for a specific reason cheer up promptly once the underlying problem is corrected. Babies with colic are not so easily satisfied; they scream and fuss no matter what parents do to comfort them. They cry not only longer but harder than do other infants, as if they were in training for some Olympic screaming event.

Causes

Over the years, colic has been blamed on just about everything, from allergies to the mother's emotional upset during pregnancy. As theories have changed, so has the focus of the problem, from the infant to the family and back again. The truth is, no one—not even Dr. Spock—really knows what causes most cases of colic. Nevertheless, research in the past few years has begun to shed some light on this vexing problem.

One popular but controversial theory is that colic results from an allergy to certain proteins in the diet, particularly milk proteins. Some recent studies have shown that giving cow's milk or milk proteins to certain infants can produce the symptoms of colic, while eliminating cow's milk from the diet can relieve such symptoms. In addition, colicky infants who are breast-fed tend to experience worse symptoms after their mothers drink cow's milk. On the other hand, several other studies have failed to show a clear-cut link between allergies and colic. Although the issue remains unsettled, many experts agree that while some cases of colic are indeed caused by an allergy to milk proteins, most cases are not.

Some theories have attempted to explain the painful abdominal spasms that are the hallmark of many cases of colic. One proposal is that colicky babies are hypertonic (that is, have too much muscle tone). As a result, they are unusually tense and restless and tend to overreact to all kinds of stimuli, which leads to the symptoms we recognize as colic. Although no one would dispute that colicky infants are tightly wound, no one has ever proved that they have excess muscle tone.

Other theories about colic have focused on the mother or the family, rather than the infant. One study performed in the 1950s concluded that colic was related to "family tension." Another study found that women who experienced anxiety or depression during pregnancy tended to have colicky infants more often than did mothers without such problems. Now that "mother-bashing" is no longer in vogue, attention happily has shifted away from parental shortcomings as the basis for colic.

Nowadays, most experts believe there are many causes of colic. Thus, some infants have milk protein allergy, some may have gas, some are overstimulated, and some may just have ornery dispositions. These differences probably explain why some colicky infants respond to certain kinds of treatment while others do not.

Coping With Colic

Colic can be a gut-wrenching experience for parents as well as infants. Anyone who has not lived through it will find it nearly impossible to appreciate just how stressful for parents a colicky baby can be. It's hard enough for parents—even experienced ones—to adjust to all the changes that a new baby brings. Yet most parents are willing, even eager, to sacrifice sleep and established routines to have a cuddly, responsive baby to nurture. What if, instead, they get a miserable, screaming bundle of gas? Their feelings range from disappointment and worry to frustration and sometimes anger. They inevitably blame themselves for their child's discomfort and even feel guilty about having negative feelings.

What is the solution? Parents of colicky infants need reassurance and support. They need to know that they did not somehow cause the problem. They need to understand that feelings of resentment toward the baby are normal under the circumstances. Finally, they need to be reminded that the baby is healthy and that this dreadful condition will eventually go away.

> **Parents of a colicky baby need to remember that their child is otherwise healthy and that this nerve-racking condition will eventually go away.**

Beyond reassurance, beleaguered parents need to get out of the house and spend some time away from the infant, even if it's just for a few hours. A movie, dinner out, or a trip to the mall can work wonders.

Treatment

Although there are as many treatments for colic as there are theories about the disorder, one of the best remedies is common sense. Even if parents and the pediatrician don't know why a given infant has colic, by trial and error they can usually find some simple ways to help relieve the infant's discomfort.

When feeding the baby, parents should try to use techniques that limit the amount of air that is swallowed. Two ways of doing this are to feed the infant slowly (preferably in an upright position) and burp the baby frequently. Between meals, a pacifier may be helpful.

Even though some colicky infants have true milk protein allergy, the majority do not. Nevertheless, many physicians will try changing an infant's formula to one that is free of cow's milk (such as a soy-based formula), just to see if it helps. If there is no improvement after about two weeks, it is usually safe to conclude that cow's milk was not the culprit.

Infants who have a great deal of abdominal pain and gas may get some relief from a warm bath or from a hot water bottle applied to the abdomen. Laxatives are usually not recommended, since they may actually cause gas to build up and make a stomachache worse. Although sedatives and antispasm medications are still frequently prescribed, there is no proof that such medications are really effective.

One of the tried-and-true ways of treating colic is to keep the baby moving. Rocking the baby, using an infant swing, going for a walk, or taking a ride in the car (with the infant in a car seat) can be soothing to the baby and may provide the parents with a few moments' peace. There is even a crib attachment that simulates a car ride. Called SleepTight, the device rocks the crib gently while imitating the sound of wind passing a closed car window. Some infants who are extra sensitive to various stimuli might not respond well to movement, however, and may prefer to be handled gently or left alone in a quiet place.

The best news about colic is that it doesn't last forever, and infants come out of it none the worse for wear. Even parents usually survive this ordeal, which gives them plenty of time to prepare for adolescence. ☐

Visiting Someone in the Hospital

Ingrid J. Strauch

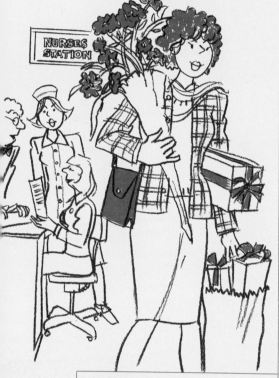

A patient's stay in the hospital can be lonely and frightening, but visits from friends or relatives can make that stay a lot less gloomy. Although a visitor may initially feel awkward about seeing a usually healthy person sick in a hospital bed, more often than not, the benefits reaped by the patient outweigh the risk of social unease.

Following a few commonsense guidelines can help ensure that a visit has its desired beneficial effect. Some of the guidelines presented here are most relevant to close family members and friends, some apply primarily to more casual visitors, still others can be equally helpful to both groups.

Before Visiting

To be on the safe side, someone outside the immediate family might first ask the patient or a close relative if visitors are wanted. The hospital switchboard can usually tell callers if an individual is not allowed visitors or has requested that no information, including room and telephone number, be given out. Some patients are just too sick to receive friends or feel uncomfortable about being seen while not at their best. Their need for rest and privacy should be respected. (However, a patient who does not want visitors may appreciate a telephone call or a card.)

How Long to Stay

If visitors are welcome, as they most often are, try to ascertain (by asking a close relative or a nurse

> **As long as a few commonsense rules are followed, brief visits from friends and relatives can help a hospitalized person maintain a positive outlook.**

or simply by observing the patient) how long to stay. The appropriate length of a visit can vary depending on the nature of the patient's illness and on the person's alertness, energy, and desires. In many cases, however, a visit should last no longer than 20 minutes. Always keep in mind the patient's need for rest and sleep. Several short visits during a hospital stay may be more comforting and less stressful than one long visit.

How long one should stay may also depend on the number of other people planning to come, since most hospitals try to limit the number of visitors at any one time. The patient can best help a friend or relative schedule a visit so that it does not conflict with other visits or with hospital procedures, but visitors should not be surprised if an X ray or lab test interrupts their stay. They may have to leave and return at another time.

Children as Visitors

Many hospitals will not allow young children to visit patients. Children are prime carriers of communicable illnesses and may be unruly or noisy. In addition, the child's health may be endangered by the possibility of contagion in a hospital. If the patient is the child's parent, however, a request may be granted to waive visitation rules.

Before arriving at the hospital, younger children should be given a clear description and explanation of what to expect. They may be scared by the strange environment and by the appearance of sick people—especially a sick relative.

Gifts

Bringing a gift is a thoughtful gesture, but make sure it is appropriate and that gifts are allowed (intensive care, coronary care, and burn units often do not allow any nonessential personal items). Traditional gifts of flowers or food may be inappropriate if the patient has a respiratory or gastrointestinal problem or is on a special diet. Phoning the nurses' station, the patient, or the patient's family before visiting could prevent such an error.

A patient who is alert and bored might like a book or magazine, some word games, or a subscription to the hospital's TV service or newspaper delivery service. A patient who left home suddenly without time to pack any personal belongings may request that a visitor bring a few practical items. In any case, company and emotional support are the greatest gifts one can offer, so a visitor should not feel obligated to bring anything else.

Exercising Tact and Discretion

While visiting a hospitalized person, remember that this is not the person's home and that you are not there to be entertained. Don't sit on the patient's bed, play with the bed controls, touch any hospital instruments in the room, or smoke (at least not without ascer-

taining that smoking is permitted). If there is another person sharing the room, that individual's need for privacy and quiet should be respected.

> **Traditional gifts such as flowers or candy may be unsuitable if the patient has a respiratory or digestive disorder.**

Try to act as you naturally would with the person you are visiting. Focus on the human being in the bed, not on any surrounding tubes, needles, or other medical equipment.

Some patients will want to talk about their illness and themselves, while others will prefer being filled in on news of the neighborhood or office, national happenings, or the

latest baseball scores—anything to take their minds off the hospital environment. If the patient wants to talk, listen. Ask if there's anything you can do to help. Be reassuring, but don't overdo it: some patients may feel that you are belittling their worries, or, if they're concerned about how others are getting along without them, that they're not needed anymore.

Visitors during a meal should not share the food on the patient's tray or eat the leftovers and should not scrape any leftovers into the trash. The nurses may need to record how much the patient eats at each meal. Likewise, if a visitor helps the patient use the bedpan, bodily wastes should not be discarded before checking with a nurse.

Special Considerations

The more severe the problem, the more medical care and observation a patient will require and the shorter the visiting hours will be. Intensive care and other special care units usually allow visits only

Some don'ts for a hospital visit.

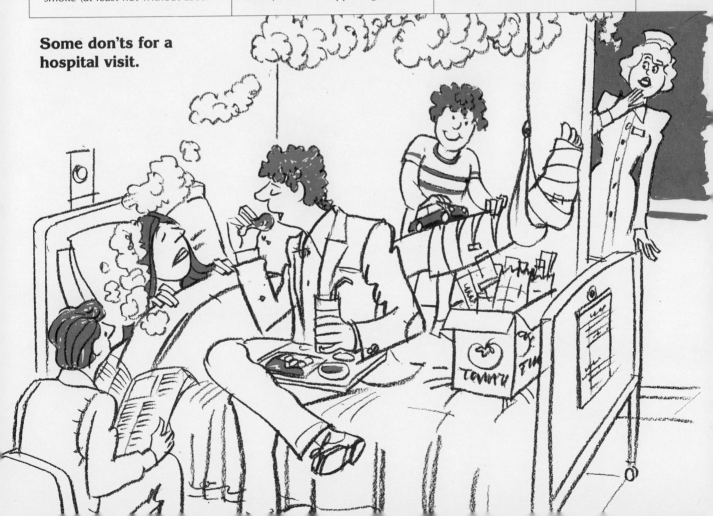

by close family members and only for very short periods of time. For both patients and visitors, the ICU may seem like a frightening whirlwind of monitors, alarms, pumps, tubes, and rushing doctors and nurses—not a restful place at all. A warm touch and a familiar voice are especially needed and appreciated by the patient in this crisis environment.

ICU patients are frequently sedated and thus confused and not

> **Only close family members are usually admitted to the intensive care unit; they should be prepared for a heavily sedated patient and bewildering life-support equipment.**

wholly aware of their surroundings. This may be disconcerting for a close relative who is not recognized, but it is no cause for panic. Visitors who know what to expect in intensive care will be better able to provide emotional support for their sick relatives. Family members should ask the nurses and doctors any questions they have about the patient's condition and treatment.

Hospitalized Children

Pediatric patients benefit from long visits with their parents, and for children aged three or younger, a parent should stay overnight whenever possible. Young children's fears of being abandoned are at a peak in this foreign environment, where they are surrounded by unfamiliar people, some of whom must examine them, draw blood samples, or give them injections. The presence of parents and other close relatives will help to reduce the child's anxiety.

Many hospitalized children seem to regress while sick: toddlers may ask for a bottle, and even older children may wet the bed. This should not be treated as bad or abnormal behavior during what is a traumatic period.

As much as possible, parents should have their children speak directly with doctors and nurses. They are the ones who really know what hurts or doesn't feel right, and they need to feel comfortable communicating with their caregivers.

Adolescents usually find phone calls and visits from friends reassuring—they need to feel accepted by their peer group even while in the hospital. Older children and adolescents most likely will welcome many visitors and bask in their popularity; a reminder to take it easy may be necessary.

Disfigurement

Patients who have undergone any type of disfigurement or whose bodily functions have changed, even temporarily, may tend to withdraw socially. They are often

> **Young children in the hospital benefit most from long visits with their parents, while older children and adolescents usually welcome telephone calls and visits from their peers.**

embarrassed by their looks or any odors, sounds, or equipment that will draw attention, and they will be sensitive to discomfort felt by others in their presence. Offers to visit may be refused until the patient adapts to the physical changes. In the meantime, letters and phone calls will remind patients that they have not been forgotten.

When meeting face-to-face with a disfigured or disabled person, commonsense rules apply: act naturally, use tact, and focus on the person, not the physical abnormalities.

> **Since a prolonged hospital stay can be stressful for those close to the patient, daily visitors should consider occasionally taking a day off from visiting to relax.**

Mental Illness

Psychiatric wards have visiting hours just like regular medical wards, but people outside the immediate family should check first with a family member or the hospital to learn whether the patient is allowed visitors and desires them.

Visiting a psychiatric patient often causes much uneasiness for the visitor, who may have no idea—or mistaken ideas—about what to expect and how to act. Speaking before the visit with one of the patient's caretakers can alleviate some of this discomfort. Just listening to the patient may be the biggest service a visitor can perform at this difficult point.

Regular visitors may be asked to bring clothing and do laundry for the patient, since psychiatric patients generally wear street clothes and the hospital cannot keep up with individual wardrobes.

Dealing With the Stress

Having a close relative or friend in the hospital can be stressful and fatiguing. If the hospital stay is prolonged, those who have been visiting every day, week after week, should consider taking a day off from visiting, especially if they know others will be there or can arrange for others to visit on that day. □

Yeast Infections

Hunter Hammill, M.D.

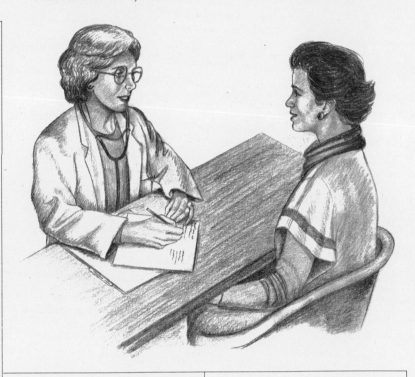

Vaginal yeast infections are usually caused by the fungus *Candida albicans*. Many women have small amounts of this fungus in their vagina and on the skin outside the vagina all the time without its causing any problems. But if conditions in the vagina change, the fungus starts to grow, a yeast infection (candidiasis) develops, and symptoms appear.

Causes and Symptoms

The harmless bacteria that inhabit the vagina usually keep *Candida*, or yeast, in check. Sometimes, however, there is a decrease in the amount of bacteria present, which leads to an overgrowth of the fungus. This can happen with the use of feminine hygiene sprays or when patients are on antibiotics. At other times, conditions in the vagina are so favorable for the fungus that yeast is able to flourish. This can happen during both menstruation and pregnancy, when hormonal changes create the perfect environment for fungal growth. Fungal overgrowth is also associ-

> **Itching and burning are the chief symptoms of vaginal fungus infections.**

ated with diabetes and with taking medications such as steroids.

The major symptoms of yeast infections are itching and burning, sometimes intense, both in the vagina and on the skin outside the

vagina (the vulva). In addition, patients occasionally have dysuria, or pain when urinating. Sometimes there is a recognizable odor, described as sour (this is in contrast to the foul, decaying odor a bacterial infection can cause). The skin may become inflamed and swollen and may even crack, causing a fissure, or small tear in the skin. There is often a white discharge, ranging from slight and watery to thick and "cottage cheesy." There also may be pain or soreness during intercourse.

Making a Diagnosis

Although vulval itching is usually caused by a yeast infection, this is not necessarily the case. Such itching can be caused by the parasite *Trichomonas vaginalis*, by pinworms (in rare cases), or by al-

lergic reactions to soaps, clothing, and so on. When a yeast infection seems the likely culprit, a physician can easily diagnose it during a pelvic examination and by looking at a sample of the vaginal discharge under a microscope.

Treatment

Once a yeast infection has been diagnosed, a variety of medications are available for treatment. Among the most commonly prescribed are the antifungal agents miconazole (brand name, Monistat) and clotrimazole (sold as Gyne-Lotrimin and Mycelex in the United States, Canesten and Myclo in Canada). These medications are available in different forms, including suppositories and creams that are inserted into the vagina once a day, preferably before bedtime, for up to two weeks. If there is irritation of the skin on the outside of the vagina, then lotion or cream also can be applied directly to the vulva.

In rare cases, an oral medication such as ketoconazole (Nizoral) is prescribed. Normally used with conditions that involve fungal infections at sites other than the vagina, ketoconazole is not the medication of first choice because, on rare occasions, it may

The standard treatment includes antifungal agents prescribed by a physician in the form of creams and suppositories.

have serious side effects such as liver disease.

Other therapies include gentian violet, available by prescription, and boric acid. Gentian violet, a solution of which is painted on the vagina, has a major disadvantage in that it leaves impossible-to-remove purple stains on clothing. It may also be far less effective than the other anti-yeast medications. Boric acid capsules, prepared by a pharmacist and inserted into the vagina, have been shown to be helpful, although this is not as well studied scientifically as other therapies. Besides boric acid, another "home remedy" is putting yogurt into the vagina to restore its normal bacterial balance. Use of yogurt in this way has never been scientifically studied, and the yogurt itself can cause irritation. Aci-jel, a vaginal jelly available on a prescription basis and used to restore and maintain the normal bacterial balance, may be a more scientific alternative.

It has been estimated that 10 percent of male sexual partners of women with yeast infections

may have *Candida*-related irritation of the urethra, or urinary channel. This alone requires no treatment. But if the partner has such an irritation on his external genitalia, he should be treated, both for his own sake and to prevent his reinfecting the woman.

During Pregnancy. Many women will have increased problems with yeast infections during pregnancy because of the hormonal changes that make the fungus grow faster. Unfortunately, it is often very difficult to get rid of the infection completely during pregnancy, and treatment of symptoms is all that can be offered. The intravaginal medications can be used, but if the infection proves stubborn, a complete cure may have to wait until six weeks after the delivery, when the hormones are back to normal. *Candida albicans* in the vagina is not associated with a risk to the fetus and is not a reason for a cesarean delivery. Rarely, babies

There is no basis in science for the belief that eating yogurt and avoiding certain foods can relieve a vaginal yeast infection.

get a minor infection or pimple on the scalp, usually treated with topical medication.

Questionable Therapies. For years there has been a debate about the effect of changes in the diet on *Candida*. Specifically, the debate has centered on whether a person can relieve a vaginal yeast infection by eating yogurt and by avoiding foods like sugar, bread, and cheese. It has also been suggested that people take one of the various oral yeast-controlling med-

ications. There have never been any scientific data to show that such things can relieve vaginal yeast infections.

Chronic Infections

In rare cases, yeast infections become chronic—the fungal over-

Strict personal hygiene in warm weather helps prevent yeast infections.

growth both is difficult to eradicate and frequently recurs. If the appropriate topical medications have been used and a patient's itch or irritation does not go away, she should go back to the doctor to verify that yeast is the cause and that no other agent is present that would not respond to antifungal medications. The physician might also suggest monitoring of symptoms in relation to the patient's menstrual cycle and sexual activity so as to rule out other causes. If a chronic yeast infection is found to be present, a longer course of treatment with the intravaginal antifungals might be prescribed. Sometimes systemic drugs such as ketoconazole may be needed as well. When the infection has been cured, any fissures or other damage to the skin resulting from long-term irritation can be treated.

There are various things chronic sufferers can do to help prevent infections. Personal hygiene, especially in warm weather, is one factor that can be controlled. Yeast tends to overgrow in skin folds (this may be more of a problem for obese patients). After bathing, a hair dryer can be used to dry the vulval area completely. Also, nylon underwear, pantyhose, and tight pants should be avoided—they keep the vulva warm and moist, which aggravates fungal problems. □

CHILD ABUSE

Henry B. Biller, Ph.D.

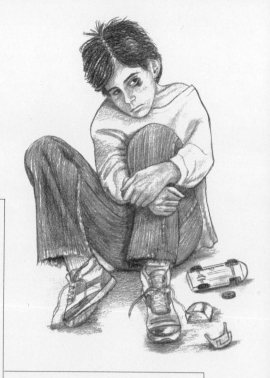

Child abuse is not just a contemporary phenomenon. But it is only since the 1960s that it has attracted widespread public concern in the United States. The catalyst was physician and educator C. Henry Kempe, who in 1962 published a landmark article in the *Journal of the American Medical Association* in which he coined the term "the battered child syndrome." With the backing of a group of like-minded physicians and social workers, Kempe pushed for a multidisciplinary approach to child abuse, going from state legislature to state legislature urging the passage of laws to deal with the problem. Kempe's efforts and the subsequent media publicity helped overcome a longstanding presumption in the United States that family violence was a private concern. The states began passing laws requiring professionals—generally teachers and doctors—to report suspected abuse, and the courts began to acknowledge that battering was a crime.

No one is quite sure how widespread child abuse really is. The number of cases reported is going up year by year (over 2 million in the United States in 1986, three times the 1976 number), but it is not clear whether this means that there are more cases, or simply that more cases are being reported. Some experts believe that for every two cases reported, there is another one that should be reported but is not. To muddy the issue further, more than half of the reported cases are declared, after further examination, to be unfounded. This does not necessarily mean, however, that the original reports were false—it may mean that social workers did not have time to investigate fully or were unable to prove anything one way or the other. One study of early 1980s cases showed that, in one year in Pennsylvania and four years in Oklahoma, roughly a third of families involved in "unfounded" complaints were found, following a later complaint, to have abused or neglected a child.

Defining Abuse

There are many different kinds of child abuse, and no single definition suffices. But experts in child welfare generally agree on the existence of four broad categories: neglect, sexual abuse, emotional abuse, and physical abuse. Neglect includes failing to give a child adequate food, clothing, shelter, or medical care, making it difficult or impossible for a child to attend school, and leaving unsupervised children who are too young to look after themselves. Any kind of sexual activity between a child and an adult constitutes sexual abuse. Emotional abuse (perhaps the most difficult kind to detect) involves chronic verbal attacks on the child or failure to respond to a child's emotional needs. Physical abuse can mean a pattern of deliberately hurting a child or the inflicting of harsh physical punishment. But even with these guidelines, physical abuse is difficult to define precisely. Because of differing values and social standards, one person's discipline may be another's physical abuse.

The kinds of child abuse that usually make the headlines involve severe physical or sexual abuse. In a notorious recent case, Lisa Steinberg, 6, the illegally adopted daughter of Joel Steinberg, a disbarred New York lawyer, and Hedda Nussbaum, a former children's book editor and writer, died from a brain hemorrhage. During Steinberg's trial (beginning in late 1988) on charges that he caused the hemorrhage by beating Lisa, Nussbaum described the chaos and violence that marked the family's daily life. Steinberg was convicted of manslaughter.

Parents are not alone in abusing children. Serious maltreatment has been uncovered in day-care centers, schools, and other social institutions. A recent case involved Margaret Kelly Michaels, a day-care teacher in New Jersey who was found guilty in the spring of 1988 of sexually assaulting 19 of her charges. Later in the year four of the people running a commune in rural Oregon (self-described as an athletic camp for Los Angeles ghetto children) were charged with flogging one of the children to death and beating and starving the others.

According to the experts, cases such as these are exceptional and give a misleading picture. Of the confirmed cases of child abuse in the United States in 1986, less than 3 percent involved serious injuries such as fractures or burns and around 16 percent involved sexual abuse. The most common type of abuse is neglect.

Causes

The causes of child abuse are complex, involving an interplay between individual, family, and social factors. No single factor is involved in every case, nor is there a particular personality pattern common to all abusive parents. Generally, however, abusive parents do have low self-esteem and feel that others are critical of them or do not accept them. When under stress, they tend to respond to their children in immature, impulsive, distrustful, and aggressive ways. Alcohol or other drug use may also contribute to parents' aggressive behavior toward their children. Moreover, many abusive parents were themselves abused as children. It must be emphasized, however, that for the most part abused children do not grow into adults who maltreat their own children. Many may, in fact, conscientiously avoid subjecting their children to the kinds of maltreatment they themselves suffered.

Society's Role. The United States has much higher rates of child abuse—as well as of murder, assault and battery, rape, and other forms of violent crimes—than do many other countries, including Britain, Canada, Sweden, China, and Japan. A comparison of the content of movies and television in these countries suggests that American society is also more accepting of violent behavior than are other technologically advanced nations.

A physical response to perceived child misbehavior is all too common in the American family. More than half of American parents at least occasionally spank, slap, or hit a child by hand, belt, or other means. Such behavior is typically not considered to be abuse unless it is so severe that it results in bodily injury to the child. The fact that physical discipline is generally thought socially acceptable contributes to the overall incidence of severe physical abuse in the United States.

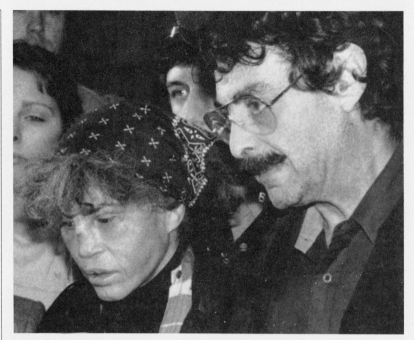

Joel Steinberg (seen here with his companion Hedda Nussbaum) was convicted of manslaughter when his illegally adopted daughter Lisa, 6, died after a severe beating.

Economic Factors. Physical abuse is found at every level of society. Some well-educated parents (Lisa Steinberg's, for example) who have prestigious jobs and are highly respected members of their communities physically abuse their children. Nevertheless, many studies have found that physical abuse—especially cases involving severe battering—is more common among families living in poverty.

Almost half of the children who are physically abused come from families who receive public assistance, and in most of these cases, there is no regularly employed adult. Child abuse rates also increase with a general rise in unemployment. It must be emphasized, however, that the majority of poor or unemployed parents do not physically abuse their children and that factors beyond social and economic pressures contribute to child abuse.

Isolation, Stress, and Single Parenthood. Poor people often feel socially isolated, and parents who feel cut off from other members of the community are more likely to physically abuse their children than parents who have a sense of emotional connectedness to other adults.

Some families suffer from many forms of stress which, in combination, are often found to be associated with physical abuse. For example, there are especially high levels of child abuse in poor households in which a single parent has sole responsibility for several young children.

In contrast, abuse is much less common in families where parents share child-rearing responsibilities. Mothers are much less likely to maltreat their children when they have the support of an actively involved partner, and fathers are rarely abusive when they have established a close relationship with the child during its infancy.

Neglect by the father within two-parent families—as well as father absence—is associated with relatively high rates of abuse by mothers. Stepfathers—or fathers who are not attached to their infants or young children—are also more likely to abuse the children if suddenly pressured into assuming parenting responsibilities. There are, however, parents who are able to maintain their self-control under very stressful conditions, as well as others who are quite abusive even when stress appears to be minimal.

Which Children Are Susceptible?

Children below the age of six are the victims of more than 60 percent of reported abusive incidents involving major physical harm and 40 percent of episodes resulting in minor injuries. Young children may be more vulnerable because they are helpless to respond to physical abuse. And the fact that they require more care and supervision than older children may make them more likely targets for adult frustrations.

Children with learning or behavior problems that make them difficult to deal with may also be more likely to be abused, although the role of such factors is difficult to assess since early and severe abuse may have contributed to the problems. Again, it must be stressed that most parents of children with such problems do not physically abuse them.

The Effects of Abuse

Even when victims of child abuse suffer no lasting physical damage, their emotional suffering is usually severe. Children who are physically abused tend to have psychological problems; they often find it hard to deal with aggressive impulses and frustration or to respond to others in a sensitive, supportive way. However, no clear behavior pattern distinguishes them from children who suffer from other types of inadequate parenting. And some people are so resilient that they can overcome the effects of abuse.

How badly a child is affected by abuse depends on many factors. Children who have a good rela-tionship with one parent usually fare better than those who are abused by both parents. Children who are rejected and neglected as well as physically abused are especially likely to have serious psychological and social problems. Children who are never physically abused but are constant targets of verbal abuse and emotional deprivation are much more at risk than are those who are occasionally physically abused but generally accepted and loved. In particular, a pattern of neglect and rejection by the father is far more likely than occasional physical abuse to lead to psychological difficulties later in life.

Helping Families

Once child abuse has been uncovered, the most promising approach to preventing further abuse is one that combines education with social support. Effective programs teach parents to use more appropriate child-rearing techniques while providing services to help them deal with other problems in their lives. Such programs might include workshops in stress reduction and financial management, job placement services, as well as marital counseling, and alcohol or drug counseling. In some cases, more intensive family therapy or individual psychotherapy for parents and children may be needed.

Therapy has not, however, been found very effective with most abusive families unless accompanied by other support services. Self-help groups (particularly Parents Anonymous) have helped many abusive adults reduce their feelings of isolation and powerlessness. Access to adequate day care can be a major factor in decreasing stress for a single parent who feels overwhelmed by total responsibility for the children. Other important services for low-income families include cooperative baby-sitting arrangements, community support groups, pooled transportation, and recreational facilities.

Educating for Prevention

Since child abuse is so often linked with neglect or rejection by the father, both treatment and preventive programs need to find ways to teach fathers about infant and child development and to get men as well as women more positively involved in their children's upbringing. Parenthood education for both boys and girls should begin as early as elementary school and should teach participants what it is realistic to expect from children at different stages in their development.

Public health programs for potential and expectant fathers and mothers can also provide information about child development and about how inadequate prenatal care can lead to physical and developmental problems for their children. These programs can also emphasize the importance of a good husband-wife relationship in bringing up children. Such insights can do much to make child rearing a rewarding experience, and greatly reduce the likelihood of abuse. □

Sources of Further Information

American Humane Association, 9725 E. Hampden Avenue, Denver, CO 80231

C. Henry Kempe National Center for the Prevention and Treatment of Child Abuse and Neglect, 1205 Oneida Street, Denver, CO 80220.

National Committee for the Prevention of Child Abuse, Suite 950, 332 South Michigan Avenue, Chicago, IL 60604.

Parents United, P.O. Box 952, San Jose, CA 95108.

Suggestions for Further Reading

BILLER, HENRY B., and RICHARD S. SOLOMON. *Child Maltreatment and Paternal Deprivation: A Manifesto for Research, Prevention, and Treatment.* Lexington, Mass., Lexington Books, 1986.

STRAUS, MURRAY A., RICHARD J. GELLES, and SUSAN K. STEINMETZ. *Behind Closed Doors: Violence in the American Family.* Garden City, N.Y., Anchor Press, 1980.

Fluoridation
A Success Story

Irwin D. Mandel, D.D.S.

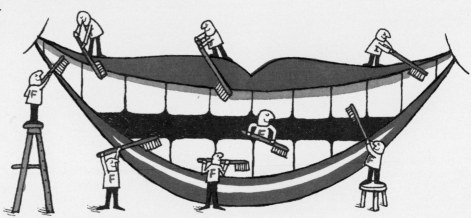

Tooth decay, which is caused by bacteria in the mouth that thrive on sugar, has plagued humankind for centuries. We have paid for the sweet life through the teeth. But the good news is that thanks largely to the widespread use of fluoride—the term refers to various chemical compounds of the element fluorine—the incidence of toothaches and tooth loss from decay is decreasing in many parts of the world. A survey released in June 1988 by the U.S. National Institute of Dental Research showed that nearly 50 percent of American children aged 5 through 17 were free of tooth decay. In 1945, when fluoride was first experimentally introduced into a public water supply in the United States, freedom from tooth decay was a rarity. Today, more than half of all Americans drink fluoridated water (and in some areas fluoride is naturally present in the water supply). Even those who use water without fluoride can derive the benefits of fluoride from a variety of products on the market.

Making Connections

At the beginning of the 20th century, a pitting and brown staining of the teeth was observed by Professor Stephano Chiaie in the area around Naples, Italy. Later, the observations were corroborated by Dr. J. M. Eager of the U.S. Public Health Service, who noted that immigrants to the United States from the region around Mount Vesuvius (near Naples) had stained teeth. In 1902, Eager published his hypothesis that the stains resulted from contamination of the local drinking water by fumes from Vesuvius or by the water's passage over the volcano's lava beds.

At about the same time, Dr. Frederick S. McKay, a dentist in Colorado Springs, was struck by the prevalence of a brown stain on patients' teeth, and he began what became a lifelong investigation of the phenomenon. He enlisted the aid of Dr. G. V. Black, the preeminent dental researcher of the period, and together they examined nearly 7,000 people in 26 communities. In 1916 they published their now-classic description of

what they called mottled enamel. Noting that the condition was more prevalent in certain geographic locations, they suggested that an unknown factor in communal water supplies was the cause and that it produced the defect during tooth development. The researchers made another observation (whose significance they did not fully appreciate at the time because of their focus on tooth appearance): despite the surface imperfections in their teeth, Colorado Springs residents had fewer cavities than residents in communities where mottled enamel did not occur.

It was not until 1931 that the techniques used for analyzing trace elements in water had become sensitive enough for chemists to establish that mottled enamel occurred in communities with exceptionally high levels of fluoride in their drinking water. (Manganese had been a prime suspect until then.) The fluoride that naturally occurs in water comes from minerals and rocks and is present in high concentrations in only a limited number of geo-

194

graphic areas around the world.

With the report of the association between high levels of fluoride in drinking water and mottled enamel—a term subsequently changed to fluorosis—in the early 1930s the U.S. Public Health Service assigned a dentist, Dr. H. Trendley Dean, to conduct a national study. Dean examined 6,000 children in 22 cities in 10 states and found that fluoride concentrations in water could be correlated with the severity of fluorosis. Severe fluorosis, with pitting, was found at fluoride levels of over 4 parts per million (ppm); brown staining occurred at 3 ppm. At 2 to 3 ppm teeth generally showed white, chalky spots, while at 1 ppm they had only occasional white flecks.

From the surveys of fluorosis, it eventually became apparent that people living in areas with higher levels of fluoride in the water had fewer cavities. In another study, Dean examined over 7,000 children between the ages of 12 and 14, in 21 cities in 4 states, who had used local water since birth. He found that children living in areas where the fluoride level was 1 ppm or greater had 50 to 60 percent less tooth decay than children in areas where fluoride was absent. At a fluoride level of 1 ppm, decay reduction was almost maximal, while fluorosis was minimal.

Fluoridation Begins

Spurred by the dramatic findings in locales where fluoride occurred naturally in the water, the U.S. Public Health Service began a series of long-term studies to see if comparable reductions in tooth decay could be produced by adding fluoride to water supplies in areas where it was not naturally present. The first fluoridation study began in 1945 in Grand Rapids, Mich., with the neighboring city of Muskegon serving as a control. Fluoride at a level of 1 ppm was added to the Grand Rapids water supply; Muskegon's natural level was about 0.2 ppm. Af-

ter 6½ years the prevalence of cavities in children 4 to 6 years of age in Grand Rapids was about half of that in Muskegon. As a result of these findings, Muskegon began to fluoridate its own water.

Studies were initiated between 1945 and 1947 in three other areas; at the end of 15 years of fluoridation at 1 ppm, the results showed children aged 12 to 14 years who had been exposed to fluoridated water for their entire lives had 50 to 70 percent less decay than children in control cities. Scientifically, the case for artificial fluoridation had been made.

Beneficial and Safe

Fluoride protects teeth from decay in two ways. First, as the teeth are developing—until about age 13—fluoride consumed as part of drinking water (or in dietary supplements) becomes incorporated in the mineral part of the tooth. This results in mineral crystals that are more stable and less susceptible to attack by acids generated at the tooth surface by the interaction of decay-producing bacteria and sugar.

Second, once a child's teeth have erupted (emerged through the gum), fluoride in drinking water is deposited on tooth surfaces by saliva. In what is called the topical effect, fluoride on tooth surfaces enhances saliva's natural ability to deliver minerals into surface and below-surface defects in teeth produced by bacteria acids. This protective process is known as remineralization.

Fluoride in toothpastes, rinses, and similar products also produces the topical effect—enhancing remineralization. Moreover, since the fluoride concentration in these products is higher than in drinking water, they can even help prevent bacteria from producing harmful acids.

Fluoride produces its maximum effect on the smooth surfaces of the teeth, especially on tooth surfaces that are next to each other. This can be particularly helpful

because cleaning between the teeth is most difficult. Fluoride is least beneficial on the biting surfaces of the back teeth, which have pits and deep fissures. To fully protect these areas, the application of plastic sealants to the teeth shortly after they erupt is recommended by many dentists.

Since the early 1950s studies have shown that the use of fluoridated water benefits adults as well as children. Tooth decay and tooth loss from decay are substantially lower for people of all ages in fluoridated communities than in nonfluoridated communities. Fluoridation also protects the roots of the teeth. People keep their teeth much longer today than in the past, and since the gums often recede as people age, the roots of the teeth—which are prone to decay—are exposed. Recent studies show that root cavities occur about 50 percent less frequently in fluoridated than in nonfluoridated areas. Clearly, water fluoridation provides lifetime benefits for everyone.

The safety of artificial fluoridation was established by the original studies and confirmed by numerous studies since. Except for minor levels of fluorosis (occasional white flecks in the enamel) in a small number of children, extensive medical testing has verified that fluoridation caused no harmful effects.

Extent of Fluoridatation

The thoroughness of the research and its dramatic results have prompted communities all over the world to initiate water fluoridation programs. Worldwide, 250 million people in some 40 countries now use fluoridated water. In Canada, 9 million people—about 35 percent of the population—consume fluoridated drinking water. The Republic of Ireland is the only country that fluoridates water nationally. Everywhere else fluoridation remains a local option.

In the United States, about 130

million people live in areas with fluoridated public water supplies. Some people have no access to a communal water supply, and about 30 percent of the population lives in communities that have opted not to fluoridate their water. While the case for fluoride's effectiveness and safety has been made scientifically, fluoridation is, for largely unwarranted reasons, still debated and resisted in some communities. Attempts are still being made by dental and public health groups, such as the federal Centers for Disease Control, to encourage these communities to fluoridate their drinking water, and grants are available from the U.S. Public Health Service to help with the cost of installation and operation of fluoridation systems. At an annual cost of only 35 cents per person, water fluoridation is the most economical way to provide fluoride protection. It has the added benefit of not requiring any special effort (such as daily use of a fluoride rinse) on the part of the user.

Other Sources of Fluoride

Several studies over the past ten years have shown that the differences in the prevalence of decay between fluoridated and nonfluoridated areas are not as great as they were in the 1960s and 1970s. This is not because water fluoridation has lost its effectiveness but rather because the widespread use of other forms of fluoride (in toothpastes, rinses, dietary supplements, and topically applied products) has had an appreciable impact on reducing decay even in nonfluoridated communities.

School Programs. In some areas of the United States (such as North Carolina and Kentucky) where community water supplies are not fluoridated, children receive fluoride through the water they drink in school. Since these children do not begin to be exposed to fluoridated water until they are about six years of age—and then only during school hours—the school water supply is fluoridated at a higher-than-average level—4.5 ppm. A number of studies attest to the safety and value of this approach; an average reduction in decay of 40 percent has been reported.

Dietary Supplements. Children 13 and under living in areas where fluoride does not occur naturally or has not been added to the water can obtain it by using fluoride drops, tablets, or lozenges or vitamin supplements that contain fluoride. These products are prescribed by a dentist or pediatrician. It is important not to exceed the recommended dosage in order to avoid the development of mild fluorosis, which has sometimes been reported when dietary supplements are given in addition to fluoridated water.

The form of the supplement depends on the child's age. Infants and young children should be given a liquid—drops placed on the tongue and swallowed, or added to water or juice. (Fluoride supplements should not be added to milk since milk can interfere with fluoride absorption.) Older children can take tablets or lozenges. Chewable tablets and lozenges bring the fluoride into contact with erupted teeth, thus providing a topical benefit.

Professionally Applied Fluoride. A dentist or hygienist can apply fluoride topically in the form of a solution or a gel. These preparations contain much higher levels of fluoride than fluoridated water and are applied once or twice a year. They are most widely used in nonfluoridated communities but can also provide some additive effect when used in areas with optimal levels of water fluoride. Few studies exist on their effectiveness in adults, but they may be of value in people with a high susceptibility to decay.

Toothpastes. Today over 90 percent of the toothpastes sold in the United States contain fluoride. The most commonly used fluoride agent is MFP, monofluorophosphate. All brands contain a level of fluoride equivalent to 1 milli-gram per gram. A milligram is the amount that would be ingested by drinking a quart of water containing 1 ppm fluoride; a gram is the average weight of the ribbon of toothpaste that most adults use for each brushing. It is advisable to use one of the brands of fluoride toothpaste that carries the acceptance seal of the American Dental Association, since that seal guarantees the product's effectiveness has been adequately tested. People of all ages can benefit from regular use of fluoride toothpaste. In areas with low levels of fluoride in water, the widespread use of such toothpaste is largely responsible for low decay rates.

Parents should brush the teeth of children too young to brush adequately themselves. A pea-sized portion of toothpaste should be used, since young children tend to swallow the paste. Even when the children can brush their own teeth, this modest amount should be used to minimize the amount of fluoride that is ingested. Swallowed toothpaste containing fluoride, when added to the fluoride ingested in drinking water, can produce mild fluorosis in the developing teeth. Once the teeth are fully erupted, however, fluorosis cannot occur.

Rinses and Gels. When children are old enough to rinse and spit out properly, a fluoride rinse can provide an additional benefit. For daily use, a 0.05 percent fluoride rinse is recommended; for less frequent use, a higher potency is needed. For once-a-week rinsing, a 0.2 percent fluoride rinse should be used. This weekly procedure is widely used in supervised programs in schools.

Adults, especially those who have a history of tooth decay, can also benefit from the use of fluoride rinses. The dentist may also prescribe a brush-on gel, with a fluoride concentration much higher than that found in regular toothpaste or suggest the use of a gel contained in a plastic tray that fits over teeth and is used at home for five minutes daily. □

Update on "Shock" Therapy

Max Fink, M.D.

Electroconvulsive therapy (ECT)—previously called, and sometimes still referred to as, shock therapy—is a treatment in which an electric current is used to produce a seizure in the brain. Such seizures have been found to have a beneficial effect on many patients with severe mental illness.

Past History

Convulsive therapy was first used in 1934, when the seizures were produced by chemical agents. Electricity was first introduced in 1938. ECT was widely used in the 1940s to treat severely disturbed patients in mental institutions, but with the introduction in the 1950s of drugs to treat mental illness, its use was curtailed. In the past decade, however, interest in ECT has been rekindled, in particular for treating "therapy-resist-

> **ECT as practiced today is very different from the ECT of a decade ago. Although shown to be safe, its use remains controversial.**

ant" cases. And because new attention has brought many changes in the procedure, ECT as practiced today is markedly different from the ECT of even a decade ago.

ECT has been shown to be effective and safe, yet its use remains controversial; it is, in effect, the stepchild of psychiatric treat-

> **ECT is considered when other therapies have failed and for those so depressed that they find life not worth living.**

ments. The fears it arouses in many may stem from misconceptions about what the treatment involves, the mystery that surrounds the way it works, or awareness of past abuses. The procedure often elicits primitive fears of electricity. Still, it seems likely that if ECT as practiced today were evaluated as a new treatment, free from its historical burdens, it would be hailed as a remarkable medical advance.

Who Should Get ECT?

ECT is a treatment for the severely ill—so ill as to require hospitalization. It is considered when other therapies have failed or when there is compelling evidence that a life-threatening situation such as risk of suicide is present. It is generally not recommended for those who are well enough to be treated at home.

ECT is effective for treating patients with major depressive illnesses (including manic-depression), schizoaffective disorder (a subtype of schizophrenia), and atypical psychosis (a psychotic disorder that does not clearly fall into other categories). It is particularly useful for patients who are so severely depressed that they

find life not worth living and for those who have psychotic ideas that are clearly inconsistent with reality.

Remarkably, ECT is also effective in treating patients with severe mania or manic delirium, who characteristically suffer from emotional turmoil and display a great deal of energy and restlessness. ECT has also benefited patients with catatonia, who suffer such severe inhibition that they appear rigid and unmoving.

Convulsive therapy was first developed for patients with schizophrenia. Although such patients still respond as well to ECT as to drug therapy, drugs are now the treatment of choice since they are easier and safer to administer.

> **Remarkably, ECT can help both patients with severe depression and those who suffer from mania.**

But schizophrenic patients who suffer from hallucinations or delusions and who are unresponsive to drugs alone may improve when ECT is added to their treatment.

ECT is also useful in some special cases, for example, in pregnant patients who are severely psychotic but who cannot take drugs because of the risk of genetic damage to the fetus. And ECT has been reported to produce good results in patients with very severe parkinsonism (a chronic nervous system disorder) for whom the standard treatments are no longer effective.

Administration and Risks

The modern administration of ECT differs markedly from earlier practice. Anesthesia and muscle relaxants are routinely used, and patients are carefully monitored. Because breathing may stop for a minute or two during treatment, oxygen is given before ECT is administered. ECT is a complex technical procedure which, like modern surgery, requires trained specialists (psychiatrist, anesthe-

> **Modern methods have sharply reduced the risks. Electric currents are controlled and patients are continuously monitored.**

siologist, nurses) and special instruments. Many institutions now require their practitioners to demonstrate proficiency before administering ECT.

In the procedure, two electrodes are placed on the patient's head. A carefully controlled electric current flows through these electrodes to the brain—typically for one to four seconds. Patients usually receive between 6 and 12 treatments, administered at intervals of two to three days.

Instruments continuously monitor the patient's heart rate, blood pressure, brain waves, degree of muscle relaxation, and oxygen level in the blood. As a result, the risk of death has been markedly reduced from the earlier rate of 3 deaths per 10,000 patients to less than 1 per 10,000.

At one time, the risks of ECT also included pain, fractures, spontaneous seizures, memory loss, and confusion. But anesthesia has eliminated the pain and the spontaneous seizures, muscle relaxants have eliminated fractures, and the use of oxygen and of a different type of electric current, as well as changes in the placement of electrodes, have much reduced memory loss and confusion. Complaints of persistent memory gaps, especially regarding events occurring in the weeks or months around the treatment period, occur in about 1 percent of treated patients today, particularly in those not treated with full attention to modern methods.

How Does ECT Work?

Although no one is certain how ECT works, there are three plausible hypotheses.

ECT may cause chemical changes in the brain. During seizures, there is an increased release of neurotransmitters (chemicals that carry messages in the brain). Many believe that these chemical changes are similar to the changes that result from antidepressant drugs, and that ECT relieves depression through the same mechanism as those drugs—that is, by correcting chemical imbalances in the brain.

ECT may reduce abnormal electrical activity. During the course of the 6 to 12 ECT treatments, it becomes progressively more difficult to induce a seizure. Some have concluded from this finding that ECT has anticonvulsant effects that help control the abnormal electrical activity in the brain sometimes found in depressed and manic patients.

> **Some researchers think ECT causes hormonal changes, others believe it works to correct chemical imbalances.**

ECT may cause hormonal changes. Severely depressed patients exhibit abnormalities in hormone functions, especially with regard to hormones secreted by the pituitary gland and the hypothalamus, the major regulatory centers at the base of the brain that influence alertness, sleep, appetite, and sexual desire. During ECT, the brain releases large amounts of peptides (compounds from which hormones are synthesized in the body) and increases peptide production. Some researchers believe that depressed patients have a deficiency in a peptide called antidepressin, which maintains evenness of mood. ECT stimulates the brain to make antidepressin, and the increase in this peptide may relieve a depressive episode.

The Need For Consent

As recently as the 1960s, ECT treatments were administered to patients without their prior consent. But in accordance with recommendations of the American

> **Before receiving ECT, patients must sign a consent document that describes the treatment.**

Psychiatric Association issued in 1978, physicians in the United States no longer administer ECT without first providing a full explanation of the procedure (including both risks and benefits) and obtaining patient consent. Whenever possible, a close relative is also asked to become acquainted with the procedure and to give consent. In many cases, patients and relatives view a videotape showing what the treatment will entail. The consent document that must be signed also contains a full description of the treatment. As with all serious illness, only in life-threatening situations may patients be treated without their consent; in the United States such emergency treatment is provided in accordance with state regulations and usually requires court intervention.

See also the feature article MANIA AND DEPRESSION. □

Children With AIDS

Arye Rubinstein, M.D.

Cases of children with AIDS (acquired immune deficiency syndrome) are occurring throughout the world. In the United States over 1,400 cases of full-blown pediatric AIDS (affecting children under the age of 13) have been recorded by the Centers for Disease Control; the total number of children infected with the human immunodeficiency virus (HIV) that causes AIDS is probably three times this number. (In Canada, where pediatric cases include children under age 15, some 40 cases have been reported.) By 1991 experts predict that the United States will have between 10,000 and 20,000 children infected with the virus and 3,000 children with full-blown AIDS.

As the number of pediatric AIDS cases grows, parents, healthcare personnel, and society at large must come to grips with this tragedy. Many children with AIDS are sentenced to death at an early age. Caring for these children entails tremendous emotional, physical, and financial burdens. In many cases the parents—because of poverty, drug abuse, or their own illness—are particularly ill-equipped to share those burdens. Yet someone must see that these children receive the best medical care possible, and the most love and support, during their short lives.

Earliest Cases

The first cases of AIDS in children appeared in the United States as early as 1978. However, these patients were not recognized as having AIDS until several years later. There were a number of reasons for the delay in diagnosis. First, many infants were born with symptoms and so had no disease-free interval—that is, they did not seem to "acquire" the disease over time. They often had recurrent infections shortly after birth, just as do infants with congenital immune system deficiencies. Second, their infections were not, in general, "opportunistic"—caused by microorganisms that are harmless in people with normally functioning immune systems. The microorganisms that cause opportunistic infections are capable of causing life-threatening illnesses only in people who lack sufficient numbers of T cells—the white blood cells responsible for controlling viral and parasitic infections and cancers. Adults with AIDS characteristically have opportunistic infections, but a large proportion of infants with AIDS are not initially deficient in T cells. Instead, they have a deficiency in B cells, another type of white blood cell that produces antibodies mainly to fight invading bacteria. As a result, the most common problems in HIV-infected infants and children are recurrent bacterial infections.

Two clues alerted doctors to a connection between what turned out to be early pediatric AIDS cases and the AIDS epidemic in adults. First, the mothers of these children also had immune system problems; the mothers of infants with congenital immune system deficiencies, on the other hand, are themselves healthy. Second,

A staff member at a New Jersey foster home for children with AIDS comforts a small patient.

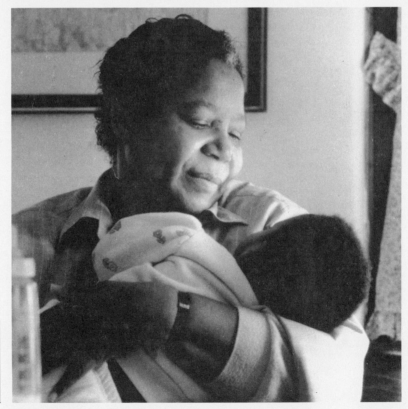

the immune system deficiencies in the mothers, although different from those of their offspring, were identical to those in adults with AIDS. Yet the definitive diagnosis of AIDS in children remained quite controversial until HIV was identified (in 1983) and new diagnostic tools were developed. AIDS is now diagnosed principally through a blood test that detects antibodies to the virus or viral antigens.

The Disease in Children

Most HIV-infected children have higher than normal levels in the blood of immunoglobulins—proteins that fight infections—yet these immunoglobulins do not protect against invading organisms. Moreover, vaccines often do not stimulate the immune system of these children to produce protective antibodies. Thus, an HIV-infected child who has been vaccinated against tetanus or measles may in fact not develop immunity to these diseases and may still acquire them. Some childhood diseases, such as measles and chicken pox, can be life-threatening for a child with AIDS.

Because of their B-cell deficiency, HIV-infected children suffer recurrent infections of the upper airways, lungs, urinary tract, and skin. They also often have bacteria in the blood, which may infect the brain and cause meningitis. Healthy children may also occasionally have such infections, but their immune systems mount a vigorous response that not only assists in overcoming the initial infection but also prevents reinfection by the same microorganism. Not so in children with AIDS. They have more severe initial infections and also can be reinfected many times by the same microorganism.

As the disease progresses in HIV-infected children, so does the breakdown of the immune system. All components of the system can be compromised, including the T cells that are not at first affected. As the immune system deterio-

rates, children suffer recurrent viral, fungal, and opportunistic infections. Two-thirds of the opportunistic infections are due to the organism *Pneumocystis carinii*, which causes an often fatal lung disease.

Children suffering from HIV infection often develop another chronic and incapacitating lung disease called lymphoid interstitial pneumonia (LIP), or pulmonary lymphoid hyperplasia (PLH). LIP/PLH is usually a relentlessly progressive disease that leads to respiratory failure.

HIV in children can affect almost every organ and system in the body. In more than 90 percent of cases the child suffers damage to the nervous system, which is apt to occur early in the course of the disease. The effect of HIV on the brain is profound; actual brain atrophy can sometimes be found in newborns. Damage to the nervous system manifests itself as developmental delay, cognitive defects, and motor abnormalities, so that children have difficulty learning to speak, sit up, crawl, and walk. In about 20 percent of children the neurological disease progresses relentlessly to dementia and/or loss of control over the limbs. In others, the disease progresses less rapidly. Some children have periods of stability, but only a few remain stable for very long.

Forms of the Disease

Studies at several medical centers of HIV-infected pregnant women and their babies have shown that there is a clear difference between the course of HIV infection in children and in adults. The majority of adults infected with HIV undergo an acute illness shortly after infection, followed by an asymptomatic phase or period of only minor symptoms, such as swollen lymph nodes, that can last for years before a full-blown case of AIDS develops. It appears that long asymptomatic phases are extremely uncommon in HIV-infected children, who generally

face early onset of symptoms and a grim prognosis.

Two major distinct disease courses in children have been recognized by the Centers for Disease Control. In the first, there is fairly early onset of opportunistic infections, before the age of two. These children rarely survive beyond age two or three. In the second course, children develop LIP/PLH. These children do not develop early opportunistic infections and may survive beyond early childhood, as long as their lung disease and accompanying bacterial infections can be brought under control. Completely asymptomatic HIV infection is rare beyond the age of five.

Even with state-of-the-art technology, doctors still cannot verify HIV infection in some sick children for more than a year after birth. One reason for this diagnostic dilemma is that in some cases where the mother is infected with HIV, her antibodies against the virus, which cross the placenta to the baby before birth, may persist for an unusually long time in the child's blood. This gives a false positive HIV blood test in an infant without the virus. With the introduction of some new diagnostic tests, doctors hope that the period of uncertain diagnosis can be shortened to the first weeks of life. Accurate diagnosis is very important if doctors wish to treat very young patients with AIDS drugs that have significant side effects.

Transmission Patterns

Many of the first cases of AIDS in children in the United States were attributed to transfusions of contaminated blood or blood products shortly after birth or later in childhood; the victims were often hemophiliacs. With the advent in 1985 of new screening tests for blood and blood products, infection by this route became rare.

Now, most children contract AIDS by what is called vertical transmission—from the mother to the child. Different studies have shown that HIV-infected pregnant women have anywhere from a 25 to 65 percent chance of transmitting the virus to their fetuses.

Many HIV-infected women are intravenous drug users—a group at high risk for AIDS because of the practice of sharing unsterilized needles. As the number of female drug abusers has increased nationwide in recent years, so has the number of HIV-infected infants.

However, more and more AIDS cases are occurring in women who are not intravenous drug users. In 1988, over 40 percent of all mothers of AIDS babies in the New York City borough of the Bronx (which has one of the highest incidences of adult female AIDS cases in the United States) claimed not to have used drugs but did admit to sexual contact with a man who was or may have been at risk for AIDS. The majority of these men were intravenous drug users, some were bisexual, and others had no known risk factors except for sexual contact with women of unknown HIV status.

Although there is strong evidence that the transmission of HIV from mother to child most often occurs in utero (while the fetus is in the womb), this is not the only way the virus may be picked up. Other potential means of infection include contact with maternal blood and fluids during delivery, breast feeding, and sexual abuse. The incidence of the last three transmission routes has not been determined but is probably small compared to in utero transmission.

Treatment

Treating AIDS patients largely consists of dealing with the bacterial, fungal, parasitic, and viral infections as they occur. Scientists are working to develop drugs that may attack HIV directly or that will boost patients' immune systems.

The only drug approved for use against AIDS is zidovudine (formerly known as AZT), sold under the brand name Retrovir. Studies are under way to determine its effectiveness in children. Prelimi-

nary results suggest that the drug prolongs children's lives and relieves some of the symptoms of AIDS, including the intellectual and neurologic damage common in children with the disease. However, zidovudine also causes serious side effects, just as it does in adults. Doctors hope that lower doses of zidovudine used in conjunction with other drugs may reduce or eliminate some of these side effects.

Another promising treatment is intravenous injection of gamma globulin, made up of antibodies harvested from the blood of human donors. The antibodies help fight the microorganisms that would otherwise cause devastating infections in young AIDS patients.

Almost as important as treating the children is providing counseling for their families. Brothers and sisters are taught to follow precautions with their ailing siblings, such as not biting and avoiding contact with blood. Infected mothers are urged to not have more children, although it is often difficult to persuade them, in order to stop the deadly cycle.

Children with AIDS are the most innocent victims of the epidemic.

Effect on Society

Considering the projection of 10,000 to 20,000 HIV-infected American children by 1991, the social consequences of this epidemic are likely to be immense. There have already been indications of how intense are the emotions raised by children with AIDS. Some children have faced rejection and harassment in their communities. In some urban areas there have been protests over the placement of homes for so-called

boarder babies—children with AIDS who have no other place to go because they have been abandoned by their parents or orphaned when the parents themselves died of AIDS. Without such group homes, most of these children languish in crowded hospital wards, straining the resources of the institutions while at the same time being unable to receive the love and attention they desperately need.

To some extent, public fear is understandable, if generally unwarranted, given the deadly nature of AIDS. However, the Centers for Disease Control recommends that children with AIDS be allowed to attend regular day care centers, nursery schools, and elementary schools, since the chance of their transmitting HIV to other children is extremely remote. (Special care should be taken with children too young to be toilet trained and too immature to avoid potentially dangerous habits like biting, which could theoretically transmit the virus.) Society will thus have to come to grips with the problem of discrimination against AIDS children, despite the apparent nonexistent risk to others.

It will also have to face the problem of thousands of poor inner-city minority families in which both parents and children are infected, especially as new treatments are developed to prolong the lives of many infected children. This population of children, adolescents, and parents will require many special services, including comprehensive medical care, day care, foster care, and residential treatment. Special counseling and educational facilities will have to be established to deal with developmental disabilities and mental retardation and to provide support for parents and siblings. The cost will be staggering. A collaboration between local, state, and federal agencies will be necessary to come to grips with this rapidly growing national tragedy. □

Hemorrhoids

Daniel Pelot, M.D.

Millions of Americans suffer from hemorrhoids, or "piles." About 80 percent of the population will develop this condition at some time in their lives, and the financial impact is considerable. According to the National Center for Health Statistics, 109,000 Americans had surgery for hemorrhoidal disease in 1986. And every year Americans spend more than $110 million on nonprescription drugs for hemorrhoids.

What Are Hemorrhoids?

Hemorrhoids are dilated blood vessels in the anal canal, the lower part of the large intestine, which controls the passage of feces. The upper one-third of the canal contains nerve fibers that are relatively insensitive to pain. The lower two-thirds, however, is lined with skin and contains nerve fibers that are extremely sensitive to pain. The lining of the entire canal contains a rich network of blood vessels that may enlarge to form hemorrhoids.

Hemorrhoids in the upper part of the canal are called internal, those in the lower part, external. Internal hemorrhoids are classified into four stages of severity: First-degree hemorrhoids are enlarged veins in the canal that bleed but do not protrude (prolapse) to the outside of the body; second-degree hemorrhoids protrude during bowel movements but recede after the bowel movement is completed; third-degree hemorrhoids will not recede on their own but can be pushed back into the anal canal by the individual, using the fingers; and fourth-degree hemorrhoids are so enlarged that they cannot be kept from protruding. (There is no classification of external hemorrhoids.)

Causes

There is some controversy about the causes of hemorrhoids. However, diet seems to be an important factor. The high incidence of hemorrhoids in Western countries, where many people eat low-fiber diets, and the low incidence among rural Africans, who tend to eat high fiber diets, suggests a relationship. Presumably, low-fiber

> **A high-fiber diet may be effective in both prevention and treatment.**

diets result in constipation, and the resultant straining during defecation ultimately causes blood vessels in the anal canal to become enlarged. Pregnancy, obesity, and a sedentary life-style are also associated with the development of hemorrhoids.

Symptoms

The symptoms of hemorrhoids may include rectal itching, pain, bleeding, and discharge, as well as protrusion. The most common complaint of people with internal hemorrhoids is painless, bright red rectal bleeding associated with bowel movements. (Rectal bleeding is also associated with other, serious diseases, so a physician should be consulted if it occurs.) Internal hemorrhoids usually do not bleed massively.

Pain is not a common symptom of internal hemorrhoids unless thromboses (blood clots), infection, or an erosion of the tissue that covers the blood vessels occurs. The pain associated with thrombosed hemorrhoids is made worse by having a bowel movement, and by sitting or walking.

Chronic prolapse of internal hemorrhoids may be accompanied by the rectal passage of mucus, causing irritation around the anus and soiling of underclothing.

Most external hemorrhoids are asymptomatic. But pain can occur if there are blood clots, and erosion of the skin that covers thrombosed hemorrhoids causes bleeding. Occasionally, excessive mucus from large internal hemorrhoids may irritate external hemorrhoids and cause itching.

Diagnosis

Many people with hemorrhoids do not have symptoms and thus may be unaware of the condition. Others who have symptoms may consult a physician. The physician will visually examine the external anal region, perform a digital (manual) examination of the anal canal, and then perform a sigmoidoscopic examination. The last usually involves the use of a flexible, fiber-optic tubelike instrument with a light source, which enables the physician to examine up to 2 feet of the lower part of the large intestine. The sigmoidoscopic examination is done because other problems—benign polyps (growths) or colon cancer, for example—may cause symptoms similar to those of hemorrhoids. Depending on the individual's age, symptoms, and family history, additional examinations may be performed to exclude other causes of bleeding.

Treatment

At-home Treatment. The bleeding, prolapse, and pain caused by hemorrhoids will usually respond to conservative at-home treatment. Taking sitz baths—sitting in a tub of warm water for 20 minutes twice daily—may decrease pain and swelling. Prescription medications such as suppositories or creams containing hydrocortisone (Anusol-HC is a common brand name) may prove effective in reducing swelling and pain. The occasional use of non-prescription suppositories and creams, such as those sold under the brand names Anusol or Preparation H, may be adequate treatment. However, if symptoms persist, or adverse side effects occur, the treatment should be stopped and a physician consulted. Stool softeners (such as the brand Colace), high-fiber bulk laxatives (Metamucil, for example), and a high-fiber diet can all be effective in both prevention and treatment since they promote regular bowel movements that are soft and do not require straining for elimination. Although most hemorrhoids respond to conservative treatment, if symptoms persist, one of the more aggressive approaches described below may be needed.

Rubber Band Ligation. The procedure known as rubber band ligation is probably the most widely used office treatment for internal hemorrhoids in the United States. Used for first-degree, second-degree, and some third-degree hemorrhoids, the procedure is performed with a special gunlike device which places a rubber band at the base of the hemorrhoid in such a way that it cuts off blood flow. Approximately one week later, the tissue sloughs off. A small amount of bleeding may occur at that time, but significant bleeding occurs in only 1 percent of cases. The technique is considered to be safe and effective, and is well-accepted by patients. Serious complications are infrequent, and anesthesia is not required. It is not, however, a certain longterm cure, since hemorrhoids tend to reoccur.

Sclerotherapy. In the procedure called sclerotherapy, which can be performed in a doctor's office, a special solution is injected into tissue at the upper part of a hemorrhoid. The solution creates inflammation and scarring, which causes the hemorrhoid to atrophy.

The procedure is effective only for first-degree and small second-degree internal hemorrhoids. The most common complaint is pain, which can occur if the injection is made too close to the skin at the lower end of the anal canal. The procedure is used widely in Britain but rarely in the United States.

Infrared Photocoagulation. A relatively recent addition to office treatments for bleeding first-degree and second-degree internal hemorrhoids and for external hemorrhoids, is infrared photocoagulation. The indications for its use are similar to those for sclerotherapy, and it works in much the same way—by causing tissue damage. A device called a photocoagulator uses a beam of infrared light to burn the tissue, subsequently causing the hemorrhoid to atrophy. Pain may follow the procedure if the photocoagulation site is near the sensitive skin in the lower part of the anal canal. Additional experience is needed in the use of this technique to determine whether it compares favorably with rubber band ligation.

Cryotherapy. In cryotherapy, a metal probe, cooled by liquid ni-

> **If symptoms persist, a choice of treatments is available.**

trogen or carbon dioxide, is used to freeze hemorrhoids. Again, the tissue damage caused by freezing results in scarring and atrophy. The procedure was a popular alternative to surgery for both internal and external hemorrhoids in the 1960s and early 1970s, but its use has greatly decreased since that time. Cryotherapy is often accompanied by significant pain, as well as anal discharge from tissue damage, and wound healing may be prolonged. In addition, sedatives must be given by intravenous injection, and local anesthesia and expensive equipment are required. Although cryother-

apy may be done as an office procedure, some physicians recommend that it be performed only in a hospital.

Laser Therapy. Several procedures that involve lasers are currently being used to treat hemorrhoids. In one technique, the laser is passed through a flexible sigmoidoscope, producing a series of burns on the surface of internal hemorrhoids. The subsequent tissue damage results in scarring and atrophy of the hemorrhoids. Another technique, termed vaporization, produces superficial burns on the surface of hemorrhoids, preventing them from protruding. A laser can also be used to remove a hemorrhoid in a manner similar to standard surgical removal.

Surgery. Surgical removal (hemorrhoidectomy) is the preferred treatment for large third-degree and fourth-degree internal hemorrhoids. It is also the best procedure when both large internal and external hemorrhoids are present. In this procedure, the surgeon cuts away the hemorrhoidal tissue, which results in long-term relief of symptoms. The procedure traditionally has been done in a hospital, with at least an overnight stay, but now some physicians are doing it in a hospital on an outpatient basis. Possible complications include bleeding, local infection, and (rarely) an abscess, or localized collection of pus.

Ultroid. A new treatment, Ultroid, is currently being used, although not extensively, in the United States. Ultroid employs probes through which low-voltage current is applied to the base of the hemorrhoid, producing a biochemical change in the blood vessels. The treatment has the advantage of working without producing burns. Moreover, it is reported to be safe and effective for all four stages of internal hemorrhoids, as well as for a combination of external and internal hemorrhoids. Experience with the technique is, however, still limited. □

Obstetrics and Malpractice

Mark Deitch

Malpractice suits and the high cost of liability insurance are problems faced by U.S. physicians in every medical specialty, but nowhere is the impact felt more deeply than in the practice of obstetrics. According to the American College of Obstetricians and Gynecologists, the average obstetrician has about a 75 percent probability of being sued at least once in his or her career—and an almost one in three chance of being involved in litigation three or more times. Even though four out of five of these malpractice suits are decided in favor of the physician, the staggering costs of the suits must be absorbed by doctors, their patients, and the health-care system at large.

Changing Field

All practicing physicians take out liability insurance to protect themselves against the possibility of a lawsuit. The premiums paid to insurance companies vary according to medical specialty: the greater the likelihood of litigation, the higher the premium. In recent years, American obstetricians have been sued so frequently and for such large amounts that since 1978 the average annual premium has soared from approximately $9,000 to close to $40,000. In some states, it exceeds $100,000 a year. On average, obstetricians pay about three times as much for malpractice insurance as other office-based physicians—and the rates keep rising.

These costs are passed along, at least in part, to the public. Fees of $4,000 or more for standard prenatal care and routine delivery are now charged in New York City and other parts of the United States. If a cesarean section (surgical delivery) is required, an additional $2,000 or $3,000 may be tacked on.

But the overall cost of the malpractice crisis goes far beyond dollars and cents. Physicians who believe that a malpractice attorney is, figuratively speaking, watching over their shoulders are more likely to practice defensively, relying on technological and surgical intervention where patience and good judgment once sufficed. For example, despite the fact that clinical studies have

> In recent years the cost of liability insurance has risen so high that many obstetricians are leaving the field.

shown that the use of continuous electronic fetal monitoring is unnecessary during normal deliveries, many obstetricians routinely employ these readout devices as a hedge against lawsuits, just in case something does go wrong.

For the same reason, cesarean sections are now commonly performed at the first sign of potential trouble—often to prevent problems that might never have materialized. Over the past decade, the proportion of babies delivered by cesarean in the United States has risen from about 15 percent to an estimated 25 to 30 percent—one of the highest rates of any nation in the world. The parallel rise of obstetrical liability premiums during the same period is no coincidence.

Shortages of Physicians

An additional consequence of the malpractice crisis is that women who fall into high-risk categories—including those with a chronic illness, such as diabetes or high blood pressure, and those who have delivered previously by cesarean section—may have some difficulty finding an obstetrician, especially one willing to give them a chance at a normal delivery rather than ordering a preemptive cesarean. Even though studies have convincingly disproved the old medical adage, "once a cesarean, always a cesarean," court-shy obstetricians know that by opting for surgery—whether or not it's really needed—they minimize the risk of a negligence suit.

Finally, and perhaps most disturbingly, a growing number of physicians are simply abandoning the practice of obstetrics. Many family practitioners no longer deliver babies as part of their services, and there is a trend among obstetrician-gynecologists to switch to less litigation-prone specialties, such as gynecological surgery. In several rural regions of the United States, there is already a shortage (and in some places, an absence) of doctors willing to practice obstetrics.

"Here in Kansas, there are only 74 physicians delivering babies west of 81 [the highway that divides the state roughly in half]," says Jimmie Gleason, a Topeka-based obstetrician-gynecologist who chairs the American College of Obstetricians and Gynecologists' committee on professional liability. "We took a survey and half the OBs in the state said they

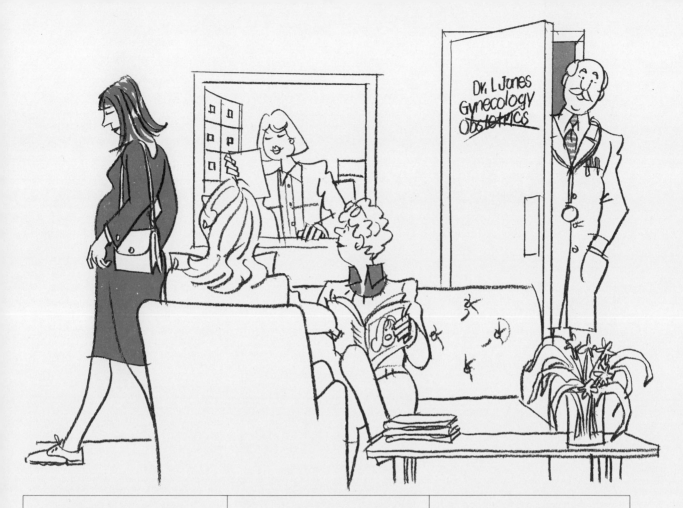

would stop [delivering babies] if premiums went up any higher. If that happened, people would have to drive hundreds of miles to get any kind of obstetrical care."

Progress Misunderstood

Why is it that U.S. obstetricians are so frequently sued? Is there something especially shoddy about the way they deliver babies that requires constant correction in the courts?

In fact, for people with access to proper medical care, having a baby is safer today than ever before. There are, of course, some clearly incompetent or negligent physicians, but by all evidence the number is small and is not unusually concentrated in the area of obstetrics. Dr. Gleason and other experts suggest that the excellent track record of contemporary obstetricians has actually contributed to the public's crisis of confidence. Unlike previous generations, for whom childbirth was al-

ways an uncertain and potentially risky event, parents today expect a perfect baby. If something does go wrong, they are less willing to accept it as an accident of nature and are more apt to blame the physician.

Many jurors, too, apparently think the same way. But the legal system may be too blunt an instrument for evaluating fine distinctions between what modern medicine can and cannot do. In a typical malpractice trial, the jury is faced, on the one hand, with the heartrending evidence of a grief-stricken family and a permanently damaged and disabled child, and on the other, with a well-to-do physician and a multi-million-dollar insurance company. Jury members are asked to sift through a confusing mass of medical statistics and studies marshaled to prove or disprove the doctor's responsibility for this tragedy. The addition of expert testimony by outside physicians, whose fees

and expenses are paid by one side or the other, rarely clarifies matters. In some states, the jurors may not be informed that the state or federal government will pick up most if not all of the child's special education and therapy bills. It isn't surprising, in these circumstances, when the jury hands down a spectacular settlement in favor of the family.

A large proportion of obstetrical malpractice cases—particularly those that are decided against the physician—center on permanent brain damage to the infant. The physician often is accused of failing to act properly or swiftly enough to prevent birth asphyxia, or oxygen deprivation to the infant during labor and delivery. (Hence, the reliance of many physicians on constant electronic fetal monitoring and on surgery at the first indication of fetal distress.) The condition cited in many of these cases is cerebral palsy, a disorder marked by lack of muscular coordination and severe speech problems. Recent large-scale studies indicate strongly, however, that cerebral palsy is rarely produced by the events of childbirth but most likely develops earlier in the pregnancy. Nevertheless, medical data of this type have a hard time penetrating the court system, and large judgments based on cerebral palsy resulting from supposed obstetrical negligence are still being handed down.

Proposed Solutions

As some authorities see it, the only adequate long-term solution to the malpractice problem is a complete overhaul of the current court system for deciding claims. In the absence of such sweeping reform, several partial solutions have been proposed for easing various aspects of the crisis. Following are some noteworthy suggestions.

Greater Hospital Involvement. The idea of hospitals paying all or part of their attending physicians' insurance premiums attracted considerable attention at a recent malpractice symposium held in Boston and sponsored jointly by Harvard University and G. D. Searle & Company, a major pharmaceutical manufacturer. The potential benefits include less financial pressure on the individual physicians and lower overall premiums, since hospitals could negotiate more cost-effective group rates. At the same time, hospitals would have greater incentive to monitor the performance of their attending physicians and to maintain standards of quality care. On the negative side, such channeling of insurance responsibilities would likely overburden the already beleaguered administrative staffs of many hospitals. Furthermore, doctors often enjoy visiting privileges at several hospitals. Any arrangement by which one facility foots a large part of a physician's insurance bill would almost necessarily limit the doctor's freedom of choice (and perhaps violate antitrust laws).

More Doctor-Owned Insurance Companies. According to Dr. Gleason, there are more than 40 physician-owned malpractice insurance companies in the United States today. By 1995, he predicts, "75 to 90 percent of all professional liability carriers will be physician-owned." Most of these companies are nonprofit, and their owners obviously have a direct personal stake in keeping premiums down. They may also offer some advantages over other carriers in screening applicants and monitoring the activities of the doctors they insure.

No-Fault Insurance Programs. The state of Virginia in 1988 instituted a no-fault system

> Some experts think that the way to solve the malpractice crisis is with a complete overhaul of the court system.

for claims involving severe neurological damage at birth. Ideally, this program would provide fair compensation to the families of brain-damaged infants without their having to prove physician negligence. The question of who is at fault—nature or doctor—is thus bypassed, as is the time, anxiety, expense, and, for the physician, stigma of a court trial. Every physician in the state contributes $250 annually to the compensation fund; those who are protected specifically under the plan (obstetricians and family doctors who deliver babies) pay $5,000 a year.

The primary shortcoming of this program is that its definition of severe neurological damage is so narrow that most candidates, including those with cerebral palsy, may not be covered. After one year, the Virginia experiment with no-fault insurance was too new and underutilized for its usefulness

to be assessed. A similar system was adopted in Florida, although doctors who do not deliver babies and who balked at paying the mandatory annual fee were challenging the law in court.

Stronger State Review Boards. Perhaps the most interesting and far-reaching reform proposal to date was developed by the American Medical Association (AMA) in conjunction with 32 national medical specialty organizations. Considering the source of the projected program, it is surprisingly pro-consumer and potentially tough on errant physicians.

Like the Virginia plan, the AMA proposal would take malpractice claims out of the courts; unlike the Virginia plan, it would retain the importance of determining fault. The body making that determination would be a beefed-up state review board or a new state agency containing medical experts, which would handle claims much the way workers' compensation cases are managed. After evaluating the merits of a claim, the board would either dismiss it or offer a settlement, which could be contested before appeals boards. Whenever compensation was awarded, the case would then be turned over to an investigatory committee with the power to discipline physicians found to be negligent.

In theory, this system would provide appropriate compensation to true victims of malpractice. At the same time it would cut down on the number of meritless suits filed by lawyers and defendants willing to gamble on a sympathetic jury. According to the AMA, the plan would lower liability insurance premiums by limiting unwarranted and excessive settlements, while enforcing tighter regulation of physicians' professional conduct.

It remains to be seen, of course, whether any or all of these proposed benefits would actually come to pass. In the meantime, several states reportedly are considering the AMA plan. □

The Right to Die

Jonathan D. Moreno, Ph.D.

Every human being has a right to die in a dignified manner. This may seem like a straightforward proposition, but it has led to a wrenching ethical debate about the medical treatment of the terminally ill, particularly in light of the vastly increased ability, through technology, to maintain heart and lung activity long after consciousness has ceased. Various considerations have entered into the debate; these include the right of a dying person or that person's family to refuse medical treatment, the cost of intensive care, the criteria for determining death, and the meaning of treatment itself.

Determining Death

The vast majority of legal jurisdictions in the United States now recognize brain death as the point at which human life has ceased, even though cardiopulmonary (heart and lung) function can be artificially sustained indefinitely. Determining when brain death has occurred is the legal responsibility of the physician. Currently, by agreement of the medical community, brain death is said to have occurred when a patient's electroencephalogram, or EEG (the measurement of electrical activity in the brain), is totally flat. Such a reading indicates that the whole brain has stopped functioning—not just the upper portion, which controls thought and awareness—for the lower brain and brain stem may continue to emit electrical impulses for some time after the upper portion has irreversibly ceased to function. (The lower brain and brain stem regulate basic bodily activities such as reflexes, sensory and motor function, and the workings of the internal organs.)

Once brain death has been established, if the heart and lungs are continuing to function only by virtue of an artificial device, medical authorities agree that the device should be removed. Conversely, when the heart and lungs continue to function without the help of machines, the whole brain is not dead, because there is evidently sufficient electrical activity in the lower brain to support respiration.

But some argue that the whole-brain standard is too severe and that when all possibility of awareness has disappeared, the individual should no longer be thought to be alive. Proponents of a less restrictive brain-death standard do not regard the continuation of basic bodily functions (known as vegetative activity) controlled by the lower brain as grounds for saying that a person is still alive. They also note that about 10,000 people in the United States are in what is known as a persistent vegetative state—a complete loss of higher brain function from which they will never recover. In a well-publicized case, Karen Ann Quinlan, who went into a coma after taking a combination of drugs and alcohol, had been in that condition for nearly ten years when she died in 1985. (Although the New Jersey Supreme Court allowed the respirator she was on to be disconnected at her family's request in 1976, Quinlan lived for years sustained by a feeding tube.)

Those in favor of easing the criteria for brain death also point out that the number of donations of precious human organs could be vastly increased if the standard for determining death were altered in this manner. This is because the organs could be retrieved from bodies that still contained enough oxygen to prevent the organs from deteriorating.

Those opposed to changing current standards warn of further confusing the general public about the point at which death occurs. They also voice concern that if standards were changed, physicians, when determining whether death had occurred, might be influenced by the prospect of obtaining viable organs.

Refusing Treatment

But what of a situation in which a dying person wants life supports removed? There is widespread agreement in U.S. law that a competent person facing imminent death may refuse medical interventions that would only prolong the dying process. This view was tested in a 1979 Florida case, *Satz v. Perlmutter*. Abe Perlmutter, a 73-year-old man, was suffering from the fatal degenerative disorder amyotrophic lateral sclerosis (Lou Gehrig's disease). Perlmutter could not move, spoke only with great difficulty, and could breathe only with the aid of a respirator. He sought to have the respirator removed, which would have made death likely within an hour; his doctors refused. The Florida Supreme Court affirmed the decision of a lower court that authorized removal of the respirator.

In reaching a decision in a case such as this, a court must balance a variety of legal and ethical factors. Legal experts agree that the state has an interest in preserving the lives of its citizens—but that this interest must be balanced

207

against dying persons' interest in determining their own fate and not having invasive procedures performed against their will. Also cited in support of an individual's legal right to resist life-extending treatment is the constitutional right to privacy.

Ethical considerations may also affect a court's decision—for example, a balancing of the benefits of continued life against the burden of unrelieved physical and psychological suffering that may mark the usually brief remainder of that life.

Family Rights and Artificial Feeding

The case of *Satz* v. *Perlmutter* involved a competent person with a terminal illness—Perlmutter himself was able to request that his respirator be removed. Frequently, however, a patient lapses into unconsciousness without having expressed any wishes about terminating life, and the family makes a request on the patient's behalf. Such requests bring up a different set of issues: Should families have the right to insist that life-sustaining treatments cease? Should "life-sustaining treatments" be taken to mean only artificial breathing devices or include artificial feeding through tubes as well? Should the same rules apply to a dying patient as to one who is permanently unconscious but not dying?

Many argue that extending the right to refuse treatment to the family of a dying person sets a dangerous precedent. They fear that relatives might decide to withhold treatment with their own interests in mind—for example, to avoid further financial or emotional cost.

Similar concerns about a decline in respect for life underlie reservations about the inclusion of artificial feeding in the medical treatments at issue. Some argue that feeding those who cannot feed themselves is a fundamental act of human compassion; hence, artificial feeding should not be re-garded as just another technique made possible by modern medicine. And in their eyes, to cease feeding those who are permanently unconscious but not dying is tantamount to an act of murder and should not be tolerated by a civilized society.

Court Decisions

Several courts have recently attempted to weigh the concerns of those who oppose withholding treatment against the rights and interests of patients and their families. In 1985 the New Jersey Supreme Court ruled in favor of the family of Claire Conroy, an elderly nursing home resident who was semicomatose and dying. Con-roy's relatives had sought to have her feeding tubes removed, even though doing so would result in her dying of starvation, perhaps sooner than she would otherwise die. Since Conroy's own wishes were unknown, the court had to find a basis for evaluating her family's request. One possibility was a so-called substituted judgment standard, in which another person decides what the incompetent patient would have wanted under the circumstances. But since the court had no information about Conroy's views on death and dying, it adopted instead a "best interests" standard, in which the benefits of continued life for the patient are weighed against the

A Sample Living Will

ARKANSAS

"TERMINAL CONDITION" DECLARATION

If I should have an incurable or irreversible condition that will cause my death within a relatively short time, and I am no longer able to make decisions regarding my medical treatment, I direct my attending physician, pursuant to the Arkansas Rights of the Terminally Ill or Permanently Unconscious Act, to withhold or withdraw treatment that only prolongs the process of dying and is not necessary to my comfort or to alleviate pain.

Other directions:

I direct my attending physician to follow the instructions of

_____, residing at

_____, as my Health Care Proxy,

to make medical treatment decisions on my behalf consistent with my wishes.*

Signed this _____ day of _____, _____.

Signature _____

Address _____

The declarant voluntarily signed this writing in my presence.

Witness _____

Address _____

Witness _____

Address _____

*If you do not name a Proxy, it is advisable to draw a line through this portion.
(See other side for Declaration pertaining to Permanent Unconsciousness)   [OVER]

burdens. The court found that Conroy's best interests would not be served by the continuation of tube feeding. In the event, however, Conroy died of natural causes before the final court ruling had been issued.

In 1980 a young woman named Nancy Ellen Jobes, who was 4½ months pregnant, was injured in an automobile accident. During an operation to remove her fetus, who had died, Jobes suffered a severe loss of oxygen to the brain and never regained consciousness. For years she survived in a nursing home in a vegetative state, sustained by feeding tubes. In 1985, Jobes's family requested that the tubes be removed. Like Conroy, Jobes had not expressed any views about death and dying on which to base a substituted judgment. But in June 1987 the New Jersey Supreme Court found that treatment decisions could be made by close family members or close friends, or—if neither were available—by a guardian. As long as these decisions were made "in good faith," the court found, they had the same weight as if they were made by the patient. Jobes's feeding tube was removed; she died in August 1987.

But the difficult legal and ethical questions have not really been settled by these court decisions, which depend on the particular facts in each case—and in any event are binding only in the state in which they are issued. A very different decision from the one in the Jobes case was reached in October 1988 by the New York State Court of Appeals, which denied a plea by the daughters of an elderly woman that she not be fed artificially. They reported that their mother, Mary O'Connor, who had been devastated by a series of strokes and was unable to communicate about any but the simplest matters, had on many occasions voiced a wish not to be kept alive by machines. But the court found that because O'Connor had not specifically referred to artificial feeding, her statements did not

meet the legal standard of "clear and convincing evidence" of her preference. This ruling implies that to be enforceable in court, a patient's preferences might have to take the form of written directives prepared in advance of an illness.

Living Wills and Proxies

Many people use legal documents prepared in advance to direct the course of their medical treatment in the event that they become terminally ill. These advance directives include the living will and the durable power of attorney. Used together, they can be a powerful expression of a person's wishes if a time comes when the person is unable to communicate those wishes.

Living wills are executed while one is still capable of making decisions, and they go into effect when the person no longer has that capacity. In general, they express the wish to forgo artificial life-sustaining measures (such as respirators or feeding tubes) if such measures would only prolong the dying process. By the end of 1988, 38 U.S. states and the District of Columbia had statutes that recognized the legal force of living wills. The statutes, which are variously called "natural death," "rights of the terminally ill," "death with dignity," and "right-to-die" laws, vary from state to state with regard to what can be covered by a living will. For example, some of them do not recognize as legal an expressed wish to remove artificial feeding tubes.

To complement the living will, many people designate—through a document called a durable power of attorney—a proxy, or surrogate, to make medical decisions on their behalf if they become unable to do so for themselves. (A durable power of attorney differs from a regular power of attorney in that the latter has force only while the person delegating authority is still competent.) The surrogate is generally someone familiar with the person's values and preferences concerning medical care of the

dying. All 50 states and the District of Columbia have statutes recognizing the validity of a durable power of attorney, although these laws were originally intended to authorize proxies to perform such activities as writing checks for the incompetent person. Since most of the laws do not explicitly address the use of the power for healthcare decisions, durable power appointments should clearly authorize the proxy to make this type of decision.

As the recent O'Connor decision in New York illustrates, the advance directive, whether it is a living will or a durable power of attorney, should be as specific as possible about treatments that should be withheld.

Fears About Euthanasia

Many oppose increased control over medical decision making by the terminally ill or their proxies because they fear that allowing such control is akin to approving a passive form of euthanasia or else because they believe it will lead to a greater acceptance of true euthanasia. Euthanasia generally implies using deliberate measures (such as the injection of drugs) to ease or hasten the death of a sufferer—which, in the eyes of the advocates of greater patient control, is different from refusing heroic measures to extend life for the terminally ill or those in a vegetative state.

Will allowing greater control by patients and family over treatment of the terminally ill create an environment in which physicians would routinely help patients die? Such a shift to active euthanasia would represent an extraordinary change in societal attitudes toward death and the physician's proper role in it, and would be unlikely to come about without a great deal of public scrutiny and debate. If active euthanasia is truly at the bottom of a slippery slope, it seems likely that we will know when we are beginning the downward slide. □

Rheumatic Fever

Milton Markowitz, M.D.

By 1980 rheumatic fever had become rare in the United States, with only 1 case annually per 200,000 population. Its complete eradication seemed not far off. Then, starting in the mid-1980s, several outbreaks occurred in scattered parts of the country. The reappearance of the disease came as a surprise, but even more surprising was its occurrence among middle-class children under good medical supervision, since in the past rheumatic fever was concentrated among the poor.

Rheumatic fever can cause crippling damage to the heart; until three or four decades ago, most cases of chronic heart disease in patients under 40 years of age resulted from one or more attacks of rheumatic fever during childhood. Indeed, rheumatic heart disease is still well remembered by older Americans, a significant number of whom carry the scars of surgery to repair damaged heart valves. Consequently, while the total number of new cases is still relatively small, the possibility of a nationwide resurgence of rheumatic fever has brought about a revival of interest in the cause, recognition, treatment, and prevention of this disease.

Villain: Streptococcus

Rheumatic fever is triggered by a streptococcal bacterial infection of the upper respiratory tract, which is usually—although not always—indicated by a sore throat (strep throat). Sore throats are one of the most common of human ailments, especially in children during their school years. Most of them are caused by viruses, but depending on the season (bacterial sore throats occur more commonly in cold months), 10 to 20 percent are caused by streptococci bacteria. Children 5 to 15 years old have the highest incidence of rheumatic fever, primarily because of the relative frequency of streptococcal infections in this age group.

While all cases of rheumatic fever are preceded by streptococcal throat infections (whether or not the patient's throat feels sore), fortunately only a small minority of strep throats are followed by rheumatic fever. What determines which patients go on to develop the disease has puzzled investigators for decades. Since rheumatic fever tends to run in families, genetic markers have long been sought. Efforts to pin down a recognizable marker have met with uncertain success. A recent candidate is a substance that has been found in the blood of a high percentage of rheumatic fever patients, but this observation needs further corroboration. Finding a genetic marker might allow doctors to identify and then provide preventive treatment to people who are at risk of developing rheumatic fever.

A throat culture is necessary to verify the presence of a strep infection, which can lead to rheumatic fever.

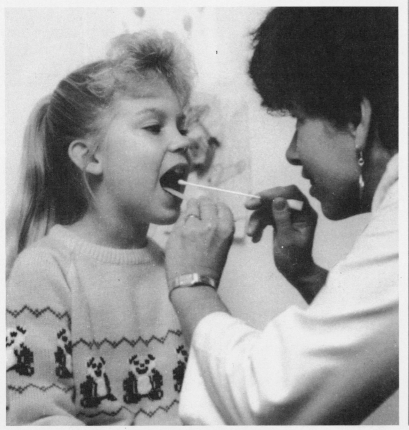

Another possible explanation for why some patients develop rheumatic fever after a strep throat while others do not is that certain strains of streptococci may be more likely to cause the disease than others. Some evidence supports this possibility, and biochemical studies are currently being conducted to determine differences between strains. The identification of particular streptococci that cause rheumatic fever could greatly simplify the development of a vaccine.

Still another gap in medical knowledge, and the most fundamental of all, is the puzzle of how streptococci set off the inflammations in different parts of the body that occur in rheumatic fever. An attack begins one to four weeks after the strep throat has subsided. At the time of the attack, streptococci cannot be found in any of the affected sites (joints, heart, nervous system), indicating that the disease is not due to the spread of streptococci beyond the throat. The most widely accepted theory is that rheumatic fever is caused by an overreaction of the body's immune system to the streptococci. Substances known as antigens on the bacteria's surface are biologically similar to antigens in human heart tissue, and researchers hypothesize that antibodies that fight the invasion of streptococci mistakenly identify the heart tissue antigen as the foreign bacteria antigen and attack the tissue, causing damage to the heart. This so-called autoimmune concept for rheumatic fever has many adherents but is still not considered fully proven.

Recognizing an Attack

Patients generally recover from a strep throat in three to five days and have no warning signs of rheumatic fever during the one to four weeks before the onset of an acute attack. An attack typically begins with a fever and severe pain and swelling in a large joint, most often the knee. The initial symptoms subside over a period of

a week, but as the affected joint improves, the inflammation starts up in another joint. It continues to jump from joint to joint in this way for several weeks, but causes no permanent damage to the joints. The joint pain and swelling usually lead parents to seek medical care for the child, and the migratory nature of the pain should alert physicians to consider rheumatic fever. Older physicians easily recognize the signs of the disease, but younger ones may not, since they have probably not seen a case during their training or practice.

The recent reappearance of rheumatic fever in the United States came as a surprise since the disease had become quite rare.

Patients often have no cardiac symptoms early in the attack unless the heart inflammation is severe enough to cause heart failure. However, most rheumatic fever patients have cardiac involvement; between 50 and 90 percent of the patients in the recent outbreaks developed signs of heart disease. Almost always, the first sign is a heart murmur that was not present previously. The murmur may already be there when the patient is first seen for joint pains, or it may be detected a few weeks later. (It may also show up in later life.) It arises from irregularities in blood flow caused by damaged heart valves. At times the patient suffers chest pain—if the outer layer (pericardium) of the heart becomes inflamed. Signs of heart failure, such as shortness of breath, may appear at any time during an attack.

In a small percentage of cases—more often in girls than boys, for a reason that is not known—rheu-

matic fever can also affect the nervous system and produce a condition known as chorea, or more familiarly as Saint Vitus' dance. The child first shows changes in behavior, such as deterioration of schoolwork (especially handwriting) and difficulty in performing simple tasks, such as buttoning clothes. Then, uncontrollable muscle contractions appear, causing facial grimacing and aimless, jerky movements of the extremities. Chorea may be the first indication or the only sign of rheumatic fever, or it may emerge after the joint inflammations have gone away. Like the joint inflammation, it is self-limited and leaves no permanent aftereffects.

The diagnosis of rheumatic fever is made the old-fashioned way: through a complete medical history, a thorough physical examination with special attention to the heart, and close observation of the patient over a period of several weeks. There is no single diagnostic laboratory test. However, testing the blood for streptococcal antibodies will reveal whether the patient has had a streptococcal infection in recent weeks. A simple test is available for judging the degree of inflammation in the heart and joints and for determining when rheumatic fever has subsided.

Treatment and Prognosis

There has been no progress in the treatment of rheumatic fever. Antibiotics have no curative effect once an attack begins. Other drugs do alleviate symptoms. Aspirin can dramatically improve fever and joint pain virtually overnight. Sedation with tranquilizers can be helpful in patients with chorea.

How to prevent permanent damage to the heart is the real challenge, and here the results of therapy have been disappointing. There is still no way to prevent damage when heart inflammation occurs. Steroids have not lived up to their early promise, although they are useful in very sick patients to help control heart failure, as are other medications (such as digitalis). Should heart failure become uncontrollable with medication, the affected valve can be surgically replaced.

The outcome of the attack spans the spectrum from complete recovery to death. The latter is rare today, although in the recent outbreaks several children's lives have probably been saved only by surgical intervention. The patient's prognosis depends on the presence and severity of cardiac involvement.

Long-term prognosis depends on the extent of residual heart disease and on whether or not the patient

The disease is triggered by a streptococcal bacterial infection of the upper respiratory tract, which is usually indicated by a sore throat.

suffers recurrent attacks. As in the initial attack, recurrences follow streptococcal infections. Once patients have had an attack, they are at great risk for recurrences unless they are protected against strep infections. Recurrences can have a devastating effect on patients who have been left with heart disease after the initial attack.

About one-third to one-half of all patients eventually develop structural abnormalities of one or more heart valves. Over time progressive scarring of the valves affected by the initial attack interferes with their opening and closing, causing either obstruction to blood flow or a leak backward between heart chambers. In either case, the heart is strained, enlarges to keep up with the demand, and ultimately fails unless

defective valves are replaced surgically.

Prevention

There are means to prevent initial and recurrent attacks of rheumatic fever, but they are imperfect and much more difficult to carry out than in diseases for which vaccines are available. Once rheumatic fever patients have been identified, at whatever stage, they should be given medication to prevent future streptococcal infections and recurrences of rheumatic fever. Patients can take a small daily dose of oral penicillin or a sulfa drug or receive a single injection of long-acting penicillin every four weeks. This regimen is required at least through childhood and adolescence.

Ideally, the goal should be to prevent the first attack. This can be achieved in many instances, but only if the throat infection is identified as streptococcal and if treatment with an antibiotic, preferably penicillin, is started promptly and carried out for a full ten days. These are two large ifs. It is often difficult to distinguish a viral from a strep sore throat without a throat culture. Once the diagnosis is established and medication is prescribed, the patient is usually free of symptoms in three to five days. As a result, many patients fail to complete the required ten days of treatment.

What can parents do now that rheumatic fever has reappeared? Should they see a physician every time a child has an upper respiratory infection of any kind? The answer is no. Some symptoms can help parents distinguish between viral and strep infections. Nasal congestion, cough, and hoarseness are caused by viruses and may be accompanied during the course of the illness by an irritated or scratchy throat. However, if the illness *starts* with a sore throat, especially if there is fever, real difficulty in swallowing, or swollen neck glands, a strep infection should be suspected and medical advice sought. If the

physician finds it impossible to distinguish between a viral and a strep infection from the appearance of the throat, a throat culture should be done; in fact, the parent should request a culture if there is a doubt about the diagnosis.

Once the diagnosis of a strep infection is established, penicillin is still the most effective drug (other antibiotics can be substituted if the patient is known to be allergic to penicillin). The most convenient method of administration is to give the child a dose of oral penicillin morning and evening for a full ten days. The child can usually return to normal activities after a few days, but the required course of treatment must be

Rheumatic fever can cause crippling damage to the heart, which sometimes necessitates the replacement of a heart valve.

completed to ensure prevention of rheumatic fever.

Doctors are uncertain why the recent outbreaks of rheumatic fever occurred. Some as yet unknown change in the streptococcus may prove to be the cause. What is clear, however, is that rheumatic fever cannot be totally eliminated with the present methods available for prevention. Many individuals who suffered rheumatic fever attacks in the recent outbreaks did not appear sick and did not suffer sore throats even though they had strep infections. Better methods are needed for screening children for strep infections. The hope of eliminating rheumatic fever lies in rekindling interest in research to explore new leads provided by the recent outbreaks and ultimately to perfect a streptococcal vaccine. ☐

What Are Dental Implants?

David C. Abelson, D.D.S.

With the proper care, your teeth can last a lifetime. However, for a variety of reasons many people lose some or all of their adult teeth. For these people, whose "permanent" teeth turn out to be not quite permanent enough, dental implants offer the chance to have replacement teeth much like their own teeth.

Dental implants are permanent devices that are attached directly to the jawbone, with artificial teeth placed onto them. Implants can support single teeth, a few teeth, or a whole series of teeth. They are an increasingly popular alternative to dentures (removable false teeth) and bridges (artificial teeth not meant to be removed but anchored only to adjoining natural teeth, not to the jaw). In recent years the designs of implants, the procedures used to install them, and the materials used to make them have so improved that implants may well be the next best thing to having one's own teeth.

Early Research

The goal of permanent replacement teeth is not a new one. Published accounts of procedures to implant artificial teeth appeared as far back as the late 1800s. The first implants were designed to mimic the form of natural teeth. They had rootlike portions that were embedded in the soft (gum) tissues and upper portions that protruded into the mouth and were sometimes covered by a fabricated crown, or artificial tooth.

The rootlike section was made of ceramic porcelain or a metal, such as lead, that was roughened or perforated to allow soft tissue to grow around or through it and hold it in place.

In the early 1900s, the first attempts were made to design an implant that would be held in place by bone growing into it. Early research also focused on materials used to make implants. The problem was finding materials that would have adequate strength and would not cause allergic reactions or be rejected by the body. A variety of materials, including ceramics, hydroxyapatite (the mineral compound that is the main component of human bone), and vitreous carbon, as well as metals such as chromium and titanium, have been used with varying degrees of success as implant fixtures. Today, the vast majority of implants are made of pure titanium—a light, strong metal—or titanium alloys; a small percentage of implants are made of ceramic materials.

Choosing Implants

Potential recipients must think about several factors when considering implants. They generally are more expensive than either dentures or bridges. Individual teeth or a small group of teeth can cost between $1,000 and $2,000, while entire sets of upper and lower teeth can cost $20,000 or more. Generally, insurance coverage is the same for implants as for bridges and dentures.

Money is not the only concern. Implants must rest in place with little use for up to a year while they are being secured by bone growing around or into them. During that time they require special care, soft foods are a must, and regular follow-up visits to the dentist are necessary. Therefore, people who choose implants must be highly motivated and must have a good deal of patience and perseverance. Physically, individuals must be in good general health and have adequate quantity and quality of bone in the jaw to hold the implant in place.

Implants are available to adults of all ages. Younger adults may want to replace individual teeth lost from accidents or other causes. But usually those who get implants are older people who have lost their teeth and have already tried dentures but had difficulty wearing them.

Types Available

Once the individual has made the decision to get dental implants, the dentist must decide which type is most appropriate. There are two general types currently available, differing primarily in the way the implant is fixed to the patient's jawbone.

The type most in favor today involves the principle of osseointegration developed by a Swedish

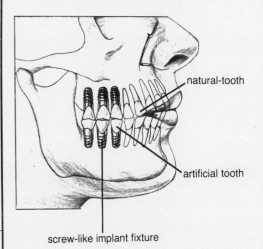

One Common Type of Implant

natural-tooth

artificial tooth

screw-like implant fixture

dentist. Solid implants (which look like screws or cylinders) are placed in holes drilled in the jawbone, and bone then grows around the implants to hold them in place. The number of implant fixtures placed depends on the number of missing teeth. The number may range from a single implant to replace a single missing tooth up to as many as six fixtures strategically placed to restore a completely toothless arch (upper or lower jaw). Generally, all the implant fixtures required are placed during a single surgical session.

Later, one or more structures that function as posts are attached to the portions of the implants that protrude into gum tissue over the jawbone, and false teeth are placed on the posts.

Research begun in the early 1960s shows that under the proper conditions the bond between implant and bone remains intact, with no detectable loosening of the implant, for many years. Osseointegrated implants made of titanium show a success rate over the course of five to ten years of better than 90 percent in the upper jaw and better than 95 percent in the lower jaw when the entire arch is treated. Long-term success rates for single-tooth implants are not available, but early indications are that they are comparable to the full-arch rates.

The other type of implant involves what is called a fibro-osseous junction between the dental implant and the jawbone. The dentist must also cut into the jawbone for these implants, but since they are blade-shaped, a slot (rather than a round hole) is made. Typically, these implants are designed with pores or vents for bone to grow into, anchoring them in place, and during the healing process, natural soft tissue—analogous to the ligament found between a natural tooth root and the jawbone—forms between the jaw and the implant. Theoretically, because of the similarity in the attachment mechanism, this type of implant may work better than

osseointegrated implants for people who still have some of their own natural teeth. Success rates, however, vary more widely than for osseointegrated implants—ranging from 55 to 85 percent over five to ten years.

Failure of an implant means that it loosens in the jawbone. Depending on the circumstances, the dentist may then try the same type of implant again or try a different type. In some cases the patient may have to revert to conventional dentures or bridges.

Regardless of the implant material or the way the implant is held in place, surgery takes place in the dentist's office. Local anesthesia is adequate, although general anesthesia may be used if the patient prefers it.

The long-term success of any implant, after it is surgically placed, depends on allowing it to remain for a period of time with minimal or no function. When osseointegrated implants are surgically placed in the bone, gum tissue is sutured back over them so that they are completely covered. If the full mouth is involved, ideally, patients should function without teeth during the healing period. Since this is usually not practical, in most cases an interim removable denture is made. When only part of the mouth is being worked on, the implant site is, if possible, left unrestored during healing. Otherwise, a temporary bridge is made. About 6 months later, for the lower jaw, or 12 months later, for the upper jaw, the implants are surgically uncovered, and the postlike portions are placed onto them. The artificial teeth are then attached, and the implant can begin to function normally.

Fibro-osseous implants differ from osseointegrated implants in that they are one-piece structures with a postlike portion already attached that extends into the mouth. They cannot be totally covered with soft tissue at the time they are installed. The postlike portion must be covered with a

temporary bridge, built shorter than the natural teeth to protect it from excessive use while the bone grows into the implant to hold it securely. After the implant is firmly fixed, the artificial teeth are cemented on.

After the Surgery

Advances in surgical techniques have greatly improved success rates for implants. However, all surgical procedures involve some element of risk. The most common complication following the placement of implant fixtures is paresthesia—a lingering numbness or tingling sensation in the surrounding tissue. Many of the sites chosen to receive implants contain bundles of nerves that may be damaged or irritated during or after the surgery. Paresthesia usually corrects itself. However, in some cases the patient will be left with permanent numbness, and there is no treatment. Other risks include accidental fracture of the jawbone or penetration of one of the sinuses during surgery, as well as infection in the bone at the implant site.

Because of the rigid requirements of the surgical technique, the dentist who places the implant must be thoroughly familiar with the proper procedures. Ideally, a surgical specialist such as an oral surgeon or a periodontist should perform the surgery. The placement of false teeth over implant fixtures is much like placement of artificial crowns over natural teeth. For this reason a dentist who is experienced in crown and bridge technique and is familiar with implant procedures should be responsible for caring for the patient after the implant is surgically installed.

To ensure long-term success once implants are in place and functional, patients must make sure the areas surrounding each implant are kept clean and healthy. This means both conscientious at-home care and regular visits to the dentist for cleanings and checkups. □

DYSLEXIA

A Reading Disorder

Natalie D. Sollee, Ph.D.

Many children who are bright and interested in learning nevertheless have difficulty learning to read because they suffer from the poorly understood disorder called dyslexia.

The dyslexic child is able to learn to read, but does so at a rate and in a way different from most children. Performance in school is often inconsistent; what is learned one day may be forgotten by the next. In some cases the child is labeled immature, lazy, underachieving, emotionally disturbed, or even retarded. If the child comes to believe these labels, self-esteem plummets. Parents often feel anxious, guilty, or depressed about the problem. In a society where the ability to read is seen as the single most important foundation for future learning and where more and more parents believe it is their duty to oversee the adequacy of their child's education, such feelings are understandable.

What Is Dyslexia?

Since the late 19th century researchers have recognized that certain children are unable to read skillfully even though they have received educational and cultural opportunities that are ordinarily adequate and even though they are developing normally in other ways. These are the children said to be suffering from dyslexia, a term based on the Greek for "defective language."

Few dyslexic children are completely unable to read. Most have a rudimentary grasp of relationships between the printed letters and the spoken word and can recognize simple words. But many of them read slowly, word by word. They may have trouble sounding out specific letters, or they may reverse letters or words, reading "d" for "b," or "was" for "saw." Their spelling, written or oral, may be poor, particularly when irregularly spelled words are involved. They may misunderstand material or have trouble remembering it correctly. They may leave out words when they are reading or substitute one word for another—saying, for example, "cat" when they're looking at the word "dog." Their handwriting may be cramped and may be almost illegible.

> **Some children are unable to develop good reading skills even though they are bright, are interested in learning, and receive adequate training.**

Parents often ask if the reading difficulty is due simply to a lag in development, which will eventually be overcome, or reflects a fixed problem, which will continue. While it is true that most children's weaker skills will improve as they develop, dyslexic children still may not be able to perform learning tasks as expected at their age and grade level. As they grow older and move into higher grades, longer and longer periods of time are required for them to master each new reading skill.

It is generally agreed that dyslexia occurs in 10 to 15 percent of the U.S. population. It is far more common in males than in females: more than three times as many boys as girls show evidence of the disorder.

What Causes It?

No one really knows what causes dyslexia, although there has been no shortage of suggestions over the years.

The pioneer in modern dyslexia research was the American neurologist Samuel Orton. In 1925 he suggested that a primary cause of dyslexia was a problem or problems in the person's visual system; words and letters, for example, might be perceived in reverse. Another possibility, in his view, was that the brains of dyslexics had not matured in the usual way. Normally, one hemisphere of the brain is dominant in the development of language. In dyslexics, Orton theorized, such "cerebral dominance" is not the case. Researchers now know that word and letter reversals are only one problem seen in dyslexic children, and that these reversals occur in only a minority of them. But the idea that dyslexia may be caused by visual problems and the idea that it may be due to lack of cerebral dominance are still important in efforts to find ways to treat the disorder.

Visual-perceptual problems under study today include those associated with tracking, or control of eye movements, and with peripheral vision (which, some researchers believe, may in dyslexics be better adapted to reading than direct vision). Other lines of investigation center on possible problems in relating stimuli received through one sense (the eye, say) to stimuli received through another sense (such as the ear); inability to remember the sequence of a series of items or events; and language deficiencies (for example, inability to break words into their component sounds). Not all of these characteristics are found in every dyslexic, however, and some dyslexics have none of them. Since many dyslexic children have relatives with reading disabilities, researchers are also exploring heredity's possible role in either directly causing the disorder or creating a susceptibility to it.

Behavior and Brain Structure

Over the past two decades, some researchers have begun to study dyslexia and possible treatments for it in terms of neuropsychology, which deals with the relationship between behavior and the physical structure of the brain and nervous system. One result has been the identification of different kinds of dyslexia, based on children's performance on batteries of tests designed to discover what their strengths and weaknesses are when it comes to learning.

These tests systematically examine such things as how a child's senses function and how much control the child has over his or her movements. They also examine the child's ability to use and understand language, organizational skills, attention span, memory, and ability to formulate ideas. Sometimes tests are given to measure "lateralization," that is, preference for use of one side of the

body or greater efficiency on that side.

Some recent neuropsychological research has attempted to localize the area of the brain responsible for dyslexia. In 1985, Norman Geschwind and Albert M. Galaburda, neurologists at Beth Israel Hospital in Boston, reported on their studies of the brains of two individuals who had suffered from severe dyslexia since childhood. During autopsies, Geschwind and Galaburda found irregularities in the arrangement of cells in the brain; almost all of these irregularities were in the left hemisphere, the area of the brain most closely associated with speech.

In spite of the increasing neuropsychological focus of the past few years, most psychologists and educators continue to believe that numerous personality factors contribute to the severity of dyslexia, including the child's feelings, self-image, and expectations for future achievement. The child who does not believe his or her efforts can be effective is not likely to respond to remedial programs or to be motivated to work hard enough to overcome the disability. Teachers, friends, and parents can influence the development of reading ability by offering important psychological support.

What Should Parents Do?

When parents suspect that their child suffers from dyslexia, they should take steps to find out if this is indeed the case and, if so, what help is available. In the United States federal law gives public school students the right to free testing for dyslexia, as well as the right to educational programs tailored to their needs. In Canada the situation differs from province to province; Ontario has a law similar to that in the United States, but elsewhere—in the absence of such a law—help may be more difficult to arrange, although it may very well be available. In both countries school systems, government agencies, and private

associations should be tapped for information.

Parents may want to consider having their youngster evaluated if the child, for no apparent reason, is generally worried about school, seems to be having difficulty with schoolwork, or has given up trying. During a teacher-parent conference, the teacher may report that the child, for unknown reasons, is not making adequate progress. An evaluation will help pinpoint the cause of the child's difficulties—whether it be dyslexia or something else—so that appropriate remedies can be devised.

Once parents have decided to have their child evaluated, they should contact the school to arrange for testing. (Testing and evaluation may also be done privately.) In addition to neuropsychological and educational testing the child should be given a physical examination. Evaluation of the home setting, a speech and hearing evaluation, and other assessments may also be done.

Under U.S. law, if the conclusion of the assessment team is that the child has a learning disability, dyslexia or any other, an educational plan is written, prescribing amounts and types of special services that must be provided for the child. These may include small-group teaching in a "resource room," individual tutoring, placement in a private school for learning-disabled children, speech or language therapy, occupational therapy, and individualized physical education. Specific teaching methods—chosen to match the way in which the child learns best—are often recommended. The plan also specifies methods for evaluating progress. Parents must give their approval before the plan is put into effect; they may oppose it and offer alternative plans during mediation sessions or in court hearings.

Looking Ahead

Given patience, encouragement, and individualized attention with appropriate educational tools, al-

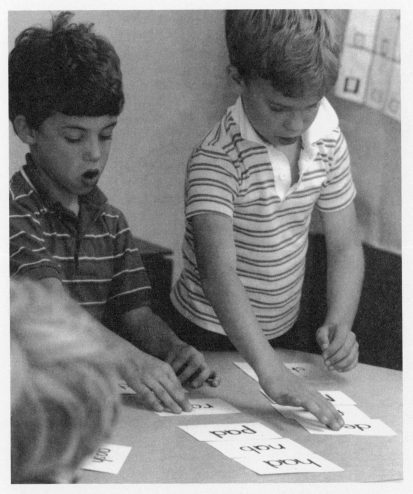

Dyslexic children may have trouble sounding out certain letters.

receiving federal funds, whether it be a public or private agency or a business.

Dyslexia does not necessarily lead to failure. Dyslexics have shown remarkable achievement in many spheres of life. Albert Einstein didn't read until age nine, and he later had a poor memory for words and texts. Thomas Edison would be recognized as dyslexic today. He didn't learn to spell or write grammatically until he was 19. Woodrow Wilson didn't read till he was 11. □

Sources of Further Information

Association for Children and Adults With Learning Disabilities (ACLD), 4156 Library Road, Pittsburgh, PA 15234.

Learning Disabilities Association of Canada, 323 Chapel Street, Suite 200, Ottawa K1N 7Z2, Ontario.

National Center for Learning Disabilities (formerly Foundation for Children with Learning Disabilities), 99 Park Avenue, New York, NY 10016.

Orton Dyslexia Society, 724 York Road, Baltimore, MD 21204.

Local branches of the ACLD and the Orton Dyslexia Society in the United States and local and provincial associations dealing with the learning disabled in Canada are also useful sources of information.

Suggestions for Further Reading

Developmental Dyslexia and Related Reading Disorders. Bethesda, Md., U.S. Department of Health and Human Services, Public Health Service, 1985.

Directory of Resources. Ottawa, Canada, Learning Disabilities Association of Canada, 1988-1989.

FCLD Learning Disabilities Resource Guide: A State-by-State Directory of Special Programs, Schools, and Services. New York, New York University Press, 1985.

Peterson's Guide to Colleges With Programs for Learning-Disabled Students. Princeton, N.J., Peterson's Guides, 1985.

SILVER, LARRY B. *The Misunderstood Child: A Guide for Parents of Learning-Disabled Children.* New York, McGraw-Hill, 1984.

most every dyslexic child can learn to read. A number of factors affect the ability to conquer dyslexia, including the age of the child when the problem is identified, the length and quality of the special services offered, the child's personality and level of motivation, and relationships with family, peers, and teachers. Indeed, how family, peers, and teachers perceive the dyslexic child and his or her problems can have a strong influence on the ultimate outcome.

Most dyslexic youngsters, however, will not become fluent and easy readers, and many will carry some lags in learning into adulthood despite years of special training. Older adolescent and adult dyslexics may suffer from low self-esteem, social failure, and performance anxiety. But they can be helped by counseling. If they wish to continue their education, or make up for lost time, there are programs in both the United States and Canada that are geared to the learning-disabled and that have offerings ranging from high school diplomas to degrees. Landmark College in Putney, Vt., teaches only dyslexics. As to legal protection other than that dealing directly with education, in Canada the Charter of Rights and Freedoms provides safeguards against discrimination. In the United States the Rehabilitation Act of 1973 forbids discrimination by any program or activity

Stocking Your Medicine Cabinet

Ingrid J. Strauch

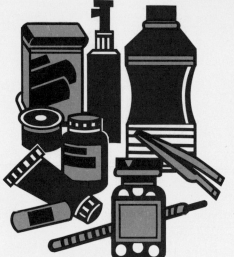

Most everyday health complaints don't require a doctor's care, but being prepared with a comprehensive stock of home medical supplies and a basic knowledge of first aid can ease the discomfort and distress that accompany even minor injuries, aches, and illnesses. Buying the necessary medications, bandages, and the like is relatively simple and not too expensive, and the peace of mind a well-stocked medicine cabinet allows has no price tag.

Drugs to Stock

Before buying any over-the-counter drugs, read the package label, paying close attention to any warning notices. If you're not sure whether a nonprescription drug is safe or appropriate for you, ask your doctor. Always follow directions for use when taking any drug, prescription or not; taking too little or too much of a drug can result in lowered effectiveness or undesired complications.

Painkillers. An effective pain-killer, or analgesic, is invaluable for relieving headaches, muscular aches, toothaches, and menstrual cramps. Analgesics also reduce fever. Common nonprescription analgesics are aspirin, acetaminophen (such as Tylenol or Datril), and ibuprofen (such as Advil or Nuprin).

The three types of pain relievers have somewhat different benefits and risks. Aspirin and ibuprofen reduce swelling and inflammation, whereas acetaminophen does not; acetaminophen, therefore, is not very effective against the pain and inflammation caused by arthritis. Aspirin and ibuprofen also sometimes upset the stomach and may interact with other drugs, while acetaminophen rarely has either of these side effects.

Households with children should also stock children's-strength acetaminophen or aspirin. However, aspirin should never be taken by children or teenagers with chicken pox or the flu before consulting a doctor; the use of aspirin for these illnesses has been linked to Reye's syndrome, a rare but potentially fatal disease.

Wound Care. While most minor wounds can be cleaned effectively with soap and water, an antiseptic like hydrogen peroxide can be used. Topical antibiotics—Mycitracin or Neosporin, for example—can prevent infection and aid the healing of minor cuts, burns, and abrasions. However, topical antibiotics, which come in ointment, lotion, spray, or powder form, should not be used on deep or serious wounds, for which a doctor should be consulted.

Skin Treatments. Mild skin irritations can be distracting and are often made worse by scratching. One of the simplest means of relief to have available is petroleum jelly, which soothes diaper rash and moisturizes dry skin. Some other products to keep on hand include anti-inflammatory/anesthetic agents and antipruritics (medications that stop itching).

An anesthetic ointment, lotion, or spray containing 0.5 percent hydrocortisone—such as Cortaid or Delacort—will reduce itching, inflammation, and irritation resulting from such sources as eczema, insect bites, poison ivy, and poison oak, as well as from reactions to soaps, detergents, and cosmet-

> **Being prepared with a stock of basic home medical supplies can ease anxiety in cases of minor illness or injury.**

ics. The ointment form is useful in relieving external genital and anal itching. Some hydrocortisone preparations also contain a lubricating agent that soothes and protects dry and scaly skin. There are also topical anesthetics that do not contain hydrocortisone; these include sunburn remedies like Solarcaine.

A calamine-based lotion, cream,

or spray—such as Caladryl or Rhuli—is a wise investment for summer. It provides quick relief from the itching and inflammation of insect bites, poison ivy and oak, and mild sunburn.

All skin products are for external use only. Before any topical medication is applied, the affected skin should be clean.

Cold Remedies. The market is replete with over-the-counter cold remedies. While none will cure a cold, the symptom relief they provide may make it easier to function during the day and sleep at night.

Antihistamines, such as Dimetane or Chlor-Trimeton, help control the sneezing and runny nose and soothe the itchy and watery eyes caused by colds and allergies. Decongestants, such as Sudafed or Duration, reduce the swelling of nasal passages, making it easier to breathe. Many cold medications combine antihistamines and decongestants (and sometimes analgesics) to alleviate several symptoms at once. These preparations—such as Actifed, Contac, or Dristan—may be available in liquid or tablet form, as nasal sprays or drops, and as vaporizing ointments and liquids for hot steam vaporizers. (Nasal sprays should be used by only one person because they can transmit infections.)

Coughs and sore throats that accompany colds may be eased by cough suppressants or expectorants. Cough suppressants, also known as antitussives, provide relief from dry, or nonproductive, coughs—the kind that irritate the

> **Medications should not be kept in a steamy bathroom but in a cool, dry storage area out of the reach of young children.**

throat but don't clear air passages or bring up mucus. Suppressants may be purchased as syrups, tablets, and lozenges. Expectorants help loosen phlegm and thin mucus and thus tend to make a cough more productive. They are often available in combination with other medications and come in syrup, capsule, and pediatric drop form. There are numerous cough medications of all types and formulations on the market; read the labels carefully to make sure you are buying the type of product you really want.

Throat lozenges stimulate saliva to soothe a dry throat; some preparations contain a topical anes-

thetic to reduce throat pain. Because many lozenges look and taste like candy, they may be tempting to children. Lozenges, like all drugs, should be kept out of reach of children.

Stomach and Bowel Medications. Products to keep on hand for digestive system problems include an antacid, an antidiarrheal medication, and a laxative. Antacids—Alka-Seltzer, Maalox, and Di-Gel are just a few examples—relieve acid indigestion or heartburn. Medications such as Pepto-Bismol or Kaopectate control diarrhea and the abdominal cramps associated with it. There are several types of laxatives: bulk-forming products (such as Metamucil), stool softeners (Correctol and Colace are common brands), and products that stimulate the bowel walls (Ex-Lax, for example). The bulk-forming laxatives are considered safest. Regular use of any type of laxative, however, can result in dependence on laxatives and should be avoided. If a digestive problem persists for several days, a physician should be consulted.

Poison Control. Some products should be kept on hand in case of accidental poisoning: syrup of ipecac to induce vomiting, activated charcoal to deactivate the poisonous substance, and epsom salts to act as a laxative. Never adminis-

MEDICINE CABINET SHOPPING LIST

MEDICATIONS

aspirin/acetaminophen/
   ibuprofen
antiseptic
topical antibiotic
petroleum jelly
topical
   anti-inflammatory/
   anesthetic
topical medication for
   itching

antihistamine
decongestant
cough suppressant
expectorant
antacid
antidiarrheal
   medication
laxative
syrup of ipecac
activated charcoal
epsom salts

DRESSINGS

Band-Aids
sterile gauze pads
gauze bandage
adhesive tape
ace bandage

UTENSILS

safety pins
blunt-ended scissors
tweezers
sewing needle
thermometers
   (oral/rectal)
hot water bottle/
   heating pad
flashlight

ter any of these drugs unless advised by a physician. Vomiting may do more harm than good if the poison swallowed was a strong acid or strong alkali or a petroleum product.

Dressings

Bleeding wounds should always receive immediate attention. Often a Band-Aid will be all that's needed to help stop minor bleeding and protect a superficial injury, and one box of assorted Band-Aids should suffice in the home. For larger cuts and scrapes, other dressings and bandages may be needed.

The most versatile type of dressing to keep on hand is 2-inch or 3-inch individually wrapped sterile gauze pads. In an emergency, a good supply of standard-sized pads is less confusing than a wide variety of assorted sizes. A roll or two of 2-inch or 3-inch gauze bandage is useful to secure the pads.

A roll of 1-inch adhesive tape, either paper or cloth, and several safety pins will be of great help in keeping bandages in place. Scissors with blunt ends should be used for removing bandages; a pair exclusively for this use should be stored with bandaging supplies.

Ice

Ice is beneficial for reducing the swelling of sprained ankles, fingers, wrists, or knees. It's a good idea to be sure that some is always available in the freezer. When applied to an injury, the ice should not directly touch the skin; it should be wrapped in a towel or placed in a plastic bag that is then covered by a towel. Ice should be applied to an area for no more than 15-20 minutes at a time. Note that ice should not be placed on burns: it may cause further damage by freezing the skin.

Other Supplies

In addition to the supplies listed above, the following items are useful to have in the home: tweezers and a sewing needle to remove splinters; an oral thermometer; a rectal thermometer in homes with children; a hot water bottle or heating pad for sore muscles; a flashlight to locate supplies if there is a blackout; an antiseptic such as rubbing alcohol to sterilize instruments; and an ace bandage to help immobilize a healing sprained joint. It's a good idea to have a first aid manual, such as *Standard First Aid & Personal Safety* written by the American Red Cross.

Proper Storage

In many homes, medical supplies are kept in the bathroom, but bathrooms get hot and steamy, and that environment may shorten the shelf life of some medications. (Read the labels on the products you buy for advice on storage; some items may need to be refrigerated.) A kitchen shelf away from the stove or a centrally located closet shelf may be better choices than a bathroom cabinet.

To prevent their accidental consumption, drugs should be inaccessible to children. Even a childproof package does not guarantee that a child will not get to its contents. If medications are locked away, all adults in the home should know where the key is kept. (Dressings, however, should always be readily available; in an emergency the time to locate a key may be lacking.)

Despite all precautions, accidental poisoning does sometimes occur. If this happens, call a poison control center or physician as soon as possible (these phone numbers should be posted by the telephone).

When to Throw It Out

Most medications expire—become less effective or actually unsafe—at some point. Drugs often have an expiration date on the label. It is advisable to check all medications in the house once or twice a year and discard any product that has reached its expiration date. Flushing pills down the toilet is recommended, so that they are not mistakenly removed from the trash and ingested.

Changes in color, odor, or consistency indicate that a product is probably too old and should be thrown out. Aspirin, for example, smells like vinegar when it goes bad. Ointments and lotions may dry up or separate, and pills may melt and stick together. Bandages and gauze pads will not expire, but their packages may crack if kept for a long time, making the dressing no longer sterile. □

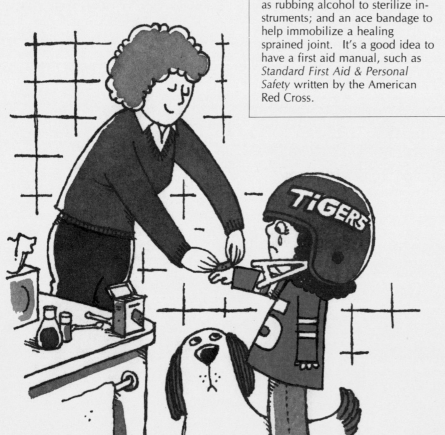

Sjogren's Syndrome

Pat Costello Smith

When Elaine Harris first experienced irritated eyes, a painful sore throat, and a general feeling of illness, she had never heard of Sjogren's syndrome (pronounced SHOW-gren's). In what she considers one of the most difficult times of her life, she consulted 11 medical specialists, trying to find the cause of her persistent eye and throat irritation, as well as the mouth sores, swollen glands, exhaustion, and other symptoms she was suffering.

Because her symptoms had many possible causes, her physicians performed numerous tests, ruling out one disease after another. Finally, many months and medical tests later, Harris learned that her troubles stemmed from Sjogren's syndrome, the classic signs of which are insufficient tears and saliva.

Sjogren's is often overlooked by physicians. But the symptoms of

Nine out of ten Sjogren's patients are women.

the disease are not minor and can seriously affect a patient's quality of life, and occasionally the disease can even be life-threatening. Since there is currently no cure for Sjogren's, treatment aims to relieve symptoms.

Dry Eyes, Dry Mouth

Dry eyes and a dry mouth have many causes, such as various diseases, aging, or side effects of certain medications. So a diagnosis of Sjogren's syndrome—often shortened to SS—must be confirmed by specific tests.

The condition is named for Dr. Henrik Sjogren, a Swedish ophthalmologist who in the 1930s identified the disorder in a group of patients with dry eyes, a dry mouth, and rheumatoid arthritis. (Rheumatoid arthritis is a chronic disease in which the linings of the joints become inflamed, leading to swelling, pain, and other problems.) Today, Sjogren's syndrome is diagnosed when a patient has any two of three features: dry eyes (technically called keratoconjunctivitis sicca), confirmed by objective tests; a dry mouth (xerostomia), also confirmed objectively; and one of the so-called connective tissue disorders, usually rheumatoid arthritis.

Like rheumatoid arthritis, Sjogren's syndrome is considered an autoimmune disease. These are illnesses in which the body's immune system, geared to defend against and attack disease-causing bacteria and viruses, mistakenly attacks the body's own tissues. In SS, white blood cells called lymphocytes attack the tear glands, salivary glands, and other exocrine glands (those that release secretions). The lymphocytes invade the glands, affecting their activity and eventually destroying them.

Elaine Harris is one of the 50 percent of Sjogren's syndrome patients who has what is called primary SS. This affects the tear, salivary, and other moisture-producing glands but is not associated with a connective tissue disease like rheumatoid arthritis. The other half of Sjogren's syndrome patients have what is known as secondary SS. Their dry eyes or dry mouth *is* associated with one of the connective tissue diseases. Besides rheumatoid arthritis, these diseases include systemic lupus erythematosus (often called just lupus), characterized by joint pain without swelling and other symptoms, and scleroderma, a condition caused by circulation problems in the small blood vessels and resulting in scarring and hardening of the skin.

Since there is currently no cure for the disease, treatment aims to relieve the symptoms.

Because Sjogren's syndrome may also affect other moisture-producing glands besides the tear and salivary glands, it can lead to dry ears, nose, and throat, as well as to dryness in the digestive tract, vagina, and skin. In severe cases, other parts of the body are sometimes involved: the lungs, kidneys, blood vessels, and nervous system. Very rarely, SS patients develop cancer of the lymph glands. In most cases, the disease does not affect a person's lifespan.

Characteristics of Sjogren's

Individuals with SS often say their eyes feel gritty, as though they had sand or a foreign body in them. Without sufficient tears, the eyes may burn, itch, redden, or fill with mucus. Sjogren's sufferers may be troubled by blurred vision and sensitivity to light. Their eyes may tire easily, especially when they

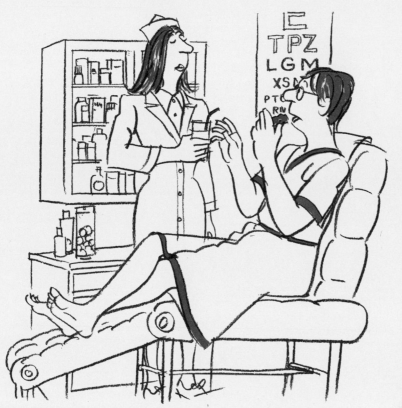

Patients typically have difficulty in swallowing a dry cracker.

Prevalence

Nine out of ten Sjogren's syndrome patients are women. Their mean age is 50. Yet people of all ages get SS, and it occurs among all races. No one is sure how many people have the disorder. A leading researcher, Dr. Norman Talal of the University of Texas Health Science Center at San Antonio, estimates that 15 percent of people with rheumatoid arthritis have secondary SS (or about 315,000 Americans) and that an equal number of people without connective tissue disease have primary SS.

People who live with Sjogren's syndrome, however, are usually less interested in numbers than in learning what their disease is, what treatments are available, and how they can live with their condition. No one knows its cause or cure (although it is thought viruses may play a role). A recent interest in research offers hope to people struggling with this chronic disease.

Diagnosis

Because SS affects various parts of the body, it is usually diagnosed by one of several medical specialists: an ophthalmologist consulted for eye problems; an ear, nose, and throat specialist, when the chief complaint is a dry mouth; a dentist consulted for a sudden outbreak of cavities; or a general practitioner, family physician, or internist, when symptoms point to an associated connective tissue disease. Individuals who suspect that they may have SS also consult or are referred to rheumatologists, who are internists subspecializing in the diagnosis and treatment of connective tissue diseases; immunologists, who specialize in disorders of the body's immune system; consultants in multidisciplinary medical centers; and special SS treatment centers (although only a few such centers exist at present).

In a simple preliminary test he calls "the cracker sign," Dr. Talal asks patients at his Sjogren's Syn-

are reading, watching television, or looking at a computer monitor.

When saliva is inadequate, people with SS have problems doing things they once took for granted: chewing, swallowing, and speaking. Food sticks to parched surfaces inside the mouth, making it necessary for individuals to drink fluids frequently while eating. With little or no saliva, SS sufferers must continually use some kind of lubricant to keep their mouths moist, often getting up in the middle of the night for a drink of water. A dry mouth causes the tongue, membranes on the inside of the cheeks, and lips to crack easily. Worse, without the protective substances in saliva, the teeth rapidly decay.

When the nose is affected, SS patients notice a buildup of crusts and scabs in the nostrils. They may have frequent nosebleeds. A dry throat easily becomes sore. The voice sounds hoarse. Dryness in the ears may lead to repeated inflammation of the middle

ear and a dry digestive tract to an irritated stomach. Bowel movements are difficult because of dryness, fatigue is common, the salivary glands may be swollen and painful, and there may be difficulty in breathing. When SS affects the sweat glands, the skin dries out. Patients then suffer chapped lips, cracked fingertips, brittle nails, and hair loss. In women, SS may attack the lubricant-secreting glands of the va-

Sjogren's is often associated with rheumatoid arthritis.

gina, causing pain during sexual intercourse.

Individuals with secondary SS suffer the joint pains, muscle weakness, skin rashes, and other symptoms of whatever connective tissue disease they have.

drome Clinic if they can swallow a dry cracker or piece of toast without drinking fluid. Invariably, patients with a dry mouth say they cannot.

Artificial tear preparations may offer relief to those who suffer from dry eyes.

To help confirm the diagnosis, both the amount of tears and of saliva can be measured by various objective tests. In one of the most important tests, a biopsy—removal and examination of tissue—is done on minor salivary glands in the lip or roof of the mouth; this can detect the invasion of telltale lymphocytes. Several types of autoantibodies—antibodies that mistakenly attack the body's own tissues—can be discovered through diagnostic blood tests.

Treatment

Once a diagnosis of Sjogren's syndrome has been confirmed, patients are usually treated by a team of physicians, including an ophthalmologist, dentist, and internal medicine specialist or subspecialist. Since there is no known cure for the disease, most treatments are aimed at relieving symptoms—which generally entails replacing lost moisture or conserving what little there is— and at preventing permanent damage to the eyes, mouth, and other tissues. Because of their serious side effects, steroids and powerful drugs that suppress the immune system are reserved for acute flareups or for those rare severe cases in which vital organs are attacked.

SS patients do well to avoid smoke and other environmental irritants, medications with drying side effects, and dry air, all of which make their symptoms worse. Many use a humidifier to add moisture to the air in their homes and, if possible, their workplaces.

For the dry-eyed, artificial tear preparations are the first line of defense. These are drops of varying viscosity, available on both a prescription and nonprescription basis. They generally must be applied a number of times a day. (Sometimes, after several months of use, the patient may become sensitive to the preservatives in a tear substitute and then must switch to another brand or to a preservative-free tear substitute.) Patients may also use a variety of gels and ointments to lubricate the eyes. Another product some find helpful is called Lacrisert—a pellet containing a supply of lubricating material that is placed between the lower eyelid and eye.

Severely dry-eyed patients resort to wearing watertight goggles called moisture chamber eyeglasses. By sealing in moisture, these specially made eyeglasses slow down the evaporation of natural and artificial tears. In extreme cases, an ophthalmologist performs what is called punctal occlusion to conserve a patient's tears. In this procedure, the doctor closes the channel through which tears drain into the nasal cavity, so that any tears the patient produces or tear substitute being used will be kept in the eye as long as possible. This can be done temporarily with plugs or permanently by cauterization.

To stimulate saliva flow, people with dry mouths chew sugarless gum, increase fluid intake, and suck on sugarless candy, a cherry pit, or even a button. Frequent sips of water and sugarless beverages, as well as use of artificial saliva, help keep the mouth moist. Drugs that stimulate saliva have many side effects and can be used only temporarily. Some patients are helped by electronic devices that stimulate saliva flow. (These devices work only in patients whose saliva glands are still functioning.) The loss of saliva leaves the teeth vulnerable to decay, making it extremely important to avoid sugar and control plaque buildup by frequent brushing, flossing, and fluoride application.

Moisturizing lip balms and skin lotions help to relieve dryness. For women bothered by vaginal dryness, a water-soluble lubricating product like K-Y Jelly may be useful.

Like others with chronic disorders, people with Sjogren's syndrome, often desperate for relief from their symptoms, must be wary of false claims of new or miracle "cures." The Sjogren's Syndrome Foundation, a nonprofit corporation, promotes research and education about the disease. Founded by Elaine Harris in 1983 as The Moisture Seekers, it is the first self-help group for SS patients, The foundation sponsors local chapters and mutual-aid groups around the United States, in Canada, and in other countries. In these local groups, patients share experiences and helpful tips, provide mutual support, and listen to experts speak on various aspects of SS.

Classic signs of Sjogren's are fatigue and insufficient tears and saliva.

The foundation also publishes a monthly newsletter for members, both patients and professionals interested in the disease. In 1989 it will publish *The Sjogren's Syndrome Handbook: An Authoritative Guide for Patients*, the first book written by medical specialists and other experts about the many manifestations of SS.

More information about Sjogren's syndrome can be obtained by sending a stamped, self-addressed, business-size envelope to the Sjogren's Syndrome Foundation, 382 Main Street, Port Washington, N.Y. 11050, or by calling the foundation at (516) 767-2866. □

Toilet Training

Michael K. Meyerhoff, Ed.D.

The one subject in early childhood guaranteed to raise parents' anxiety level is toilet training. While it is being contemplated and carried out, nothing seems to have higher priority or greater importance. Nevertheless, the process can be surprisingly smooth and simple as long as readiness is respected and relaxation is the rule. Although "training" is the term typically used, what really takes place is "education," and the easiest and most effective way to educate children is to teach them what they want to learn when they want to learn it.

Many parents want to have their child trained early. They may feel pressure from friends and relatives or be worried about meeting enrollment requirements for preschool. Or they may just be tired of dealing with dirty diapers. However, no matter how eager, or how determined and methodical, a mother and father may be, their efforts are likely to result in frustration and failure—and even prove counterproductive—unless they hold off until the child is mature enough to handle the situation and can be recruited as an enthusiastic partner.

When to Begin

Successful toilet training requires that children have the physical capacity to control both bladder and bowel. Some children may appear to have been trained extraordinarily early, but what really happened is that their parents simply learned to whisk them away to the bathroom in the nick of time. True training cannot take place until children recognize the sensations immediately preceding urination and defecation, are able to constrict their sphincter muscles accordingly, and can get to the

> **Toilet training can go smoothly if the child is ready and the parents are relaxed.**

bathroom, undress, climb on the potty or adapter seat and then relax their sphincter muscles so that elimination can take place.

This is a complex set of activities, and children cannot be rushed into mastering all the elements. The development of sufficient internal control rarely occurs before 18 months of age, and the majority of children still do not have it by their second birthday. By the time all the other necessary skills come along as well, many children are approaching their third birthday, and some will already have passed it. Given the variety of skills involved and the great differences in the rates at which children develop, indications of readiness—at the very least, signs that a child recognizes when he or she is about to wet or soil the diaper—coming anywhere between two and four years of age should be considered well within the normal range.

Motivational factors are also important. Children approaching their second birthday are developing a sense of self, and they delight in exercising their personal power. For several months this shows itself in a tendency to say "no" to virtually any request. Thus, there is a good chance two-year-olds will not be willing to follow toilet-training instructions. It is a good idea to wait until later, when they will be more civil and will be actively seeking parental approval.

During the third year of life children begin to engage in a great deal of role play and fantasy behavior, regularly imitating their parents and otherwise expressing a desire to grow up. Also, as they become more interested in out-of-home activities and play with other children, walking around in dirty diapers and going through the fuss of being changed become sources of discomfort and distress for them. Waiting for such sentiments to kick in makes a lot of sense.

Differences and Dangers

Girls usually are toilet trained a bit earlier than boys, and for both sexes bowel control ordinarily precedes bladder control. However, individual patterns of development are so variable, and the contributing factors so complicated, that one child's readiness at a certain age is never an accurate gauge by which to assess or worry about the readiness of playmates or of a brother or sister, even a twin.

Waiting to begin toilet training may mean more work for parents and more money spent on diapers. But starting too soon can have serious psychological consequences. Inappropriately early attempts can instill a sense of failure in the child that may have long-lasting, deleterious effects on self-esteem. In addition, they can create feelings of anxiety about the entire process that will make later attempts more difficult and may even result in regressive tendencies that can emerge as late as the teen years. Starting too soon can also cause extra stress for the parents. Tragically, parental frustration over unsuccessful toilet-training tactics is a principal trigger for child abuse.

How to Proceed

Toilet training is a learning process, not a disciplinary action.

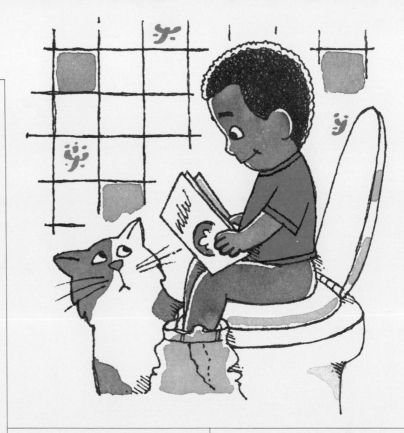

When children seem to be approaching readiness, it is a good idea to help them gradually become comfortable with the different aspects of the experience. Encourage them to say when they are about to go (or at least when they *are* going). Identify relevant body parts and functions. It might help to have the child accompany a parent or older sibling of the same sex to the bathroom or practice sitting on the potty chair or adapter seat while still clothed.

Once a child has displayed adequate awareness of bodily urges and familiarity with the appropriate procedures, the next step is to provide ample opportunities for all this new knowledge to be put to use. At a time during which elimination tends to occur (for example, half an hour after a meal or upon waking from a nap), the child can be taken to the bathroom, assisted in undressing and getting seated, and told that from now on the toilet should be used instead of the diaper. The child should be accompanied at all times, be treated with patience, and be praised for any progress—no matter how small. Children should not be forced to stay seated, and shaming or punishing them for noncompliance or imperfect performance should be avoided. Toilet training usually takes several days and sometimes requires a couple of weeks.

Problems and Precautions

A child may appear to achieve success but then suffer an "accident." It is important not to overreact to this. The child may well feel worse than anyone else. By matter-of-factly cleaning up and then suggesting going to the toilet "to see if there's any more," one can keep the accident from being blown out of proportion and help put the child on track.

Occasionally, a child may threaten an "accident" to obtain, say, a toy or extra attention. Parents definitely should not give in, nor convey the impression

that the accident produced the desired effect. Responding casually to the mess and involving the child in its cleanup will deny him or her the satisfaction being sought and, in addition, should provide sufficient punishment without allowing toilet training itself to become an issue.

Full regression is another matter, and it usually indicates a deeper emotional problem. A death in the family, prolonged separation from a parent, and the arrival of a new sibling are common causes. With such regression it is a good idea to go back to diapers for a while so as not to make the situation worse. Although it may be necessary to "start all over again" at some later point, as long as the child has not been made to feel ashamed, fearful, or resentful, toilet training should be considerably easier the second time around. If sibling jealousy seems to be the source, talking about the disadvantages of being a baby while simultaneously suspending some "big kid" privileges may assist in speeding up the process.

It must be noted that difficulty in training, accidents, or regression

may very well be due to a physical problem. Diarrhea can cause a lack of control, and constipation can produce a lack of cooperation. Allergies and infections can also cause the best efforts of parents and child to be defeated. Therefore, if a child shows excessive resistance to training, seems unable to achieve success despite apparent readiness and willingness, or suffers repeated, unexplained accidents or unexplained regression, a visit to the pediatrician is in order.

Recommended Reading

Parents preparing their children for toilet training, or seeking to motivate them during the process, may find it helpful to read them special books about the subject. The following are a few especially appropriate choices:

ALLISON, ALIDA. *Toddler's Potty Book.* Los Angeles, Price, Stern, Sloan, 1985.
FRANKEL, ALONA. *Once Upon a Potty.* Woodbury, N.Y., Barrons, 1980 (boys' version), 1984 (girls' version).
LANSKY, VICKI. *Koko Bear's New Potty.* New York, Bantam, 1986.

Detecting Cancer Early

Susan S. Lichtendorf

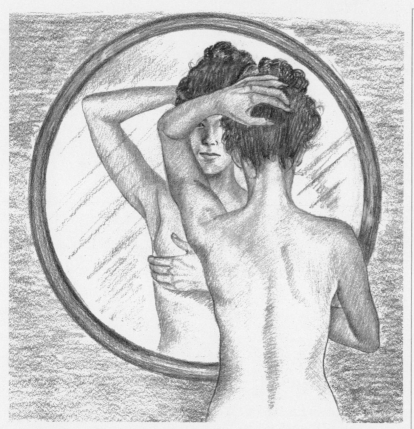

people who are basically healthy.

That early detection is a goal worth achieving is strikingly clear. The American Cancer Society estimates that of the half-million Americans who die of cancer each year, some 178,000 might have been saved through early detection and prompt treatment. For example, for colon cancer the chance of being cured—which usually means being free of the disease five years after diagnosis—

Many deaths from cancer could be prevented if the disease were detected in an early stage.

is almost 90 percent if the disease is found in an early stage. The chance of cure drops to 40 percent if the cancer is found in a more advanced stage. When breast cancer is detected before it has had a chance to spread, the chance of five-year survival is almost 100 percent; once the cancer has spread, the rate drops to 60 percent.

Beyond lifesaving potential, early detection may allow for less traumatic treatment. A woman found to have an extremely small, early breast tumor may have only the cancerous portion of the breast removed and be spared the ordeal of a mastectomy, in which the entire breast is removed.

In some instances, screening tests can uncover precancerous conditions that can be treated and cured before cancer develops. The Pap test—which involves laboratory analysis of a sample of cells from the cervix, taken by the

Right now—without waiting for new medical discoveries—it is possible to prevent a greater number of deaths from cancer. The key is finding the disease early, when it can be most easily and successfully treated. Early detection is a goal that can be achieved for several of the major forms of cancer because of the availability of simple diagnostic tests and do-it-yourself procedures. Knowing some of the major warning signs of different types of cancer and having the checkups and screening tests recommended by cancer specialists can actually mean the difference between life and death.

Benefits of Early Detection

Early detection works because of the way cancer becomes established in the body. In cancer, there is uncontrolled growth and spread of abnormal cells. The process begins in a limited number of cells in a particular place in the body. If those cancerous cells can be found where they began to grow, before they have had a chance to invade and destroy surrounding tissue and ultimately to send malignant cells to other, more distant sites in the body, the chance of successful treatment is measurably better. Early detection is designed to do just that—to find cancer while it is still localized, in physician during a pelvic examination—can indicate precancerous cervical changes usually treatable with office procedures. A doctor's checkup can lead to the detection and removal from the colon of a particular kind of polyp, or growth of tissue, likely to evolve into cancer. No single blood test is useful for screening asymptomatic people for the common adult cancers.

A Question of Age

Certain types of cancer become more common with age, and people over 40 should have more frequent and more extensive screening tests. But cancer can occur at any age; the accompanying tables give recommended tests for various age groups.

Cancer can also strike children. The signs of childhood cancer may be difficult to recognize because they can have many other explanations. At some time most children bruise, complain of headaches, limp, vomit, lose some weight, or seem overly tired. While there can be many explanations for a loss of energy, weight loss, or bruising, there is always the faint possibility of leukemia. While a limp might be the result of a minor sports injury, bone cancer is a slight possibility. For parents, the key to dealing with that kind of frightening chance is to make sure that their children have regular medical checkups and to call a physician's attention to persistent symptoms or unusual behavior.

Tests for Women

Women need to be concerned about breast and uterine cancer. In the case of breast cancer, they can themselves help look for early signs of the disease.

Breast Cancer. Beginning no later than age 20, women should perform monthly breast self-examinations. Breast cancer is the most common cancer among women, and 90 percent of all tumors are found by women themselves. In the examination—which should be done about a week after the men-

---

CANCER CHECKUPS FOR WOMEN

Age	Action
Teens +	Annual pelvic examination and Pap test for those who are sexually active or have reached age 18; after a woman has had normal Pap tests and pelvic examinations for three consecutive years, Pap tests may be performed less frequently at the physician's discretion.
20-40	Monthly skin self-examination; monthly breast self-examination; breast examination by physician every three years; cancer-related checkup, including complete physical examination, every three years. Between ages 35-39, baseline mammogram. Continue regular Pap tests.
40 +	Annual digital rectal examination for colorectal cancer; annual breast examination by physician; mammogram every one to two years; for women at risk of endometrial cancer, tissue sampling at menopause; annual cancer-related checkup. Continue regular Pap tests, monthly self-examinations.
50 +	Mammogram every year; annual blood stool test, as well as annual digital rectal examination; procto examination every three to five years after two initial normal tests one year apart. Continue regular Pap tests, monthly self-examinations, annual checkups.

Source: American Cancer Society

---

strual period, when breasts are smallest and easiest to examine—a woman should be alert to any lump, thickening, or change in the breasts or any discharge from the nipples; such symptoms should be discussed with a physician, who may decide to do further tests. Most lumps are *not* cancer.

In addition to self-examination, a woman should have her breasts examined by a physician every three years until she is 40 and annually after age 40. Between the ages of 35 and 39 a woman should also have a baseline mammogram, which can be used for comparison with mammograms taken in the years ahead. A mammogram is a low-dose X-ray picture of the breast that is one of the most important means of early cancer detection, since it can find tumors too small to be felt. A mammogram should be taken every one or two years when a woman is in her 40s, annually from age 50 on.

Uterine Cancer. Over the past 40 years, deaths from uterine cancer (including cancer of the cervix and endometrium, or lining of the uterus), once the number one cancer killer of American women, have declined by more than 70 percent—because of the Pap test and regular checkups. Pap tests, primarily for the detection of cervical cancer, are recommended once a woman has reached age 18 or has become sexually active. Health experts have disagreed as to how often Pap tests are needed. However, the American Cancer Society and the American College of Obstetricians and Gynecologists in early 1988 agreed on the following guidelines: Women should have annual Pap tests and pelvic examinations until they have had three consecutive normal results. After that, at their doctors' discretion, they can have the tests done less frequently.

As a woman grows older, her risk of endometrial cancer increases. Since the Pap test is only about 50 percent effective in detecting this kind of uterine cancer, it is recommended that at menopause, women at risk have a sample of endometrial tissue taken—this is done in an office procedure—and analyzed to look for cancer cells. Depending on the patient, the doctor might schedule future biopsies. (See the accompanying list of risk factors for various types of cancer.)

Tests for Men

Testicular cancer is one of the most common cancers in men between the ages of 15 and 34. Survival is close to 100 percent if cases are detected early, but many men are unaware of the need to perform a monthly self-examination of the testes. The self-examination should be done after a warm shower or bath, when the scrotal skin is relaxed. Men should look for any slight enlargement, lumps, or change in consistency, and anything unusual should be checked by a physician.

Prostate cancer is the third most common cancer in American men. Some 85 percent of patients whose cancer is discovered early survive; the rate drops to 48 percent if the cancer has spread. For early detection, men over age 40 should have an annual rectal examination done by a physician.

Other Cancers

For both women and men, the risk of colorectal cancer increases with the passing years. Colorectal cancer is the second most common cancer, behind lung cancer, in the United States. Early detection involves three things. From age 40 on, everyone should have an annual digital rectal examination, a quick and simple procedure done by a physician. After the age of 50, all people should have an annual test for blood in the stool. Persons over 50 should also have proctosigmoidoscopy, in which the physician examines the rectum and lower colon by means of a lighted tube. This procedure, done in the doctor's office, should be performed annually at first, then once every three to five years

for people who have had two consecutive normal annual exams.

Most cases of skin cancer are highly curable. However, one kind—malignant melanoma, which strikes 27,000 Americans every year—can be fatal. Early detection is critical in curing ma-

CANCER CHECKUPS FOR MEN

Age	Action
Teens +	Monthly testicular self-examination.
20-40	Monthly skin self-examination; cancer-related checkup every three years, including complete physical examination. Continue monthly testicular self-examination.
40 +	Annual digital rectal examination for colorectal cancer, prostate cancer; annual cancer-related checkup. Continue monthly self-examinations.
50 +	Annual blood stool test, as well as annual digital rectal examination; procto examination every three to five years after two initial normal tests one year apart. Continue monthly self-examinations, annual checkups.

Source: American Cancer Society

lignant melanoma since it almost always spreads. Adults should examine all skin surfaces on a monthly basis. New moles or growths that are irregularly shaped or colored, as well as a sudden change in an existing mole, should be called to the attention of a physician.

Checkups and Warning Signs

The recommendations for different screening tests at different intervals can be confusing. To simplify matters, experts recommend having a cancer-related checkup every three years between the ages of 20 and 40, and annually thereafter.

A cancer-related checkup for healthy people without symptoms should include the diagnostic tests noted in the accompanying tables. In addition, there should be physical examination of the mouth, thyroid, skin, and lymph nodes, as well as of the testes and prostate in men and of the ovaries in women. The checkup should allow sufficient time for the doctor and patient to talk about diet, cigarette smoking, family history, and risk factors (including occupational health hazards). Self-examination techniques should be taught.

Between checkups—indeed, at any time—alertness to physical changes is mandatory. Cancer may or may not be present—very often it is not. But if it is, the earliest possible diagnosis is essential. Be on the lookout for the following warning signals of cancer, and see a doctor if you recognize any. (Note: the first letters spell out the word "caution.")

• Change in bowel or bladder habits
• A sore that does not heal
• Unusual bleeding or discharge
• Thickening or lump in the breast or elsewhere
• Indigestion or difficulty in swallowing
• Obvious change in a wart or a mole
• Nagging cough or hoarseness

The early detection guidelines presented here are for the general population. Within that population are people at higher-than-normal risk of developing particular forms of cancer. High risk is not a decree that one will develop

RISK FACTORS FOR MAJOR FORMS OF CANCER

Risk factors and what to do about them should be discussed with a physician. Having a particular risk factor does *not* mean you will get cancer. The degree of correlation between specific risk factors and cancers differs.

Bladder Cancer
Higher incidence in men; cigarette smoking; exposure to chemicals used in rubber, petroleum, photographic, and leather tanning industries.

Breast Cancer
Increases with age beginning at 50; personal or family history of breast cancer; never had children or had first child after age 30.

Colorectal Cancer
Personal or family history of colorectal cancer or colorectal polyps; history of inflammatory bowel disease. Diet high in fat and/or low in fiber may be a causative factor.

Leukemia
Excessive exposure to radiation or certain chemicals (benzene, for example). Linked with some hereditary disorders like Down's syndrome.

Lung Cancer
Currently smoke cigarettes; past history of smoking for 20 or more years; industrial exposure to substances like asbestos, particularly for smokers. Passive smoking and prolonged exposure to radon may contribute to risk.

Oral Cancer
Use of cigarettes, cigars, pipes, smokeless tobacco; excess use of alcohol.

Ovarian Cancer
Risk increases with age, with highest incidence in women between ages 65-84. Other possible risk factors include never having had children; history of breast, endometrial cancers.

Pancreatic Cancer
Risk increases with age, with highest incidence between 65-79; cigarette smoking. Other possible risk factors include chronic pancreatitis; diabetes; cirrhosis; high-fat diet.

Prostate Cancer
Risk increases with age and is most common over 65; especially common among American blacks. Other possible risk factors include high-fat diet.

Skin Cancer
Excess exposure to sun; fair complexion; industrial exposure to coal tar, pitch, creosote, arsenic compounds, or radium.

Testicular Cancer
Highest incidence in men between ages 15-34; history of undescended or late-descended testicles.

Uterine Cancer
For cervical cancer: early age at first intercourse; multiple sex partners; genital warts.
For endometrial cancer: highest incidence is between ages 55-69; late menopause; history of infertility or failure of ovulation; obesity; prolonged estrogen therapy.

Source: American Cancer Society

cancer. Rather, it should be regarded as an indication that more intensive health checkups and appropriate preventive measures are necessary. It is especially important that people at risk for lung cancer stop smoking, and while everyone should avoid excess sun, elderly, fair-skinned people should be especially careful because they are at high risk. (See the accompanying risk factor list.)

As in any other field of medicine, advice about cancer detection changes and is sometimes controversial. Just a few years ago, some health experts enthusiastically advocated annual checkups for all adults, annual Pap tests for every woman, and annual procto examinations for all people over 40. These recommendations have changed largely because the costs of such widespread screening seem to far outweigh the potential benefits. Some doctors may, however, recommend more frequent screening for their patients than outlined in the general guidelines here.

Many people may have fears about the process of cancer detection. Perhaps a particular test will hurt. And many women fear that the radiation used in mammography might itself cause cancer—although in actuality the X-ray doses are so low that the risk is almost nonexistent. Beyond this, perhaps the most important fear that needs to be overcome is the fear that cancer will be found. But ignoring the need for testing does not mean that cancer, if it is present, will go away. On the other hand, undergoing testing and thereby possibly detecting cancer early may save your life. □

Chicken Pox

Raymond B. Karasic, M.D.

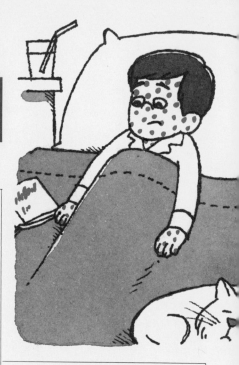

Chicken pox may be the last of the great childhood rashes. While effective vaccines have reduced the chances of catching measles, rubella (German measles), and other important illnesses, chicken pox remains as common as ever. But its days are numbered—a vaccine to prevent it is just around the corner.

Pox Vobiscum

Chicken pox, also called varicella, is an extremely contagious disease that is best known for its distinctive, itchy rash. Although no one is sure why the disease is called "chicken pox," some experts believe that the blistery skin rash was named after the chick-pea.

The illness is caused by the varicella-zoster (V-Z) virus, a member of the herpesvirus family. People catch chicken pox by being exposed to the airborne viral particles that are shed from the skin blisters (and probably also the respiratory passages) of infected individuals. Once the virus enters the body via the throat or surface of the eye, it takes about 14 days to complete its journey to the skin and cause the rash. Chicken pox is so catching that if a susceptible person comes in close contact with the disease, he or she has more than a 90 percent chance of wearing spots within the next few weeks. Patients with chicken pox are contagious from roughly one day before the rash starts until about a week later, when all of the blisters have dried up.

Almost everyone who recovers from chicken pox develops protective antibodies that make an individual resistant to a later attack by the V-Z virus. The good news, therefore, is that second bouts of chicken pox are extremely rare; the bad news is that once the symptoms of chicken pox subside, the V-Z virus doesn't just go away. Instead, it tends to remain inside the individual forever, lying dormant in clumps of nerves (called ganglia) next to the spinal cord and brain.

As is true of other herpesviruses, the slumbering V-Z virus can be reactivated at a later time by certain infections, cancer, or other stresses. Once reawakened, the virus travels along nerve endings from the ganglia back to the skin, where it causes a localized, often painful rash on the trunk or face known as herpes zoster, or shingles. Because this rash is chock-full of active V-Z virus, herpes zoster is highly contagious (and can cause chicken pox in people exposed to it). Fortunately, most people who get chicken pox never develop shingles.

Symptoms and Signs

The hallmark of chicken pox is the distinctive-looking rash. In fact, the disease is usually easy to diagnose on the basis of the rash alone.

The rash progresses through several stages. It begins as small red spots and bumps, which quickly evolve into the typical watery blisters with red halos that are often described as "dewdrops on rose petals." The rash, which is usually very itchy, can occur anywhere on the body's surface, although it tends to be most concentrated over the central portions of the body, such as the trunk, face, upper arms, and upper legs. As new blisters continue to appear in batches over the next five to seven days, older ones begin to dry up and form crusts, or scabs; as a result, the rash contains a motley mixture of red bumps, blisters, and crusts. The scabs fall off in about one to three weeks and, if left alone, usually heal without scarring. On the other hand, vigorous scratching of fresh scabs can dislodge them prematurely, resulting in permanent scars.

The majority of children with chicken pox experience mild fever (less than 102°F) or none at all. The fever may be accompanied by headache, poor appetite, and just plain not feeling well.

Problem Patients

For most healthy children, chicken pox is more of a nuisance than a serious illness, and complete recovery is the rule. However, certain groups of patients are prone to develop a more serious case of the disease.

Individuals who manage to escape the infection as children can catch chicken pox when they become adults. The disease is generally a more serious problem in grown-ups than in children. Adults who are afflicted commonly have high fever, general body aches, and a widespread rash. They are also more prone to complications.

Young babies, like older children, usually have no trouble coping with chicken pox. However, infection of a pregnant woman with the V-Z virus can have dire consequences for her developing fetus or newborn infant. If the virus attacks the fetus, it can cause birth defects involving the eyes, limbs, and nervous system. If the mother comes down with chicken pox just before delivery, her newborn is at risk for developing a severe case of chicken pox. Luckily, both kinds of situations are extremely rare.

Patients whose immune systems have been weakened by certain malignancies (such as leukemia) or medications (such as steroids and anticancer drugs) are also at risk for an unusually severe case. In such patients chicken pox is a life-threatening condition. It is associated with high fever (sometimes reaching 105°F) and an extensive rash that can cover the body from head to toe. Without a working immune system to keep the V-Z virus in check, the ambitious virus can invade internal organs, such as the liver and lungs, or the nervous system. Before the advent of effective antiviral medications such as acyclovir (brand name, Zovirax) to combat the virus, as many as 15 out of 100 children with such severe chicken pox died; fortunately, nowadays the mortality rate is much lower.

Complications

Although most children with chicken pox sail through their illnesses without a hitch, complications can arise. Skin infections occasionally develop when bacteria that ordinarily live on the skin invade the chicken pox blisters or scabs. The problem is seldom serious and is usually treated with antibiotics.

A rare complication of chicken pox is encephalitis, or inflammation of the brain. The most common form of encephalitis associated with chicken pox involves the cerebellum, the part of the brain that controls balance. As a result, affected individuals typically stagger when they try to walk and generally have trouble with their coordination. As frightening

as this complication can be, it usually disappears over several days without any special treatment. More severe forms of brain inflammation can also occur, but luckily they are very rare.

Reye's syndrome, affecting children and adolescents, is an uncommon but serious complication of chicken pox, influenza, and other viral illnesses. It causes swelling of the brain and accumulation of fat in the liver. The illness usually begins with severe vomiting and sleepiness, which can progress rapidly to coma. Although no one knows what causes Reye's syndrome, there is some evidence that taking aspirin during the preceding bout of chicken pox or flu may increase the chances of getting it. Until the possible role of aspirin is clarified, it makes sense for children and teenagers to avoid taking aspirin during chicken pox or flu-like illnesses.

Although chicken pox seldom causes pneumonia in children, adults and individuals with impaired immunity are much more likely to contract it. Patients with pneumonia often need to be treated in a hospital.

Treatment

Most cases of chicken pox can be treated with tender loving care and a little time—generally a week or so. Bed rest usually is not necessary unless the patient is exceptionally sick. Since itching tends to be the most bothersome symptom, medications that coat the skin—such as calamine lotion—can be soothing. If lotions alone don't relieve the itching, oral antihistamines may do the trick. It is also a good idea to cut the fingernails short, especially in young children; this may keep the child from digging at the rash and thus prevent scarring. Fever, headache, and body aches can be treated with an aspirin substitute like acetaminophen.

Traditional antibiotics are not used to treat chicken pox since they do not work against viruses. The newer antiviral drugs like acy-

clovir are also not given to the average chicken pox sufferer but are usually reserved for the most severe cases.

Preventing Pox

Throughout history, chicken pox has been as much a part of growing up as pimples, and just about as welcome. But thanks to recent medical advances, it may soon join the ranks of once common infectious diseases, like polio, that have become nearly extinct.

There are two different ways to immunize a person against chicken pox. One approach is to give a blood product called varicella-zoster immune globulin (or VZIG), which contains antibodies against the V-Z virus. Since the protection lasts only for a few weeks, VZIG is used primarily to prevent infection in patients with weakened immune systems who are accidentally exposed to the V-Z virus.

More permanent protection could be provided by a vaccine—and in fact, a vaccine to prevent chicken pox may soon be approved by the Food and Drug Administration for use in the United States. Already in use in Japan, where it was developed over ten years ago, the vaccine contains an attenuated (weakened) virus that makes a person immune to the V-Z virus without causing disease. The vaccine works extremely well in healthy children and very well even in those with serious underlying conditions like leukemia. Unfortunately, it is not nearly as effective in adults.

There is still debate in the medical community over whether to try to immunize all American children with the vaccine at around 15 months of age (when they get their measles, mumps, and rubella shot) or to restrict its use to patients with faulty immune systems. Most experts currently favor the first approach, which means that once the vaccine becomes available, children will have to find other excuses besides chicken pox for missing school. □

Safety at the Salad Bar

Ingrid J. Strauch

Salad used to be a simple matter: some iceberg lettuce, a few radishes or raw carrots, and salad dressing. At its most exotic, some croutons were sprinkled on top. Not anymore. With the advent of self-service salad bars in restaurants, take-out food establishments, and even some grocery stores, "salad" has evolved into a complex production of raw, cooked, and preserved vegetables, fruits, pasta and seafood concoctions, Jell-O, meat, cheese, stuffed grape leaves, sushi, and garnishes too numerous to mention. Some salad bars include hot foods as well, such as stir-fried combinations, fried chicken, egg rolls, macaroni and cheese, meat loaf, and barbecued ribs.

As more and more people seek healthful and nutritious foods when they eat out, salad bars have become increasingly popular. While the mile-long salad bar may make lunch more healthful—as well as more fun—it also creates many opportunities for bacteria to contaminate the food, which can be exposed to varying temperatures and air-borne pollutants for several hours. Because most of the harmful bacteria that may be found in food are colorless, odorless, and tasteless, a consumer cannot always know by looking, smelling, or tasting which, if any, items in a salad bar have been contaminated. There are, however, steps that can be taken to minimize the chances of contracting a case of food poisoning.

Things to Look For

Temperature. The temperature at which food is stored and served is of utmost importance. One fact to remember is that it is dangerous to eat food that's been kept between 40°F and 140°F for more than two hours (with the exception of foods that are normally stored at room temperature). Bacteria thrive and multiply most successfully in this temperature danger zone.

Of course, when purchasing food from a salad bar, you won't know the exact temperature or how long it has been there. Therefore, try to choose a busy salad bar where food must be replenished regularly—or you may be getting yesterday's leftovers. Beyond that, note the relative hotness or coldness of food when eaten immediately after purchasing it. Beware of items that reach room temperature quickly. If the cold section of the salad bar is kept cold with ice, notice whether the ice seems to have been replenished recently or is allowed to melt completely, possibly causing food temperatures to rise to dangerous levels. There should be condensation on metal containers holding cold food and steam rising from hot food. Finally, eat the food soon after purchasing it, especially in the summer.

Mold and yeast. Two obvious signs of food deterioration are mold or slime resulting from yeast infection. While mold and yeast themselves rarely cause illness, their presence may indicate that the food has been kept too long in

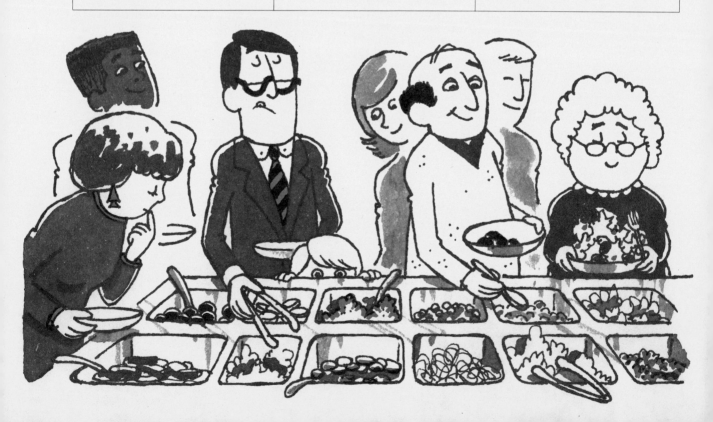

conditions that are favorable for possibly harmful bacteria.

Choosing Safe Foods

Raw vegetables and fruits are usually safe choices at the salad bar. Make sure raw produce looks crisp and clean and is kept in the refrigerated section of the serving area. Any fruit or vegetable that is wilted, has begun to turn brown around cut edges, or is mushy or limp has probably been kept too long or stored improperly. Although eating old produce may not cause sickness, the food's flavor, texture, and color will be unappetizing, and its nutritional content will have decreased.

Other usually safe selections at the salad bar include items that do not normally require refrigeration, such as nuts, seeds, and dried fruits. These items will become stale and dusty, however, if kept too long.

Canned vegetables and fruits are generally free from bacterial growth, since commercially canned food is processed under strict sanitation rules. But once the cans are opened and the food is displayed in the salad bar, it is susceptible to spoilage, just like fresh produce. Beware of brown spots, signs of mold or yeast, and bad odors. Preserved vegetables, such as pickles, rarely harbor harmful bacteria.

Salad bar items most susceptible to contamination are meat, poultry, fish, shellfish, milk products, tofu, eggs, gravies, pasta salads, and cooked vegetables, or any composed salad containing these ingredients. Contrary to popular belief, commercial mayonnaise itself is not likely to cause food poisoning: it is full of acid flavorings that inhibit bacterial growth. Foods served in a mayonnaise dressing are thus to some extent protected from harmful bacteria. However, they may still be susceptible to bacterial growth.

In addition, bacteria can be easily spread to less susceptible foods if utensils are not cleaned between uses. For this reason, each item in a salad bar should have its own serving utensil, and customers should be careful to put back utensils where they found them.

Cleanliness

The general appearance of a restaurant or store and its workers may give valuable clues as to the conditions under which food is prepared and stored. There should be a protective hood, or "sneeze guard," over the salad bar to prevent customers from breathing directly on it. The serving area should be kept clean, and there should be an attendant who wipes up spills regularly with a clean rag. The attendant should discard misplaced items; returning them to their serving containers can cause cross contamination.

Note the appearance of employees. Their hands should be clean, and long hair should be tied back or in a hair net. They should not eat or smoke on the job, nor should they be working with uncovered food if they have an obvious illness or one that causes coughing or sneezing. When replenishing salad bar selections, they should use plastic gloves or utensils to handle the food, being careful to use a separate utensil for each item. Notice also the behavior of the other patrons: Are they smoking, coughing, or sneezing over the food? Are they using their hands to serve themselves? If conditions are not optimal, it might be a good idea to take your patronage elsewhere.

Common Food-borne Illnesses

When storage, preparation, and serving conditions are not right, microorganisms waste no time invading food, as evidenced by the millions of cases of food-borne illness Americans suffer each year. One of the most common is salmonellosis, which results when *Salmonella* bacteria infect food, usually meat, poultry, eggs, fish, and milk products. Only heating food to 150°F or higher will kill the bacteria—cold does not kill them—so beware of cooked salad bar items that appear underdone.

Staphylococcal food poisoning is usually caused when the *Staphylococcus aureus* bacterium is transmitted to food by infected individuals, often kitchen workers. The bacteria produce toxins that flourish in foods such as meat, eggs, and milk products and are resistant to high temperatures.

Perfringens food poisoning is caused by *Clostridium perfringens*, a widely occurring bacterium that is easily destroyed by heat but produces spores that can withstand conditions that kill the bacteria. It is commonly found in soups and stews.

Storing food at room temperature is a major problem with all of these bacteria. Any bacteria that have not been killed during cooking will multiply rapidly if the food is not kept cool or hot enough.

In addition to toxic bacteria, some foods may be infected with worms or their larvae. The most familiar parasitic roundworm in the United States is *Trichinella spiralis*, which causes trichinosis. Infection results from eating undercooked meat, particularly pork, that contains the larvae.

Flies and cockroaches are never welcome near food. The mere sight of a fly or roach on food is enough to dissuade most people from eating it; these insects can act as transmitters of disease.

Most cases of food poisoning are characterized by nausea, vomiting, and diarrhea that clear up spontaneously within one to seven days. The severity of the symptoms depends in part on the bacteria involved, and treatment generally requires no more than resting and replenishing fluids. If you suspect a case of food poisoning, contact a doctor when symptoms are severe or when the victim is very young, old, or has a chronic illness. If you think an illness was caused by food eaten at a restaurant or bought at a delicatessen, phone the local health authorities and file a report. Your call may save others from the same fate. □

IMPOTENCE
A Treatable Problem

Marc Cendron, M.D., and Philip M. Hanno, M.D.

Impotence, a term derived from the Latin word for "power," is defined as the inability to achieve an erection sufficient for sexual intercourse. Over the centuries, difficulties with erection—and the anxieties and insecurities generated by such a problem—have been described in both the lay and medical literature. This topic has received even more attention in the last 20 years. With increasing awareness of the problem, a better understanding has developed of male sexual function—and dysfunction.

At the same time, new forms of diagnosis and treatment have been developed. The study of impotence is one of the most active fields in urology. It is now felt that almost any man who visits a doctor complaining of some form of sexual dysfunction can be diagnosed properly and treated satisfactorily, so that virtually all patients can resume satisfying sexual relationships.

Normal Sexual Function

In order for a man to engage in sexual intercourse, erection must occur. This involves the interplay of the nervous system, the blood vessels, and hormones. These mechanisms can be described as follows: Erection occurs when various nerves produce changes in the blood vessels in the penis. Blood accumulates in the penis, causing it to become engorged, rigid, and elevated, and able to penetrate the vagina. The male hormone testosterone, produced by the testes, is necessary for all this to occur. Sperm and secretions from the prostate gland and seminal vesicles (located near the bladder) are then deposited into the urethra (the tube that carries urine from the bladder). Ejaculation occurs when involuntary muscular contractions expel semen down the urethra and out of the penis; this is usually accompanied by orgasm and is followed by detumescence (the return of the penis to its nonerect state).

Possible Causes of Impotence

An estimated 10 million American men suffer from impotence. The incidence in the general population is estimated to be about 5 percent in the fifth decade of life, increasing to 35 percent by the seventh decade and 60 percent in the eighth decade. There are several possible causes.

Psychological causes contribute to about half of all cases of impotence. Such factors as stress, anxiety, and depression play important roles here. Often a man whose impotence has a psychological basis may be impotent only in certain circumstances—with one sexual partner, say, but not another.

Anatomic causes include congenital abnormalities of the genitals, a condition called Peyronie's disease (a disease affecting middle-aged men that is marked by the development of scar tissue in the penis, causing pain and curvature during erection), and priapism (prolonged, painful erections that are not associated with sexual desire and that result in scarring of the erectile tissues). Infections of the genital tract may also cause pain on arousal or ejaculation and can add to sexual dysfunction.

Atherosclerosis (hardening of the arteries) can affect the blood vessels of the penis as well as the vessels elsewhere in the body and will decrease the amount of blood flow available to produce an erection. Known risk factors for atherosclerosis, such as smoking and high blood cholesterol levels, can, over the years, cause impotence.

Neurologic diseases can also interfere with sexual functioning. Multiple sclerosis is an example. Tumors or injuries affecting the nervous system can lead to impotence as well.

Other diseases may cause impotence. Diabetes, which often affects nerves and blood vessels, and kidney failure are the conditions most commonly responsible. In addition, diseases that affect the level of different hormones account for 10 percent of cases of impotence; these are usually caused by disorders of the pituitary gland, which stimulates the testes to produce testosterone.

Certain drugs and medications interfere with sexual function. Blood pressure medications, antidepressants, estrogen pills, amphetamines, barbiturates, and sedatives can inhibit erections, as can alcohol and certain drugs like cocaine and marijuana.

Finding the Cause

Doctors trying to determine the cause of a patient's impotence will generally start with a careful history of the patient's problem, which may include certain possibly associated sexual problems, such as premature ejaculation, inability to ejaculate, and decreased sexual drive. A thorough physical examination may give the physician clues to the causes of the patient's impotence, such as underlying diseases. Blood tests can indicate if there are hormonal deficiencies, such as low levels of testosterone.

Recently, several new diagnostic techniques have been developed. One is the monitoring of nighttime erections; if a man has erections during sleep, his impo-

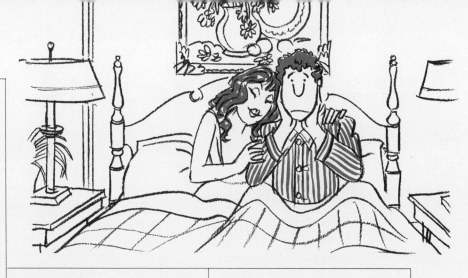

tence most likely has an emotional basis. The doctor also may test penile blood pressure and pulse, perform penile arteriography (injection of a dye followed by an X ray to study the penis's blood supply), and X-ray the erectile tissues (a procedure called cavernosography). Psychological tests may also be given.

Treatment

Many psychologically based sexual problems will disappear with simple reassurance by the physician and with time. Rare are men who have never experienced an episode of erectile dysfunction at some point in their lives. Where psychological therapy is necessary, it may include formal marriage counseling and sexual therapy by trained specialists. Sex therapists William Masters and Virginia Johnson, using techniques of behavior modification, report that their patients have up to 80 percent improvement in sexual function over a two-week course of treatment. In most such treatments, the patient is taught to recognize performance anxiety and to practice so-called desensitizing techniques, such that the sexual experience is not looked upon merely as one where intercourse is the ultimate endpoint. Once the patient is able to relax and is relieved of pressures to perform sexually, he gains confidence and in most cases can resume normal sexual relations.

Hormone therapy, in the form of testosterone injections or pills, is often helpful when the patient has below-normal or low-normal blood testosterone levels. Any underlying diseases should be treated to allow restoration of normal sexual function. Under the doctor's guidance, patients may stop taking medications possibly responsible for their impotence, and they should discontinue practices that may interfere with erections, such as drinking and smoking.

Recently, a new form of non-surgical treatment has become popular: the pharmacologic injec-

tion program. Patients directly inject into the penis a combination of two medications that increase the blood flow to the erectile tissues. Such treatment may be useful in patients with impotence resulting from neurologic causes or from minor atherosclerosis and in men with psychologically based impotence that cannot otherwise be cured.

Surgery and Implants

Surgery is usually necessary when a patient's impotence cannot be treated by other means. Patients whose impotence is caused by blocked blood vessels to the penis may undergo vessel reconstruction, bypass surgery, or both. In bypass surgery, undamaged blood vessels are grafted into the area to bypass the blockage.

One of the most exciting advances in the treatment of sexual dysfunction is the development of surgical implants to create an erection. There are two types of penile implants: rigid or semirigid prostheses and inflatable prostheses. The rigid or semirigid devices consist of a pair of flexible silicone rods that are surgically placed inside the penis, producing a permanent degree of rigidity that is capable of vaginal penetration. The newer semirigid implants have a metal center rod that enables the patient to bend the penis, so that it can be easily concealed.

The inflatable penile prosthesis, which allows for both an erect and flaccid penis, is more complex. It is generally composed of a pair of cylinders placed in the

penis, a reservoir of fluid usually placed behind the abdominal muscles, and a pump system usually placed in the scrotum; the three components are connected by tubes. (Newer models are self-contained and consist only of inflatable cylinders implanted into the penis.) The patient is able to achieve erection easily by squeezing the scrotum to activate the pump; fluid from the reservoir is then forced into the cylinders, making the penis rigid. The penis is returned to its flaccid state when a release valve on the side of the pump is pressed. These prostheses can be easily concealed and allow for more controllable erections. Partner satisfaction is reported as excellent. However, the devices are quite costly and subject to mechanical malfunction, which occurs over time in 10-20 percent of patients.

All types of penile prostheses have their drawbacks. They are foreign objects introduced into the body and their presence may cause infection. This occurs in approximately 1 percent of patients (5 percent of people with diabetes). Also, when the devices are placed in the penis, normal erectile tissue must be destroyed; consequently, if the devices must be removed, the patient will never be able to obtain a normal erection. A small number of patients complain of pain in the penis requiring removal of the device. Regardless of these problems, the advent of safe, reliable penile prostheses has revolutionized the treatment of impotence. ☐

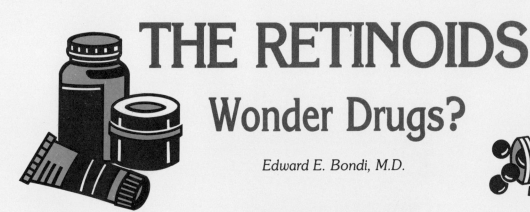

THE RETINOIDS
Wonder Drugs?

Edward E. Bondi, M.D.

The retinoids are a group of drugs derived from vitamin A (retinol). Their impact over the past decade in the treatment of an increasing number of skin diseases has greatly changed the field of dermatology, and their benefits in the future may extend far beyond that field. Almost daily, new discoveries are being made about the possible uses of these drugs. Early studies suggest that the retinoids can affect the process of aging, and they appear to be beneficial in the treatment and prevention of some types of internal cancer. Most currently available retinoids are toxic in high dosages and have a variety of other side effects—some quite serious. But scientists are working to synthesize new, safer, and more effective retinoid drugs.

Early Investigations

The new and exciting discoveries about retinoid treatment evolved from experimental and clinical observations that initially seemed inconsequential. Possibly because vitamin A in large amounts was known to produce dry skin, dermatologists in the 1940s began to experiment with its therapeutic effects in oily-skinned acne patients. Because large amounts of vitamin A caused a scaling off of the dead outer layer of the skin, it was also tried in the treatment of skin diseases that cause a thickening of that layer, such as psoriasis and ichthyosis. Finally, early animal studies had shown that large amounts of vitamin A could inhibit

> **Some side effects of retinoids taken orally can be quite serious, including birth defects.**

the formation of chemically induced skin tumors; thus, researchers thought the vitamin might have an anticancer effect.

Unfortunately, high oral doses of vitamin A proved to be toxic, as was demonstrated by the deaths of early Arctic explorers who consumed polar bear liver, which is rich in the vitamin. This meant that the benefits of systemic vitamin A (affecting the whole body) that had been hypothesized could not be obtained without unacceptably high, potentially toxic doses.

An obvious solution to this dilemma was to have patients apply vitamin A topically to the skin rather than ingest it. However, vitamin A applied topically to both normal and diseased skin had absolutely no effect. This finding led researchers to propose that the therapeutic effect of systemic vitamin A must stem from its breakdown into another product once inside the body. Further investigation revealed that the major naturally occurring breakdown product of vitamin A was vitamin A acid, called tretinoin. It then seemed logical to test the effects of vitamin A acid topically on skin disease.

The results were exciting. In the early 1960s, benefits of topical vitamin A acid were reported in skin conditions such as ichthyosis and actinic keratosis (a sun-induced thickening of the outer layer of the skin with the potential to transform into a type of skin cancer). A 1969 study reported dramatic benefits of tretinoin in the treatment of acne. (Tretinoin is now available by prescription in the United States under the brand name Retin-A and in Canada under the brand names StieVAA and vitamin A Acid.)

Further Research

Although topical tretinoin had significant benefits, it also had limitations. It was irritating to the skin, and the topical application of any medicine to the entire skin surface (for diseases such as psoriasis) is impractical.

The next logical step was to find a safe systemic retinoid for use as an oral medication. When ingested, tretinoin, like oral vitamin A, is severely toxic to the liver. Chemists therefore set out to produce new forms of vitamin A that could be ingested without harming the liver. This led to the production of isotretinoin (now sold under the brand name Accutane). In addition to being much less toxic than tretinoin when taken orally, isotretinoin also greatly suppresses the production of sebum, the oily substance secreted by sebaceous glands in the skin. In the late 1970s researchers documented the dramatic benefit of oral isotretinoin in the treatment of severe cystic acne. The retinoid era had begun.

While dermatologists were widely proclaiming the miraculous effects of isotretinoin for acne, chemists were busy producing other retinoids. Etretinate (sold under the brand name Tegison) was the next therapeutically significant retinoid to be developed. Although it only mildly suppresses sebum production, it has a strong effect on diseases characterized by thickening of the skin, like psoriasis. Etretinate was also shown to normalize the process by which skin cells mature during their migration from the site of their origin in the base of the epidermis to the site of their death at the surface of the skin. This effect suggested possible future benefits in the treatment of skin cancer. It also made clear that each retinoid had its own unique effects on the body. Unfortunately, tests would subsequently show that each new retinoid had risks as well.

Side Effects

The benefits of the retinoids as yet cannot be separated from a host of side effects, some merely annoying, some potentially quite serious. Although the severity of each adverse effect varies with each retinoid, the list of problems is roughly the same for the different derivatives of vitamin A taken orally. Chapped lips and dry skin are experienced by all patients taking these drugs. Severe dry eyes and even blurring of vision is experienced by some patients, as well as a temporary decrease in nighttime vision.

Retinoids taken orally have also been shown to affect fat levels in the blood. During treatment, patients experience an increase in the levels of fats that raise blood cholesterol and a decrease in the level of high-density lipoproteins, which help remove excess cholesterol from the blood. Over the long term, these changes would increase the risk of stroke and heart disease. Fortunately, the

Using Retin-A

Since scientists demonstrated in early 1988 that applying tretinoin (Retin-A) to the skin can diminish some signs of aging and make the skin smoother and rosier, use of the drug—available only by prescription—has soared. Retin-A does have some side effects, such as skin irritation and redness and an increased sensitivity to sunlight. Steps can be taken to diminish these problems.

- Begin therapy with the low-strength, mild, 0.05% Retin-A cream formulation.
- Make sure all make-up is completely removed and the skin is clean before applying Retin-A.
- Apply sparingly to dry skin (wait 15 minutes after washing face).
- Avoid application to sensitive areas such as the eyelids and corners of the mouth.
- Use a moisturizer to minimize the dryness and irritation caused by the drug.
- If skin inflammation is severe, it may be necessary to skip some doses of the drug, which is ordinarily used daily.
- Once daily applications of 0.05% Retin-A cream are tolerated, the stronger 0.1% formulation can be substituted.
- Apply a sunblock before going outdoors, even if it is overcast.
- Avoid prolonged exposure to the sun even if a sunblock is used.
- If you have a sunburn, do not use Retin-A until the redness is completely gone.

changes in fat levels are temporary; the levels return to normal when patients stop taking the retinoid. However, when extended retinoid therapy is considered, for

diseases such as psoriasis or cancer, this complication becomes a major concern.

As mentioned before, high oral doses of vitamin A and its derivatives are potentially toxic to the liver. Patients taking any kind of retinoid thus need to have liver function blood tests done repeatedly during therapy and should discontinue the drug if there is any evidence of liver damage. Patients taking oral retinoids for long periods of time can also develop bone spurs and calcified ligaments and can suffer stunted bone growth and decalcification of bones.

Most disturbing of the oral retinoids' side effects is their potential for causing birth defects. Children born to mothers taking retinoids have had severe brain, heart, and skeletal abnormalities, and many die shortly after birth. Pregnant women therefore must not take any of the retinoids, nor should a woman become pregnant while the drug remains in her system. The drugs do not cause lasting genetic damage; once they are out of the body, it is safe for a woman to become pregnant. However, etretinate may be stored in the body for such long periods that it may never be safe for a woman who has taken it to become pregnant. There is no evidence that the topical retinoid tretinoin causes birth defects, but discontinuation of its use during pregnancy is still generally recommended.

Although doctors have long known that retinoids can produce birth defects and government agencies and drug manufacturers have issued widespread warnings to that effect, hundreds of babies have been born with birth defects caused by retinoids. The U.S. Food and Drug Administration in 1988 considered withdrawing Accutane and other retinoids from the market. It stopped short of that action—but did require Accutane's manufacturer to take stronger measures to prevent its use by pregnant women, measures that included placing a photograph of a deformed infant on the drug's warning label and requiring doctors to obtain a signed consent form from patients indicating that they are aware of the drug's dangers and will take steps to avoid pregnancy.

Retinoids and Acne

Isotretinoin, or Accutane, taken orally, is widely recognized as the most effective treatment available for severe cystic acne, which can leave disfiguring scars. Acne completely clears in many patients, and almost all see dramatic improvement as a result of the drug. Furthermore, about half of patients experience a prolonged, sometimes permanent, remission after they stop taking Accutane. The mechanism by which the drug produces this prolonged remission is unclear. Although the drug reduces the skin's sebum production by 80 percent, sebum production rapidly returns to pretreatment rates after Accutane is discontinued. Why the acne doesn't rapidly return is a persistent puzzle.

The lower the dose of the drug used during the standard five-month treatment period, the more likely it is that acne will reappear after treatment. However, even patients taking lower doses usually enjoy a disease-free interval of more than a year. When the acne returns, they can be treated again with Accutane.

Treating Psoriasis

Severe psoriasis is a skin disease characterized by patches of itchy, red, thickened skin covered by silvery scales. It is sometimes complicated by arthritis, and individuals can develop life-threatening forms of the disease that involve either widespread flare-ups of pustules (pus-filled skin eruptions) or inflammation over extensive areas of the skin. The oral retinoid etretinate is widely recognized as an effective treatment for all forms of psoriasis and is most beneficial in treating the life-threatening pustules and widespread inflamma-

tion. Unfortunately, etretinate is not a cure—it produces only a partial and temporary remission. Furthermore, it persists for years in the body, increasing the risk of side effects. The hunt for a safer, more effective retinoid for psoriasis continues. The experimental drug acitretin, which is currently being tested for the treatment of psoriasis, is more rapidly excreted from the body and thus promises less long-term toxicity.

Cancer Research

Because early animal studies suggested that vitamin A worked against lung, bladder, and skin tumors, it was logical to test retinoids in the treatment and prevention of human cancer. Skin

> **Daily application of Retin-A cream can produce cosmetic improvement in aging skin.**

cancer can be observed and evaluated without any invasive procedures and so offers an ideal model for the testing of different treatments. One study involved patients who, because of heredity or exposure to chemicals, had a marked propensity to develop malignant growths on the skin. When these patients were treated with oral isotretinoin, only 8 percent of their existing skin cancers regressed. More importantly, the study documented a marked reduction in the tendency to develop new skin cancers during the treatment period, although this preventive effect did not persist after the retinoid therapy was discontinued.

Scientists hope that in humans, as in animals, retinoids will have a protective effect against internal cancers. Studies involving bladder cancer, leukemia, and other forms of internal cancer are already in progress. Johnson &

Johnson is testing a new retinoid, fenretinide, for the prevention of breast cancer.

Another new retinoid, arotinoid ethyl ester, has been shown in animal studies to have an extremely potent antitumor effect. And Hoffmann-La Roche has developed a topical form of isotretinoin (called Isotrex) that has been shown to have anticancer effects; it is still experimental. There is little doubt that the most effective retinoids for cancer therapy in the future will be different from the retinoids used in acne and psoriasis today.

Retinoids and Aging

Public opinion surveys repeatedly show that for many people, one of the most distressing parts of getting older is *looking* older. It is not surprising, then, that no aspect of the retinoid revolution has engendered more excitement than the promise of benefits for aging skin. The reports in 1988 that the topical application of tretinoin, or Retin-A, could produce cosmetic improvement in aged skin have resulted in wide use of the drug. In both animal and human studies, tretinoin appears to reverse signs of aging caused by the sun, wind, chemicals, and other environmental factors.

The drug will not reverse what is called intrinsic aging—the inherent tendency of cells to change and slowly deteriorate over time. Nevertheless, human studies have shown that the daily application of tretinoin cream can effectively remove age spots, precancerous growths, and even fine wrinkles, while improving overall skin texture and making the skin rosier. In short, this topical retinoid restores a more youthful appearance to the skin.

These antiaging effects of the topical retinoids appear to be only the beginning. Already, early studies with oral retinoids have yielded similar antiaging results. There is now a real possibility of a safe and effective antiaging pill in our future. □

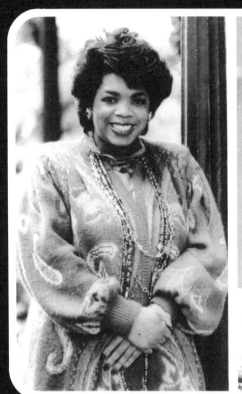
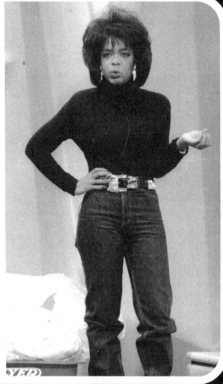

HEALTH AND
MEDICAL NEWS

Aging and the Aged

Undergoing Surgery • New Findings on Alzheimer's Disease • Exercise and Aging

Surgery in the Elderly

Age alone should not prevent older people from undergoing serious operations. Two recent studies lend supporting evidence that overall health and nutritional status, as well as age, are important considerations in determining whether elderly people should undergo surgery.

The need for surgery is the reason for hospital admission of 30 percent of patients over 65 years of age in the United States. Although the risks of surgery are greater for the elderly than for younger people, age alone is not the only risk factor. Many older people have chronic ailments that add to the risks. However, more and more patients in their eighth, ninth, or tenth decades of life are successfully undergoing operations of all kinds, including serious ones.

A report published in late 1988 looked at patients between 70 and 89 years of age who underwent open-heart surgery on an elective basis. Most had coronary artery bypass surgery to restore adequate blood supply to the heart. (In the procedure, a blood vessel is taken from elsewhere in the body and grafted to a coronary artery to reroute blood around a blockage in the artery.) Other patients underwent heart valve replacement, and a few had both of these procedures done. The investigators compared the outcomes of patients between the ages of 70 and 79 with those of patients between the ages of 80 and 89. They found that the older group had no increased risk of dying or of suffering postoperative problems. This suggests that age alone may not be a reason for deciding against open-heart surgery.

Another report published in 1988 looked at the outcome of 100 patients 80 years of age or older who underwent open-heart surgery in the years 1976-1987. Most of the patients had coronary artery bypass surgery, many required replacement of one of the heart valves, and some had both of these procedures performed. Before surgery, 90 percent of the patients had severe symptoms, such as chest pain and shortness of breath, that did not respond to other medical treatment, such as medication or the techniques of angioplasty or valvuloplasty (in which narrowed heart arteries or valves, respectively, are widened). The investigators found that 71 percent of the patients survived the surgery and immediate postoperative period. All of the survivors were relieved of their preoperative symptoms. At greatest risk of dying in the early postoperative period were those patients who had surgery on an emergency basis, had suffered a heart attack prior to surgery, were malnourished, or had severe symptoms while at rest. In studies conducted with younger patients, these same factors have been shown to play a significant role in survival rates after open-heart surgery.

Alzheimer's Disease

New insights into the possible causes of Alzheimer's disease raise researchers' hopes of eventually developing effective treatment and a means of prevention for this as yet incurable illness. Alzheimer's disease accounts for 40 percent of all cases of dementia—a decline in intellectual function that interferes with an individual's daily living—in the United States. Alzheimer's, which affects one in seven Americans over age 65, is diagnosed when all other possible causes of dementia have been ruled out. Memory loss is the most prominent early symptom. It is eventually accompanied by one or more of the following: impaired judgment, personality changes, and other disturbances of higher functions, such as speech and motor activities.

Alzheimer's may affect both sides of the brain symmetrically or only one side. Depending upon which part of the brain is affected, patients may have different behavioral patterns and disorders in language or movement. About 30 percent of patients have slowed or absent motor responses, body rigidity, changes in posture and gait, or jerky movements. The fact that patients have many different characteristics and an array of symptoms has led to speculation that Alzheimer's may have several causes and, in fact, may be several different diseases with similar characteristics. In keeping with this supposition, subtypes of Alzheimer's have been identified and singled out for study, including familial Alzheimer's disease, a form that runs in families.

A Genetic Cause? Researchers have postulated that one or more genes are responsible for familial Alzheimer's, which is characterized by early onset and rapid progress and could account for 10 to 20 percent of all Alzheimer's cases. A number of years ago, scientists believed they had found a link between familial Alzheimer's and an abnormal gene located on chromosome 21. However, recent studies of groups of families, conducted by other researchers, failed to show the connection to this particular chromosome. In addition, scientists have reported findings that suggest that other genes may also be linked to the cause of Alzheimer's disease.

The genetic defect found on chromosome 21 suggested a relationship between Alzheimer's and Down's syndrome, a genetic disorder caused by an extra copy of chromosome 21. After age 35, Down's patients begin to show the clinical symptoms of Alzheimer's. Their brains show the same type of abnormalities that are seen in people with Alzheimer's—an overabundance of protein accumulations called plaques and a buildup of tangled fibers. Investigators have found that the plaques are made of a material called beta-amyloid and have possibly located the gene responsible for its production on chromosome 21.

Infectious Transmission. Research conducted at Yale University and reported in 1988 provided increased evidence for suggestions that Alzheimer's disease may be linked to an infectious agent—perhaps a type of virus. The hypothesis was tested by injecting into the brains of laboratory hamsters white blood cells drawn from nine healthy relatives of Alzheimer's patients and two individuals with early signs of the disease. Some of the animals developed brain degeneration after about a year. When brain tissue from the affected hamsters was injected into a new set of hamsters, the second set developed brain degeneration even more rapidly. It remains unclear, however, whether this is truly an infectious type of transmission or the result of some other process that leads to similar brain tissue changes. An infectious-type transmission of Alzheimer's has never been demonstrated in humans. The Yale researchers emphasized the tentative nature of their report and the need for further study to substantiate their findings. They pointed out that there is no evidence of Alzheimer's being transmitted in humans through blood transfusions.

People of any age can enjoy participating—and competing!—in active sports. Old in years but still going strong, Ruth Rothfarb, 84, and John Kelley, 77 (left), get set to run a 5-mile event for senior citizens. The oldest competitor in the 1988 Summer Olympics, Durward Knowles, 70 (right), finished 19th in the yachting Star class.

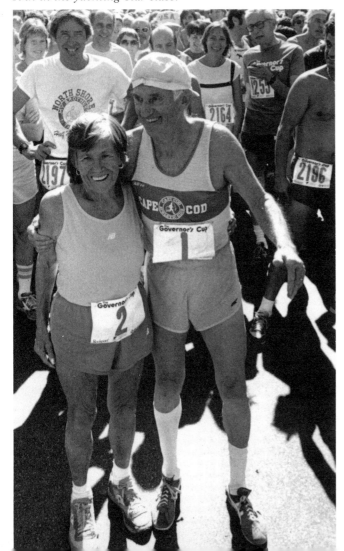
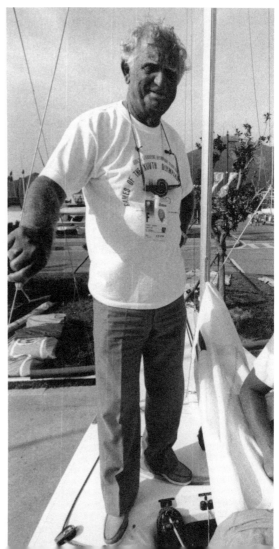

Exercise and Aging

More and more studies are showing that the stereotype of the elderly as frail and sedentary need not be a reality. Through exercise, older people can maintain strength and fitness. Exercise has many benefits for people of all ages, including an increase in functional capacity and an enhanced sense of well-being. Of particular interest to older people is the evidence that physical activity may prevent or slow down some of the physical and mental changes that were once thought to be part of "normal" aging—such as loss of muscle mass, narrowing of the coronary arteries, and slower reaction times.

Current research supports the idea that exercise may prevent or help control some chronic health conditions. Recent studies show that blood pressure is lowered in elderly people who participate in exercise training programs. It has also been shown that older people who exercise adequately have less coronary artery disease than those who are sedentary.

Exercise has been shown to improve the body's ability to regulate levels of blood sugar by helping cells utilize insulin more efficiently. Exercise has long been recommended to people with diabetes as a means of controlling their disease, if combined with diet and other life-style changes. Because the form of diabetes that begins in middle age is often associated with excess body fat, exercise may help prevent the onset of the disease by keeping an individual's weight down.

Osteoporosis, a condition characterized by loss of bone density, occurs in both men and women as they age and is often seen in individuals who are relatively inactive. When severe, it may result in fractures of the hip and spine. But research has shown that weight-bearing exercises, such as walking or jogging, increase bone mass and may prevent or slow the progress of osteoporosis.

Intellectual and psychological benefits can also be obtained from exercise. Physical activity has been shown to reduce anxiety, tension, and depression, with effects lasting for hours after exercise. Fitness training programs and increased stamina can improve self-esteem, especially among those with doubts about their physical capabilities. It has been suggested that ongoing exercise programs play an important role in preventing the decline in speed of mental processing that occurs with aging. There may also be improvement in brain function in sedentary individuals who start to exercise.

Exercise programs can be started at any age, even by individuals who have never been active. However, before beginning any exercise program, older people should be sure to have a physical examination and discuss their plans with their doctor. In addition, for many older people a very gradual buildup of activity is necessary. But given its numerous benefits and ability to improve the quality of life, a carefully planned exercise program based on individual needs and restrictions may be the most important prescription a physician can give to an older adult.

See also the feature article Choosing Long-Term Care.

PAUL R. KATZ, M.D.
IRIS. F. BOETTCHER, M.D.

AIDS

New Knowledge About the Virus • New Drugs and Treatment Strategies • Concern Over Discrimination

Acquired immune deficiency syndrome continues to capture much of the spotlight in the public health arena. Recent months could be characterized as ones of steady progress in both research and control, without major breakthroughs. Despite feverish activity on many fronts and increased understanding of the disease, successful tools for prevention and treatment remain elusive.

Virus Characteristics

There has been recent concern that more than one virus causes AIDS. In the United States the disease is caused by the human immunodeficiency virus type one—or HIV-I, hereafter referred to as HIV. Of some concern to most AIDS investigators is the question of whether a significant threat is posed by a similar virus, the human immunodeficiency virus type two (HIV-II), which was recently discovered in West Africa. Does it pose a serious threat of causing AIDS, and is it spreading throughout the world? The fact is that although occasional cases of immune deficiency do appear to develop in people who are infected with HIV-II but not with HIV, and one such case has been diagnosed in the United States, the newer virus does not seem to have as great a potential for producing an immune deficiency syndrome. Therefore, at present there does not seem to be justification for studying HIV-II with the same urgency as HIV. But health experts will watch HIV-II closely to determine whether, after more incubation time, it actually causes AIDS.

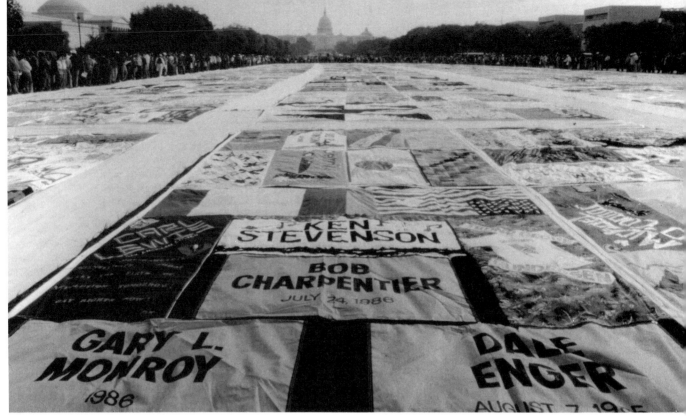

An enormous quilt made up of panels commemorating those who have died of AIDS was displayed at an October 1987 gay rights demonstration in Washington, D.C., and then sent on a 20-city cross-country tour in 1988.

They will also monitor the second virus to see whether it spreads around the world.

Much of the news from research on HIV continues to be discouraging. Evidence is accumulating that it is not rare for some people to be infected with HIV for more than a year before their bodies produce antibodies to the virus; current tests for AIDS detect these antibodies in the blood, rather than the virus itself. Early evidence suggests that the virus finds a way to "hide" in immune system cells in such cases. The immediate concern is the safety of donated blood and blood products used for transfusions.

Future Prospects

The June 1988 international meeting on AIDS in Stockholm, Sweden, did not produce much optimism for the near future. The outlook for people infected with HIV is still bleak, despite some progress in drug treatment. Health officials in New York City estimate that only 15 percent of those with full cases of AIDS will survive five years or more.

It is still not known whether all of those who become infected with HIV will eventually develop AIDS. The majority of people in the United States who are infected with the virus still have no symptoms. Some groups, such as those from 2 to 21 years of age, seem to develop the disease more slowly; very young chil-

dren (under the age of 2) appear to develop it more quickly. Studies of some of the first people in the AIDS epidemic known to have been infected with HIV reveal that the majority have gone on to develop full-blown cases of AIDS, and the majority of them have died. Estimates of the proportion of HIV carriers who will eventually develop AIDS range from 50 to 100 percent, but nobody really knows.

Projecting probable rates of infection and the actual number of AIDS cases in the future, and even estimating the prevalence of HIV infection at present, is difficult. In 1988 health officials debated over the number of people in the United States who have the virus. The U.S. Centers for Disease Control estimated that up to 1.5 million people were infected, whereas a study by the Hudson Institute, a private research organization based in Indianapolis, concluded that the number was closer to 3 million. One of the year's biggest AIDS flaps occurred when sex researchers William H. Masters and Virginia E. Johnson published a book claiming that "the AIDS virus is now running rampant" in the heterosexual community. They also concluded that about 3 million people in the United States are infected with HIV. The scientific community soundly rejected their claims, partly on the basis of the poor method of sampling used.

Internationally, estimates of the number of people with HIV infection are increasing rapidly. One new estimate suggests that about 500,000 people are infected with HIV in Brazil alone. Another study projects that there will be at least 450,000 cumulative cases of AIDS in the United States by the end of 1993. (As of March 1989 the United States had over 88,000 cases of AIDS; Canada had over 2,500 cases.) One organization estimated that worldwide, one new person becomes infected with HIV every minute. In the United States a new AIDS case is reported about every 14 minutes. Preliminary data suggest that about 3 in 1,000 American college students are already infected with the virus.

Despite the large number of Americans probably infected with HIV, few people use protective measures in casual sexual relationships—a disturbing finding. A recent study reported that the use of condoms by Americans remains low, and an increasing percentage of unmarried women are having unprotected sexual intercourse despite the dangers of acquiring HIV.

Modes of Transmission

Researchers in 1988 found that under certain conditions HIV may be more easily transmitted to men. A study in Africa found that men had a greater risk of acquiring HIV upon exposure if they had a venereal disease that caused genital ulcers (such as syphilis or herpes), perhaps because the ulcers provide a means of entry for the virus. The same study also found the risk of transmission higher in uncircumcised than in circumcised men, regardless of whether they had genital ulcers. Researchers suspect that the foreskin may allow the virus to survive longer on the skin, giving it more time to enter the body.

New cases of HIV infection among healthcare workers, apparently acquired from needle sticks, appeared in 1988. The American Medical Association felt compelled to affirm that physicians are obliged to treat AIDS patients regardless of the danger, which remains quite low in American hospitals. But one U.S. study from Baltimore found that over 5 percent of adult emergency room patients at an inner-city hospital tested positive for HIV, so the potential for inadvertent transmission of the virus is real.

AIDS or HIV infection in newborn babies is a rising concern. One study in New York City found that 1 in 77 newborns had HIV antibodies in their blood. This does not necessarily mean the babies were infected with HIV; they might have picked up their infected mothers' antibodies to the virus, and the antibodies could persist for some time. However, a sizable proportion of babies showing antibodies at birth are actually infected with the virus. Presumably, they will eventually die of the disease. (*See also the Spotlight on Health article* CHILDREN WITH AIDS.)

Developments in Treatment

Using two drugs to fight HIV may be more effective and cause fewer side effects than using only one. The drug zidovudine (sold as Retrovir and formerly known as AZT) has been shown to extend the lives of and improve the quality of life for some AIDS patients. But a large proportion of those using the drug suffer severe side effects, such as nausea, vomiting, and anemia. In one trial, patients receiving alternating one-week treatments with zidovudine and another drug, dideoxycytidine (ddC), have shown striking improvement for over a year and do not show the usual ill effects of those using zidovudine alone. One reason these and similar drugs may be effective is that they appear to stop the reproduction of HIV in macrophages. These large immune system cells are important targets of HIV (along with other white blood cells called T-4 lymphocytes). Macrophages also may transmit HIV to the brain, which can be severely damaged by HIV infection. Other combinations of anti-AIDS drugs are also being studied.

In March 1989, researchers announced that some strains of HIV showed resistance to zidovudine in patients who had taken the drug for more than six months. Such resistance could explain why some AIDS patients' conditions deteriorate after months of treatment with the drug. No changes in treatment were recommended, but researchers suggested that treatment schedules that alternated drugs might slow the development of the virus's resistance to them.

In recent months the U.S. Food and Drug Administration (FDA) made two experimental drugs more widely available to treat *Pneumocystis carinii* pneumonia (PCP), which afflicts and ultimately kills many AIDS sufferers. In August 1988 the FDA relaxed its rules on the drug trimetrexate, allowing it to be used by patients who do not respond to either of the two FDA-approved drugs to treat the pneumonia. (Some months earlier the agency had allowed the drug to be used by seriously ill patients, but only if they experienced dangerous or life-threatening reactions to the other available drugs.) Under previous policy, the FDA allowed experimental drugs to be released to patients only if the drugs showed some effectiveness in trials. In the case of trimetrexate, the agency released the drug even though official studies had not yet shown its effectiveness.

Another drug made more widely available to treat PCP was pentamidine. The drug had already been approved for use in injectable form, but in February 1989 the FDA allowed it to be used as an inhaled aerosol after it showed promise in treating and actually preventing PCP. The new FDA decision allows not only those who have already suffered one bout of

PCP to use the drug, but also people who have no symptoms of AIDS but who have T-cell ratios that have fallen to the point where they are likely to acquire opportunistic infections like PCP. (Opportunistic infections are those that rarely affect healthy individuals but can be life-threatening in people with impaired immune systems.)

In March 1989 the FDA decided to allow the experimental drug ganciclovir to be used by AIDS patients for eye infections. Though not approved for marketing at that time, the drug was the only one available for treating cytomegalovirus infections. The virus usually does not harm healthy people, but it often causes serious illness in AIDS patients and blinds them when it attacks the eyes. After protests from AIDS patients and their advocates, the FDA reversed a December 1988 decision to restrict the drug's use until further tests were completed on it.

In November 1988 the FDA approved genetically engineered alpha-interferon to treat Kaposi's sarcoma, a rare kind of cancer that sometimes afflicts AIDS patients. In February 1989 the drug was also approved for that use in Canada. Alpha-interferon is a hormone-like substance similar to ones naturally produced in the body in minute quantities. The first drug approved to treat Kaposi's sarcoma, it works best in people in the earliest stages of the disease, causing a significant reduction in the size of tumors. Patients taking the drug in trials lived about a year longer than those who did not take it.

Testing and Needle-Exchange Programs

Progress was reported in 1988 in the development of better screening and diagnostic tests for HIV. Several new tests are being developed that are thought to be more accurate and sensitive than the current tests and that could be on the market soon. Several companies are even developing mail-in or home HIV antibody tests. The U.S. Postal Service, however, is concerned about transporting biological material that might be infected with HIV. There are also concerns about the impact test results could have on people who do not have professional counseling when they receive the results.

One of the hottest debates in recent months concerns giving intravenous drug users clean needles in exchange for their dirty ones in the hopes of reducing the risk of AIDS transmission. Drug users, who can contract AIDS by sharing contaminated needles, make up a growing proportion of AIDS patients. A few cities are experimenting with such programs, and some others are distributing bleach or disinfectants to drug users so that they can clean their needles.

Risk of Discrimination

One of the major problems created by AIDS is discrimination against people with the disease and those infected with HIV. The president's AIDS commission and a panel appointed by the National Academy of Sciences both concluded in reports released in June 1988 that people with AIDS and HIV carriers are at increased risk for discrimination. Such people face the possibility of being denied jobs, housing, insurance, and medical care.

A review of 53 national and international opinion surveys agreed with the reports. The review found that most Americans foresee that the control of AIDS will require some loss of individual privacy and possibly even some restrictions on civil rights. The surveys suggest that many Americans—although a minority—see AIDS as a deserved punishment for offensive or immoral behavior, would refuse to work alongside someone who had AIDS, would support the right of employers to fire such workers, and would take a child out of school to avoid contact with a classmate with AIDS. A sizable minority would also exclude AIDS patients from their neighborhoods and would give landlords the right to evict such persons. On the other hand, the respondents by a strong margin opposed discrimination in access to hospital care for

In the hope of slowing the spread of AIDS, New York City in late 1988 began the first government-sponsored program in the United States to offer free needles to intravenous drug users, who make up the largest number of newly reported AIDS cases in that city. A Health Department counselor shows a needle and the AIDS prevention packet being distributed; the packet contains materials for cleaning needles, information on how AIDS is spread, and condoms.

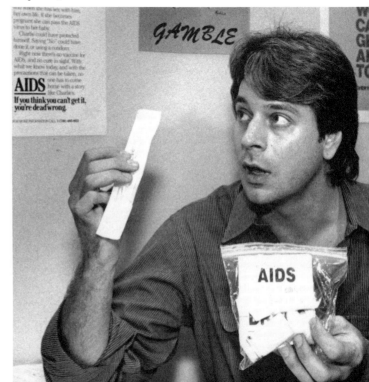

AIDS patients. Given these findings, the call by the president's commission and National Academy of Sciences panel for a federal antidiscrimination law appears justified.

The two reports also criticized the government's sluggish response to the AIDS epidemic and suggested that increased federal funds were necessary to fight it. Although the Reagan administration virtually ignored the reports, Congress in October 1988 passed the first major legislation to deal with the AIDS epidemic. The law directed more than $1 billion over a three-year period toward testing, research, and education but remained silent on issues of confidentiality and discrimination.

Some of the nation's leading companies and organizations agreed to a new ten-point "bill of rights" for workers infected with HIV. However, a study discovered that most health insurance companies screen applicants for evidence that they might be infected with the virus. The justification they give is that their insurance costs are much higher for those individuals. Such activity is contrary to guidelines of the National Association of Insurance Commissioners, and some states are taking steps to assure that such discrimination does not occur.

See also the Health and Medical News article WORLD HEALTH NEWS. JAMES F. JEKEL, M.D., M.P.H.

Bioethics

Funding Cutoff for Fetal Tissue Research • Right-to-Die Plea Rejected • Who Owns Human Tissue? • Minors and Abortion

Fetal Tissue Research

Ethical Questions. The debate over the use of human fetal tissue in research continued in 1988 and 1989. Such tissue has several advantages over adult tissue in medical applications. It grows rapidly, is easy to freeze and store, and if used in transplant operations, is less likely to be rejected by the host's immune system. Fetal tissue transplants show some promise in treating conditions such as diabetes and Parkinson's disease and other neurological disorders.

Much of the controversy surrounding the use of fetal materials in medical science stems from the fact that the tissue must be retrieved from the results of induced abortions. (Because it dies so quickly after the death of the fetus, fetal tissue is almost impossible to obtain following miscarriages.) Critics argue that widespread use of fetal tissue might justify an abortion for some women or even encourage a woman to become pregnant and then have an abortion in order to donate—or sell—such tissue; it is also argued that research made possible by the destruction of a human fetus has an immoral taint. Some proponents, on the other hand, contend that the use of fetal tissue to benefit the gravely ill can redeem the tragedy of an abortion by giving it some positive consequences. They also point out that there is no evidence to suggest that abortion will be encouraged by this practice.

Federal Funding Ban. Pending consideration of these questions, the U.S. Department of Health and Human Services (HHS) declared a moratorium in April 1988 on federal financing of new research involving the transplantation of fetal cells. (The ban did not extend to other experiments involving human fetal tissue.)

The assistant secretary of health appointed a 21-member committee of experts to examine the scientific and ethical issues. That panel, which met in September 1988, recommended that the use of fetal tissue for transplants be continued, but under stringent ethical guidelines. These include ensuring that no physician involved in an abortion is associated with a research project that uses the fetal tissue later on, that no payment for the tissue is made to the woman having an abortion, and that the woman is not allowed to designate a donor for the fetal tissue. An advisory body of the U.S. National Institutes of Health urged adoption of the panel's recommendations, but as of early 1989 no action had been taken by HHS.

Ethics Regulatory Body. In a related development, the Reagan administration surprised the scientific community by announcing in July 1988 that the Ethics Advisory Board of the Department of Health and Human Services would be reappointed. The board was created in 1974 in response to concerns about the possibility of abuses of human fetuses in the laboratory, then dissolved in 1980 when the President's Commission on Ethical Problems in Medicine and Biomedical and Behavioral Research was examining similar issues. But after the commission finished its work, the Ethics Advisory Board was not reappointed.

A reconstituted board could provide federal leadership in developing policies on ethically acceptable research involving fetal tissue. However, it will probably be some time before the new Ethics Advisory Board is actually appointed. The Department of Health and Human Services plans to revise the board's charter and to solicit comments from the public on the new charter before designating board members.

Right-to-Die Case

In a decision that ran counter to the trend in other states, New York State's highest court ruled, 4 to 3, in October 1988 that an elderly woman's artificial feeding tube could not be removed based on the assertions of her daughters that she would prefer to die. The patient, Mary O'Connor, had suffered a number of strokes and could not respond to any but the simplest questions. Her daughters argued that, in caring for several terminally ill relatives, their mother had often stated her wish not to be kept alive artificially and thus be a burden to her family.

But a majority of the New York State Court of Appeals judges found that O'Connor's statements were not specific enough to meet the standard of "clear and convincing" evidence. She had not said that a particular type of artificial therapy—feeding through tubes—was what she would want withheld if she were terminally ill. The decision meant that O'Connor would continue to be fed through a tube running through her nose to her digestive tract.

The court minority and outside critics of the decision contended that the articulated standard was too strict, since it seemed to require highly specific written statements, drawn up in advance, and to reject reports of less formal expressions of preference. (*See also the Spotlight on Health article* THE RIGHT TO DIE.)

Who Owns Human Tissue?

In November 1988 the California Supreme Court agreed to rule on the case of John Moore, a Seattle businessman who claimed he had a right to share in profits derived from his spleen tissue after his spleen was removed as part of his cancer treatment. The court's action has again focused attention on the central philosophical question raised by Moore's 1984 lawsuit: Do human beings lose commercial control of their organs when those organs are removed from their bodies?

When John Moore's leukemia was treated in 1976 at the University of California at Los Angeles Medical Center, Moore did not know that some of his spleen tissue would be used in UCLA research laboratories. The use of human and animal cells in research is a long-standing practice, and since such use presents no risk to patients, they are not told about it. But Moore's tissue was instrumental in producing a cell line—a culture of cells with uniform characteristics—that the university subsequently patented. The cell line was used, in turn, to help develop a new drug that controls white blood cell count and may be useful in the treatment of leukemia and of immune disorders like AIDS. The possible commercial value of products

derived from the cell line has been estimated to be as high as $3 billion. Moore sued the university, Dr. David W. Golde (the oncologist who treated him), and others, claiming that his rights to his tissue continued and that therefore he should share in any profits that resulted from the sale of products developed from it.

Many medical researchers fear that if Moore's suit is successful, new bureaucratic obstacles will be set up that would slow the pace of research using human body parts.

Anencephalic Infants

In 1988, Loma Linda University Medical Center in California decided to suspend a program that had kept alive newborns with a lethal brain defect called anencephaly (absence of all or most of the brain) long enough to make their organs available for transplant. The program was instituted because of a shortage of tiny organs for transplant to infants who would die without them. Anencephalic infants rarely live longer than one or two weeks. Some of their vital organs, such as the heart, liver, and lungs, may be initially unaffected by their condition, but as these infants die, their organs are slowly deprived of oxygen; by the time death occurs, the organs are no longer suitable for transplant.

To avoid this problem, the Loma Linda group (acting with parental consent) placed a number of anencephalic infants on respirators, so that oxygen would continue to perfuse their organs. The program called for testing the infants after one week to see if they met technical criteria for brain death. If they did, they would be declared legally dead and their organs made available for transplant; if not, the respirator would be turned off, the infants would be allowed to die naturally, and their organs would no longer be eligible for donation.

From the outset, the program raised serious ethical questions, since keeping a human being alive only for the sake of another was regarded as a pronounced departure from normal standards of medical ethics. Furthermore, scientific disagreements arose about the adequacy of tests for brain death in anencephalics.

In announcing the suspension of the program, the university alluded to these medical and ethical problems. In any event, the effort had met with disappointing results: of the 12 anencephalic babies in the program, only one had met brain death criteria within the required time, and no recipient could be found for his organs. (In October 1987 an anencephalic infant's heart was transplanted at Loma Linda into a newborn boy, but the donor was a baby girl who had been maintained on life support systems in Ontario and not at Loma Linda.)

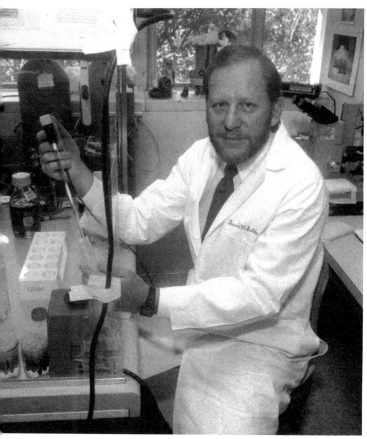

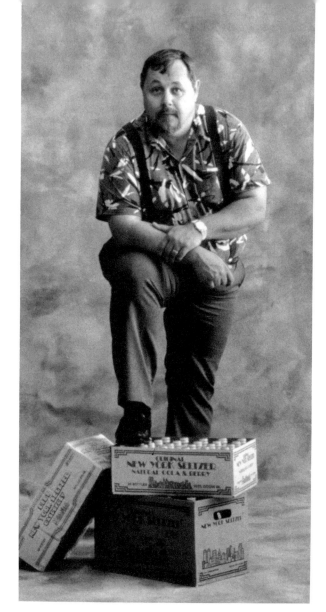

John Moore (right) is suing his oncologist, Dr. David Golde (left), and others for rights to products developed from his spleen tissue after his spleen was removed during successful treatment for leukemia. At issue is the question of who owns human tissue removed from the body.

Extending Organ Life

A most serious problem with regard to acquiring human organs for transplants is that the organs are rarely usable for more than 36 hours after they have been removed from the donor's body. Heart tissue, for example, begins to deteriorate after only four hours. Since an appropriate recipient is not always immediately available, or the organ may have to be transported a long distance to reach a desperately ill person, the lifesaving potential of organ donation is severely limited. Sometimes an ethical dilemma arises because the neediest patient is just far enough away to create doubts that the organ will survive, while another patient who is not in imminent danger is nearby. But now a new device that greatly extends the usable life of organs such as hearts, kidneys, and livers may resolve some of these problems.

A group of scientists at the University of California at Irvine have developed an apparatus about the size of a television set that can keep a heart beating for up to 24 hours. It does this by pumping a blood substitute through the heart and by maintaining favorable electrical, chemical, and physical environments, controlled by a computer. The process slows the heart rate to about ten beats a minute through cooling, which ensures that the tissues do not suffer from lack of oxygen. The device has been successfully tested with the hearts of sheep, pigs, and dogs. Similar principles may be applicable to other organs.

But as is so often the case with potentially lifesaving medical technologies, the device raises a new set of ethical problems. One problem is that its effectiveness with human hearts must be tested; however, there are currently no U.S. government rules on the use of viable human organs in research. Another problem is that if human hearts could be preserved long enough for shipment across international borders, a black market could develop. These ethical issues may prove more difficult to resolve than the remaining technical problems.

Minors and Abortion

In August 1988 a federal appeals court upheld a Minnesota law that requires girls under the age of 18 who want an abortion either to notify both parents or to obtain special approval from a state judge. Minnesota is one of 25 states that require parental notification or consent to a minor's abortion.

The 1981 Minnesota law provides that minors who do not obtain special judicial approval give 48 hours notice of the abortion to both parents, even if the parents are no longer married to one another. The federal court's majority opinion stated that restrictions on access to abortion by minors (such as notifying parents in advance) are not unconstitutional so long as "an appropriate judicial bypass" (in this case, approval by a judge) exists. The dissenting judges argued that the law could cause trauma for pregnant teenagers, especially those from broken homes, and that previous U.S. Supreme Court decisions have not supported a requirement that both parents be notified.

Opponents of the law have appealed the case to the Supreme Court. In the past the Court has struck down laws that either gave parents a veto over a decision to have an abortion or required notification with no alternative (such as judicial appeal). But it has ruled in favor of laws that required family consultation.   JONATHAN D. MORENO, PH.D.

Bones, Muscles, and Joints

Improved Treatment for Trauma Patients • Advances in Imaging Techniques

Treating Trauma

Recent improvements in orthopedic surgical techniques have greatly improved survival and recovery prospects for victims of trauma—an injury inflicted by a physical agent against the body. Trauma results in 100,000 deaths and 10 million disabling injuries in the United States each year. It is the leading cause of death in America in people under the age of 30. This health problem robs society of many young people before they reach their productive years, and treatment for such injuries constitutes a major healthcare expense in the United States. Because many patients with severe traumatic injuries have skeletal injury, they usually need orthopedic surgery.

Complications of Fractures. Unstable fractures—those that are apt to move out of position during the healing process—can cause a variety of complications in trauma patients, including life-threatening lung problems. Multiple fractures of the long bones of the legs and arms can cause a syndrome called fat embolism, in which fat released from the marrow of the broken bones is transported in the blood to the lungs and the brain. This can cause breathing and brain disorders and can lead to death. A condition called adult respiratory distress syndrome (ARDS) can be caused in part by skeletal trauma. Skeletal trauma, by preventing a patient's movement, can significantly interfere with pulmonary (lung) care and can lead to the worsening of ARDS and to pneumonia.

Unstable long bone and pelvic fractures can also be a source of continued bleeding. Because hemorrhaging can cause death in trauma patients with such injuries, the injured area must be immobilized immediately and steps taken to control blood loss and to prevent shock.

Improvements in orthopedic surgical techniques and implants, including more aggressive steps, can help prevent these complications. Surgically fixing the broken bone with plates or rods allows the patient's care to be directed toward cardiovascular, pulmonary, nutritional, and rehabilitative concerns, which are the important predictors of the patient's ultimate survival and function.

Fractures of Leg Bones. Fractures of the tibia, the major bone in the lower leg, are usually treated by immobilizing the area in a cast. An open, or compound, fracture of the tibia—in which the broken bone tears and protrudes through the skin—is often best repaired with devices called external fixators. These consist of an external frame with connecting pins that penetrate the skin and bone above and below the fracture. This immobilizes the fracture, yet allows access to the wound for appropriate care.

Many fractures of the thighbone, or femur, can be fixed in place with a rod inserted in the marrow cavity. This effectively stabilizes the fracture, allows soft tissues (cartilage and ligaments) to heal, and enables the patient to move about freely, with improved hip and knee motion. Over the last several years use of such rods has become widely accepted. As a result, even infection-prone compound fractures of the femur, which previously were treated with traction (a rope-and-pulley device that pulls on a fracture to hold it in place), now may be best fixed with the insertion of stabilizing rods.

Pelvic and Hip Fractures. The treatment of pelvic and hip fractures has significantly improved through changes in surgical instruments and advances in surgical approaches, techniques, and methods of immobilizing fractures. These severe injuries often result in pain, deformity, and death. They are often associated with massive bleeding that is not easily controlled by surgery. Simply opposing the raw, fractured bone surfaces—pressing them back together in their original position—to decrease the potential space for bleeding, and immobilizing the bone with an external fixator, represent major advances in the care of pelvic injuries. Plates and screws applied to the pelvis through large surgical incisions allow the pelvis and the hip socket to be reconstructed and repaired in such a way as to improve both the early rehabilitation and the long-term prospects for successful function.

Spinal Injuries. There have also been improvements in the surgical treatment of patients with spinal injuries resulting in paraplegia (paralysis of the legs) or quadriplegia (paralysis of the arms and legs). Improvements in spinal surgical implants (rods, screws, and plates), especially for the upper and lower back regions, have contributed to a more rapid rehabilitation of patients with severe fractures. This appears to lower the risk of complications and to allow the patient to cope more rapidly with the disability instead of languishing in bed for months waiting for the fracture to heal. Some patients with incomplete spinal cord injuries and ongoing compression of the spinal nerves from displaced bone or disk material may improve from surgery to relieve pressure on the nerves.

Fractures of the Upper Body and Extremities. Surgical treatment of fractures in the upper body is important for long-term functioning. Realigning bones in hand, wrist, forearm, and elbow fractures is especially critical for good recovery. Fractures in and about the elbow and fractures of displaced bones of the forearm require surgery, but many fractures of the wrist can be treated with nonsurgical realignment and pinning procedures (surgically installing metal pins through broken bones and the plaster cast to hold them in place). Surgical care of hand fractures has recently gained popularity, but frequently, fractures of the hands and fingers can be treated well with nonsurgical realignment or pinning procedures to allow healing.

Improvements in Imaging

Major gains in two separate areas of imaging have significantly improved physicians' ability to diagnose and treat musculoskeletal problems.

Magnetic Resonance Imaging. A relatively new technique that is becoming more widely used is magnetic resonance imaging (MRI). In MRI, an extremely high magnetic field and radio waves are used to stimulate the hydrogen atoms in the patient's body. The stimulated atoms emit signals that are processed by a computer, which creates an image of the body part being studied. MRI provides detail of soft tissue structures that other imaging techniques do not. It also does not expose patients to X rays, which carry the slight risk of causing cancer if given repeatedly, or to dyes, which cause allergic reactions in some patients. X rays, while they clearly visualize structures such as the spinal cord, spinal disks, cartilage in the knee, and the muscles and tendons about the shoulder, require dyes for viewing some structures and always expose patients to radiation.

Until recently, the only method available to provide images of the contour of the spinal cord, nerve roots, and contents of the spinal canal was myelography. This procedure involves injecting a dye into the spinal fluid and taking a series of X rays. MRI in some cases is rapidly demonstrating greater sensitivity and specificity than myelography in diagnosing and evaluating problems in spinal structures—all without the risks involved with the injection of dye and X-ray exposure. The full impact of this technique has yet to be determined, but in some situations MRI has actually replaced myelography.

In the hands of professionals experienced with it, MRI has impressive accuracy in evaluating the cartilage and ligaments of the knee. An X-ray dye test for joints called arthrography and a surgical diagnostic technique called arthroscopy (in which a fiber-optic instrument is inserted into the knee joint to allow a physician to view it) may not be necessary in some patients when the information needed can be supplied by MRI. The removal of risks of reactions to X-ray dye or to anesthetics (used to numb joints in arthroscopy) makes MRI a safer diagnostic tool for investigating mechanical problems of the knee.

Diagnosing shoulder problems has also improved with MRI. Doctors can have a difficult time diagnosing a relatively common condition of middle age called a rotator cuff tear—a tear in one tendon of the short muscles that help extend and rotate the shoulder. Even when a physician is suspicious of and looking for a rotator cuff tear, the standard shoulder arthrogram offers limited information. This can be a major drawback, since although many small rotator cuff tears improve without surgery, large tears frequently cause a severe shoulder arthritis that cannot be treated with the reconstructive technique of total shoulder arthroplasty. (Arthroplasty requires a normal rotator cuff to achieve reasonable shoulder function.) MRI is more accurate than an arthrogram in diagnosing a rotator cuff tear and its size, and MRI better helps the doctor to decide whether surgical or nonsurgical treatment would be most beneficial.

CT Scanning. Computerized tomography (CT scanning), in which a computer constructs a three-dimensional image of a body structure from X rays taken from many different angles, is a technique that in recent years has begun to find its way out of research laboratories and into various medical applications. The standard pictures available from X rays require physicians to mentally construct a three-dimensional image from a two-dimensional one to give them an accurate picture of an injury. This three-dimensional visualization is especially important in planning surgery to repair complicated fractures of large joints, such as the hip socket and the knee. Computers, using information provided by CT scanning, can create three-dimensional models of body structures that can be rotated and expanded. Portions of the structures can even be removed to allow the surgeon to see inside the joint. In difficult bone reconstructions, this technique allows the surgeon to hold, manipulate, and try fixing these models before actually attempting a complex procedure on the patient. At present, this technique is used infrequently, for unusually complicated cases, and may never be used routinely. But as the technology becomes more available, it will probably improve patient care.   ERIC L. HUME, M.D.

Brain and Nervous System

Preventing and Treating Stroke • Cocaine, Speed, and the Nervous System • Update on Parkinson's Disease

Stroke

Stroke is the third leading cause of death in most developed countries, behind only heart disease and cancer. Although the incidence of stroke has been falling steadily in the United States since the early part of this century, about 450,000 Americans have strokes each year, and 150,000 of them die. Over the past several decades, enormous progress has been made in understanding the causes of stroke as well as in recognizing individuals who are particularly at risk. Unfortunately, progress has not been as rapid in the treatment of stroke, and there has been some controversy over the best ways to prevent it, with a common operation, long thought to be a valuable preventive, coming under increasing scrutiny. A number of recent studies, however, have identified several promising new treatments.

Causes. A stroke is an interruption of the blood supply to a part of the brain. Most strokes occur when an artery supplying blood to the brain is blocked by a blood clot, either one that has traveled from another part of the body or one that has formed inside an artery supplying the brain. Other strokes occur when an artery within the brain or on its surface bursts. All strokes lead to the death of some of the brain's nerve cells, and the parts of the body controlled by those cells stop functioning—the results can include partial paralysis; impairments in speech, understanding, memory, movement, or visual perception; and behavioral changes.

Various factors are known to increase an individual's stroke risk. The most important is high blood pressure (hypertension). Diabetes, cigarette smoking, obesity, a high-fat diet, and a family history of certain diseases each confer additional risk. It has been widely assumed that controlling hypertension would lower the risk of stroke, and indeed, the steady decline in stroke incidence has been largely attributed to the aggressive treatment of hypertension. Until recently data directly confirming this assumption were lacking, but a number of studies have now confirmed that control of high blood pressure is very effective.

The role of oral contraceptives (birth control pills) in causing stroke has also been clarified recently. In the early 1960s, shortly after the introduction of birth control pills, physicians began seeing increasing numbers of complications such as blood clots in the legs, heart attacks, and strokes. By the late 1960s it seemed clear that the dose of estrogen in the contraceptives was the most important factor in determining risk, and after the dose was greatly reduced, the risk of complications was likewise substantially lowered. In fact, the risk with current versions of the pill compares favorably with the risk of neurological complications from pregnancy itself. This has been very reassuring to women now taking birth control pills. However, until recently it was not known whether women who took high-dose estrogen pills in prior decades would have a greater risk of stroke in later life. A recent study provides reassurance on this point as well. It concluded that the risk of stroke and other complications involving blood clots falls to normal shortly after a woman stops taking oral contraceptives.

Cigarette smoking in women who also take birth control pills has been found to greatly increase the risk of stroke and other complications. Several recent studies have confirmed that both cigarette smoking and heavy consumption of alcohol (more than four drinks a day) are risk factors for women who have never taken oral contraceptives and for men. Stopping smoking, even late in life, seems to lower the risk of both heart attack and stroke.

Debating Prevention. From 10 to 15 percent of individuals who suffer strokes have a warning symptom beforehand. The warning may be loss of vision in one eye for a few minutes, temporary double vision, difficulty with speech, weakness of an arm or leg, or abnormal sensations in one or another part of the body. These brief warnings are called transient ischemic attacks, or TIAs. The importance of TIAs as possible precursors of stroke has been recognized for the past 30 years, and it is now known that sometimes—but not always—proper treatment after a TIA can decrease the risk of stroke. However, over the past five years there has been enormous controversy over what proper treatment is, for the information available has not always provided a clear answer.

The most controversy has centered on the surgical procedure called carotid endarterectomy. By the mid-1980s this procedure had become the second most commonly performed vascular operation in the United States (coronary artery bypass surgery being the first). It involves opening a carotid artery (the two carotid arteries, which run up the front of the neck, are major suppliers of blood to the brain) and removing a buildup of fatty deposits that narrows the artery and increases the risk of stroke if a blood clot lodges in the narrowed area. Since 1986, growing criticism of carotid surgery has led to a substantial decline in the frequency of the operation. For while it is clear that in many patients strokes have been prevented by carotid surgery, it is also clear that the surgery itself may lead to a stroke in some individuals. It has been suggested that, at least in part, the problem may be a lack of expertise on the part of some surgeons. While it is clear that the operation should not be done by an unskilled surgeon, it is not clear whether the benefits outweigh the risks when a skilled surgeon performs the operation in a sophisticated neurological center, with the help of expert neurological anesthetists, neurological critical care specialists, and experienced cardiovascular consultants. To answer this question, a clinical trial has been organized by neurologists at the University of Ontario. The study, which is ex-

pected to take five years, will enroll 4,000 patients at 40 medical centers in the United States and Canada and follow them carefully to determine whether carotid surgery is of benefit. Until the study is completed, the surgery should be reserved for carefully selected patients with severe narrowing of the artery.

There has also been considerable debate among physicians about the proper dose of aspirin to prescribe as a preventive. The mainstay of drug therapy for the prevention of stroke for the past decade, aspirin suppresses substances, produced by the body, that cause blood vessels to constrict and blood platelets to aggregate, or clump together, causing clots to form. Unfortunately, aspirin also suppresses another substance that normally serves to dilate blood vessels and to prevent platelet aggregation. Because of this dual action, there has been a good deal of debate about the optimal dose of aspirin to be used in the prevention of stroke (and of other conditions in which blood clots play a role). In recent years, doses have ranged from four adult aspirin, or 1,300 milligrams, daily to as little as 300 milligrams every other day. None of the studies over the past decade has provided a definitive answer to the dosage question. Analysis of these studies does seem to indicate, though, that lower doses may be sufficient to lower the risk of stroke, as well as being perhaps somewhat safer. Another unresolved question under study is why aspirin seems to be more effective in men than in women. (*See also the feature article* ASPIRIN.)

The connection between heart disease and stroke is receiving increasing attention. Since the fatty deposits that can block the arteries in the neck and within the skull, helping precipitate a stroke, also tend to occur in the coronary arteries, stroke and symptoms of heart disease often go hand in hand. The extent to which this is true is only now becoming clear. For instance, it is now known that 6 out of every 100 patients with transient ischemic attacks of the brain die each year, with 5 of those deaths being due to heart disease rather than stroke. In fact, two to three times as many TIA patients die every year as do patients with known heart disease but without TIAs. Therefore, individuals with TIAs should have a careful evaluation of their risk for a heart attack as well as a stroke, and a program of medication, diet, and exercise should be carefully supervised by the patient's physicians with an eye to preventing both.

Minimizing the Effects. It has traditionally been thought that, when an individual has a stroke, little can be done to limit brain damage—that the brain is very intolerant of loss of blood supply and its nerve cells die in any area where circulation is lost for more than just a few minutes. However, it has recently become clear that nerve cell death does not occur immediately. This raises the possibility that what happens in the brain after the blood supply is lost might be reversed or altered in such a way as to minimize neurological damage. Research is underway on just this question: Can the devastating effects of stroke be minimized once the stroke has started?

One promising experimental approach involves holding down the level of glucose (a form of sugar) in the blood. Doing this may limit damage after a stroke by decreasing the metabolic needs of nerve cells. This discovery may lead to the clinical practice of avoiding glucose injections shortly after a stroke begins. A second promising approach involves drugs. In animal trials two groups of drugs appear to be protective when given an hour or two after a stroke has begun. They are calcium channel blockers (already widely used in the treatment of heart disease, hypertension, and migraine) and NMDA blockers. Both act to decrease the metabolic and electrical activity of nerve cells, thereby protecting them from injury. Human trials of these drugs are expected to begin shortly.

The evolution of treatment for stroke is closely paralleling progress in cardiology, where a number of new drugs have dramatically changed the treatment of heart attacks and greatly improved survival rates over the past several years.

Cocaine, Speed, and the Nervous System

Whenever a new illicit drug appears on the scene, serious physical, psychological, and neurological con-

---

"TONGUE-TIED BUT NORMAL-NOTIONED"

Severe cerebral palsy and the ability to write a prize-winning book may not usually be regarded as compatible, but they are in the case of Christopher Nolan. Nolan, who was born in Ireland in 1965, can see and hear, but he cannot talk and has little control over his movements. Confined to a wheelchair, he is completely dependent on his family for physical needs. Mentally, however, it is a different story.

Shortly after Nolan's birth—during which he suffered a period of asphyxiation, and brain damage—his family realized that his body might be mute and helpless but his mind was not. Over the years, they developed a language of eye signals. Also, beginning at age 11, when Nolan began taking a drug that helped control the muscle spasms in his neck, he has been able to type using a pointer strapped to his forehead, but someone, usually his mother, must stand behind him and support his chin while he works.

In this fashion Nolan has written two books. He describes the first—a critically acclaimed 1981 volume of poetry called *Dam-Burst of Dreams*—as "my nomadic-memory's minted musings." The second, released in the United States in 1988, is his autobiography, *Under the Eye of the Clock*.

Both books display a bold and distinctive style and an ability to coin metaphors and use words in unconventional ways that have led critics to compare Nolan with James Joyce. In the autobiography, the 1988 winner of Britain's presti-

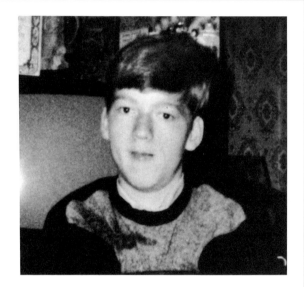

gious Whitbread Prize, Nolan uses the third person to write about himself with remarkable objectivity.

The book tells of his struggle to use his acute intelligence as he made his painful way from a school for the handicapped to ordinary high school to Dublin's Trinity College, dealing with the hypocrisy, intolerance, and pity of society toward such as he—"crass crippled man dashed, branded, and treated as dross in a world offended by their appearance."

Unable to forget all those others who are "tongue-tied but normal-notioned" and never found a way out of their prison, Nolan has one overriding ambition: "to find a voice for the voiceless."

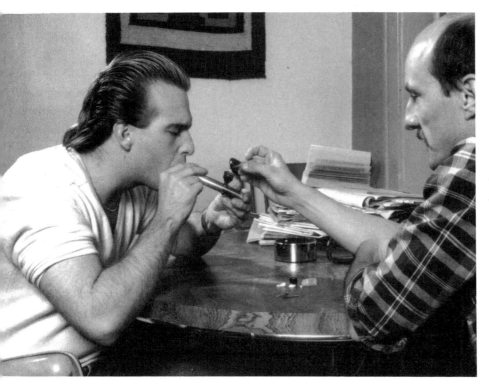

Physicians are reporting serious and permanent neurological consequences from cocaine use, including strokes and prolonged seizures. The new problems are the result of the wide availability of crack, a smokable form of cocaine that is absorbed very rapidly into the bloodstream.

sequences soon follow. Recent experience with cocaine, especially crack, and with methamphetamine, or speed, has shown that these drugs are no exception.

Cocaine. In 1985 the U.S. National Institute of Drug Abuse estimated that 30 million Americans had used cocaine, that 5 million were taking it regularly, and that thousands were trying it each day for the first time. Since those estimates appeared, crack, a smokable form of cocaine, has become more widely available and can be found everywhere, from large cities to small towns. When cocaine is smoked, it is absorbed very quickly into the bloodstream, where it rapidly reaches very high concentrations. This appears to lead to a high incidence of neurological and psychiatric complications.

For centuries it has been known that conventional cocaine, even in low concentrations, can lead to sudden death, and now heart attacks, heart rhythm abnormalities, and shock are well-recognized complications. In addition to these effects, changes in personality, disorientation, alterations in sleep patterns, and seizures have long been known to occur because of changes in the nervous system. For the most part, these complications were thought to be infrequent and, in the case of the nervous system, usually reversible. Now, however, it is clear that crack has permanent—and serious—neurological consequences.

Neurologists from all areas of the United States have begun to report cases of several kinds of stroke and severe and prolonged seizures in patients who have used crack. For instance, physicians at the Harbor-UCLA Medical Center in Los Angeles reported several common as well as uncommon kinds of stroke in 14 patients seen over a two-year period. They observed stroke in the spinal cord, a very unusual occurrence (leading to rapid onset of paralysis from the neck down), as well as strokes in more common locations such as the brainstem and the area of the brain called the cerebral cortex. TIAs were also observed. What was especially striking was that many of these complications occurred instantaneously after crack was consumed, sometimes immediately after the individual used the drug for the first time. The exact mechanisms causing these neurological effects are unknown, but it is likely that wide fluctuations in blood pressure or heart rhythm abnormalities underlie at least some of them. They appear to be as unpredictable as they are devastating to the individual.

Speed. Another drug whose effects are well-known to neurologists is methamphetamine, or speed. This drug was widely abused in the United States in the 1960s and 1970s, when diet pills containing methamphetamine were diverted from legitimate use to the illicit market or abused by those for whom they had been legitimately prescribed. Abuse of methamphetamine largely disappeared after physicians began restricting its prescription and the U.S. Food and Drug Administration applied additional controls.

Observers of the illicit drug scene on the West and East coasts have now begun to see an increase in the use of "street speed," most of which is illegally produced in small laboratories.

Methamphetamine and cocaine share a number of properties, including similar adverse psychiatric and neurological consequences and effects on the heart. Therefore, as the use of methamphetamine grows, it is very likely that cases of stroke, sudden death, and seizures similar to those accompanying crack use will be observed.

Methamphetamine also has other, more insidious properties. In particular, its chronic use in moderate or even small amounts, either swallowed or inhaled, can lead to changes in personality, a state of disorientation, and a prolonged state of paranoia that closely resembles paranoid schizophrenia. Even very experienced physicians can mistake the psychosis associated with methamphetamine for true schizophrenia. Though this psychosis is reversible, a number of long-term changes in personality, cognitive ability, and emotions have been observed with methamphetamine, making the drug particularly dangerous.

Update on Parkinson's Disease

In Parkinson's disease the brain fails to produce enough of a chemical called dopamine that carries messages between nerve cells in the brain. As a result, the patient loses some control over movement, tending to shake, to be unable to initiate movement, and to feel "frozen." Depression and deterioration of memory and thought processes each affect about 25 percent of Parkinson's sufferers. In 1987 there was great excitement over the seeming promise offered by a new treatment for Parkinson's disease—implantation of cells from the medulla (or inner portion) of the adrenal glands into the brain. The medulla produces small amounts of dopamine. Frequent press reports recounted the success of this surgery in patients in Mexico, China, Cuba, Europe, and the United States. By 1989, however, the optimism had largely been dashed by additional and more specific information about the patients who underwent these operations.

In the United States, about 125 patients with severe Parkinson's disease received implants from their own adrenal medullas. These operations were conducted in about a dozen university medical centers. Though some patients apparently benefited, the improvement was not striking, nor was it sustained, contrary to the early promising reports from Mexico. In addition, a number of the patients died, or had very serious complications, following surgery, indicating that the operation was not nearly as safe as many had hoped. A similar lack of success was reported in Sweden.

Because of these poor results, the technique has largely been abandoned outside of research centers.

Nevertheless, much has been learned by physicians from this limited use of transplant surgery. For instance, more is now known about the effect of adrenal cells on the brain, and it is hoped that more can be learned about how this effect is produced. Researchers are attempting to isolate the various chemical factors that travel from one cell to another and can influence the growth of the nervous system. Such a factor might be injected or implanted in the brain instead of the adrenal cells themselves.

Also, it might be possible to use cells from other sources, for instance cells grown in a laboratory culture or fetal brain cells (fetal tissue grows quickly and is less likely than other foreign tissue to be rejected by the recipient's immune system). The first implants of fetal brain tissue in Parkinson's patients in the United States were performed in late 1988; similar operations had previously been done elsewhere. So far, fetal tissue implants in humans have had no more success than adrenal tissue implants, although in animals fetal tissue is much more successful.

HAMILTON MOSES III, M.D.

Cancer

Progress Against Cancer • Prevention and Early Detection • Treating Early Breast Cancer • Biological Weapons Against Cancer

Progress Against Cancer

The latest U.S. cancer statistics from the National Cancer Institute (NCI) show mixed progress. Between 1950 and 1985 the incidence of all types of cancer combined rose 37 percent (this figure is for whites, the only group for whom incidence data are available for the entire period). During the same years, death rates decreased for all races for all age groups up to 55. When lung cancer, the leading U.S. cancer killer, was excluded, death rates decreased for all age groups up to 85. But mortality rates among the older age groups have been slowly increasing in recent years (and more than three-fourths of cancer patients are over age 55), and mortality rates for lung cancer for all age groups combined increased steadily between 1973 and 1985.

Currently in the United States, about half of all cancers are cured. The NCI believes that universal application of the latest knowledge about prevention and treatment would further reduce cancer deaths by 50 percent. Since the National Cancer Act of 1971 established a national cancer program, there have been many new discoveries about how a normal cell becomes cancerous. In late 1988 scientists reported the successful transplantation of the major elements of the human immune defense system into mice. Such work, plus the National Institutes of Health's plan to map, identify, and define all the human genes, hold out hope of unprecedented progress in understanding cancer. For now, though, prevention and early detection remain the best ways to significantly decrease U.S. cancer incidence and death rates.

Prevention and Early Detection

In the area of prevention and early detection, the NCI continued its focus on changing the nation's health behavior. The importance of chemoprevention continued to grow, and the dangers of radon as a cancer-causing agent were well-publicized.

Changing Behavior. According to the 1987 National Health Interview Survey, conducted by the NCI and the National Center for Health Statistics, Americans are not doing what it will take to meet the NCI's goal of halving the cancer death rate in America by the year 2000. The survey—the results of which were released in 1988—found that the use of smokeless tobacco, which causes cancer of the mouth, esophagus, and larynx, has increased dramatically, especially among young white men. According to the surgeon general's 1988 report on smoking, nicotine, found in all forms of tobacco, is a powerfully addicting drug, with an addiction process similar to that in drugs such as cocaine and heroin. This may help explain why, although smoking rates have declined over the last 20 years, about 30 percent of Americans 18 and older still smoke. (*See also the Health and Medical News article* SMOKING.)

The Interview Survey also showed that while the majority of Americans are aware of the link between cancer and diet, they are not sure how to set about meeting the NCI's dietary recommendations—such as reducing fat intake to 30 percent of total calories and increasing fiber intake to 30 grams a day. And although most people have heard of pap tests, mammograms, and blood stool tests for different types of cancer screening, most do not know when and how often to have these tests done.

Chemoprevention. Work is progressing in the area of chemoprevention, the use of chemical agents to prevent cancer or to reverse early precancerous changes in cells. One agent being explored is beta-carotene, a compound in carrots, squash, and other vegetables that is converted into vitamin A in the body. The Harvard Medical School and Brigham and Women's Hospital in Boston are in the midst of a study of beta-carotene that will follow 22,000 physicians until 1990. Initial research indicates that beta-carotene may reduce the incidence of lung cancer. Vitamin A and beta-carotene are also the subject of research on preventing oral cancer.

Researchers are experimenting with another form of vitamin A, retinoids, as a preventive for skin cancer. Participants in a recent study, all of whom were suffering from a hereditary condition called xeroderma pigmentosum that causes skin cancer, were treated with one of the retinoid drugs, the oral prescription medication isotretinoin. Treatment resulted in a significant decrease in the number of skin cancers. (Isotretinoin, sold under the brand name Accutane, is currently used to treat severe cystic acne.)

Tamoxifen, a synthetic antihormone, is also a candidate for chemoprevention. Tamoxifen is thought to slow cancer by sticking to special estrogen "receptors" (called positive receptors) on cell surfaces. When tamoxifen occupies these receptors, the hormone estrogen cannot enter and stimulate the cells to grow. Tamoxifen is one of the most effective and least toxic drugs for women whose breast cancers grow when they are stimulated by estrogen. (Only some breast cancers do.) The Wisconsin Clinical Cancer Center is currently studying 160 women with positive estrogen receptors who have recovered from early-stage breast cancer to see if tamoxifen prevents the development of new tumors.

Radon. The U.S. Environmental Protection Agency (EPA) issued a warning in September 1988 that cancer-causing radon gas may be seeping into homes across the country. One out of three U.S. homes may be affected. Radon is an odorless, colorless, radioactive gas that occurs naturally in soil and rocks. It seeps into homes through small cracks in building foundations and is dangerous when it accumulates in enclosed spaces. The EPA recommended that all homeowners test basements and lower floors for radon using inexpensive charcoal canisters. If high levels of radon are found, the problem can be remedied by sealing cracks in foundations and installing pipes to vent the radon outdoors, where it can dissipate. Radon is estimated to cause 10 percent of all lung cancers.

Adjuvant Therapies

Progress has been made on several fronts regarding adjuvant therapies, those used in combination with cancer surgery. Recent strides include understanding why cells become resistant to several of the different drugs used in chemotherapy after exposure to only one drug. There has also been work on using chemotherapy to prevent a recurrence of disease after surgery for early-stage breast cancer, as well as on refining biological response modifiers—naturally occurring substances that help the body fight cancer.

Research into adjuvant therapies, like all cancer research, is dependent on clinical trials to test new treatments before making them available to the general public. The pace of cancer research could increase significantly if more patients took part in these trials. In 1988 the NCI began a major effort to increase participation. One tool being used is a computerized database called PDQ (Physician Data Query), which provides information on which clinical trials are accepting patients. Physicians can purchase access to PDQ, have database searches done through medical libraries, or gain access through their own computers. Patients whose doctors do not use PDQ can call the NCI's Cancer Information Service at 1-800-4-CANCER to have a search done.

Multidrug Resistance. A fundamental question in chemotherapy is why some types of cancer quickly become resistant to the powerful combinations of anticancer drugs that are used. Scientists are exploring a number of mechanisms that might be responsible for drug resistance. One is gene amplification, where the cancer cell makes multiple copies of genes that code for a protein, called P-glycoprotein, that acts as a pump to push the drugs out of the cell. Another mechanism is the accumulation of the detoxifying protein glutathione, which diminishes a drug's ability to kill the cell. Scientists have reported progress in understanding these mechanisms and are working on drugs that can overcome resistance with fewer toxic side effects than the drugs developed so far.

Chemotherapy for Early Breast Cancer. The NCI took a bold step in May 1988, when it sent a letter called a clinical alert to thousands of physicians who treat cancer patients. The letter contained data from three studies, on adjuvant treatment for breast cancer patients, before the studies had been published in medical journals (which means they have been reviewed carefully by journal editors and advisers). NCI officials said they had followed this unusual course because the results of the studies were so important they should be made known immediately. The studies indicated that all breast cancer patients should have chemotherapy or hormonal therapy (like tamoxifen) following surgery, even if there was no evidence that the cancer had spread to their lymph nodes. While women whose cancer has spread to the nodes are routinely treated with drugs after surgery, standard treatment for other breast cancer patients—about half

of all newly diagnosed cases—had generally included only surgery and radiation therapy. The three studies cited by the NCI—and a fourth, conducted in Europe—were published in *The New England Journal of Medicine* in February 1989.

Biological Response Modifiers. The past five years have seen phenomenal progress in the understanding of why normal cells turn into cancer cells, how the body fights cancer, and what role biological response modifiers can play in that fight. Biological response modifiers are substances that the body's immune system produces naturally to fight infection or abnormal cells. They can be produced outside the body in large quantities through genetic engineering. One biological response modifier showing unusual promise is interleukin-2, a substance that helps tumor-fighting cells to grow. Researchers at the NCI have been isolating from the tumors of cancer patients small numbers of what are called tumor-infiltrating lymphocytes, which are white blood cells that are particularly effective at penetrating and killing cancer cells. After these cells are removed from the patients, they

In 1988, George H. Hitchings and Gertrude B. Elion became the first scientists to win the Nobel Prize in physiology or medicine for work on cancer treatments.

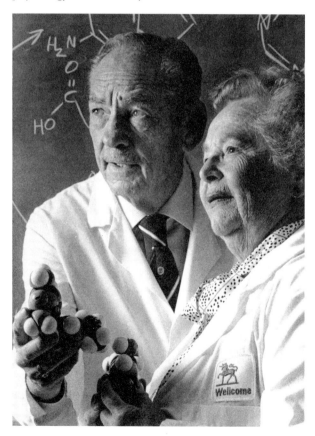

are cultured (grown in the laboratory) for 30 days with interleukin-2—increasing their numbers by billions—and then injected back into the patient. The procedure has helped shrink tumors in about half of the 25 patients treated so far.

Researchers are interested in following these reinjected cells in patients whose tumors do not shrink, to find out if the cells are dying too quickly or losing some of their tumor-killing properties. With current techniques the cells can be followed in the body for only three or four days, but in January 1989 the U.S. government approved the researchers' plan to transplant foreign genes into the cultured tumor-infiltrating cells before they are reinjected into the patients. The cells with the new genes will serve as "markers" that the researchers will be able to follow to keep track of the reinjected cells. This is the first time the federal government has approved the transfer of cells containing foreign genes into humans. However, at the end of January a suit to block the transplant was filed by a group opposed to genetic research.

Nobel Prize

In 1988, for the first time, the winners of the Nobel Prize in physiology or medicine included scientists working on cancer treatment. Gertrude B. Elion and George H. Hitchings, Ph.D., began working together in 1945 to discover how normal human cell growth differs from that of bacteria, parasites, viruses, and

---

A BOOK FOR KIDS WITH CANCER

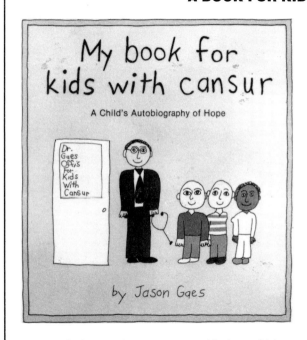

In 1984 at age six, Jason was diagnosed as having Burkitt's lymphoma, a form of cancer that is quite rare in the United States. Because it spreads quickly, Burkitt's lymphoma is usually fatal, but after two years of rigorous treatment, Jason emerged from his ordeal cancer-free. He has since had no recurrence.

In *My Book for Kids With Cansur*, Jason describes his fears, his experiences with hospitalization, and the treatments he received, including chemotherapy, radiation, and surgery. "Sometimes keymotharupy makes you sick and you throw up," he writes. "Sometimes you looz your hair from it but you can wear hats if it bothers you." He gives advice on how to cope with being afraid: ". . . if your scared of blood tests have your Mom or Dad cover your eyes." But he adds, "If you get cansur you might as well not even be afraid cause your probly not even going to die anyway."

Finally, he reassures the reader, ". . . when you feel real bad its ok to cry sometimes. It doesn't mean your a baby and Dr. Karen says sometimes it makes you feel better." Jason includes his telephone number in case any of his readers want to talk to him. He plans to become a doctor "who takes care of kids with cansur."

Being a kid isn't always easy, and being a kid with a potentially fatal disease like cancer takes an extra dose of courage and hope. Jason Gaes of Worthington, Minn., not only survived cancer, but wrote a book to help other children deal with the disease and to let them know that not all youngsters with cancer die. Published in Jason's own handwriting, spelling, and style—and illustrated by his brothers, Tim and Adam—*My Book for Kids With Cansur* is both heart warming and frank without being either sentimental or morbid.

My Book for Kids With Cansur is available for $11.95 from Melius & Peterson Publishing, Inc., P.O. Box 925, Aberdeen, SD 57402-0925; toll free telephone number 1-800-882-5171. A portion of the proceeds goes to the American Cancer Society.

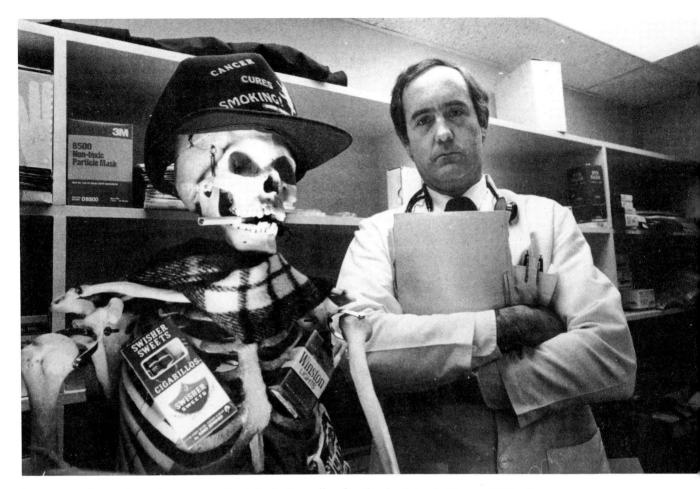

In a personal crusade against cancer, Dr. John J. Cannell, a family physician in Beaver, W.Va., has refused to take on new patients who smoke; prominent in his office is a human skeleton decorated with tobacco labels and antismoking warnings.

cancer cells in the hope of finding ways to selectively kill these disease-causing life forms in humans. Their work led to the development of new drugs for the treatment of many diseases, including leukemia. (Sir James W. Black shared the Nobel Prize for his work on drugs that block receptor molecules on cells.)

Cancer Research Prizes

The General Motors Cancer Research Foundation's 1988 awards went to four cancer researchers. Dr. Alfred G. Knudson, Jr., of the Fox Chase Cancer Center in Philadelphia won one prize for contributions to understanding of the causes and ultimate prevention of human cancer. Dr. Yasutomi Nishizuka of Kobe University in Japan was awarded his prize for basic science contributions to cancer research. Professor Sam Shapiro of the Johns Hopkins University in Baltimore and Dr. Philip Strax of the University of

Miami shared a third prize for contributions to the diagnosis of early breast cancer.

Genetics and Cancer. In 1971, Dr. Knudson developed a model explaining how both genetics and environment may cause retinoblastoma and Wilms' tumor, rare childhood cancers. Recent studies have verified Dr. Knudson's theory that there exist certain anticancer genes, or anti-oncogenes, that protect against the disease. (Genes that play a role in the development of cancer are called oncogenes.) The lack of or destruction or damage of anti-oncogenes can cause cancers such as retinoblastoma, which is a tumor of the eye. Both hereditary and nonhereditary retinoblastoma, it is now known, involve the same anti-oncogene. It may be missing entirely or inherited in a damaged state, leaving the child susceptible to cancer if further damage occurs. Or it may be inherited intact, with environmental damage later causing cancer.

Dr. Knudson's work also includes understanding of

why some families seem to be prone to cancer and identification of genetic factors that may relate to other forms of cancer. He was a pioneer in such work, and other scientists have gone on to apply his theories. In colorectal cancer, for example, long known to be more common among people with a parent or sibling who had this type of cancer, researchers suspect that the causes of the cancer include the actions of an abnormally transformed gene (the oncogene) and the failure of certain anti-oncogenes to function. A University of Utah study released in 1988 found strong evidence that about one-third of white Americans inherit a gene or genes that increase their susceptibility to developing colon and rectal cancers. The researchers concluded that this genetic susceptibility interacts with environmental factors to cause the cancers. For those with colon or rectal cancers in the family, early and regular screening and prevention is the best protection.

Molecular Signals Within a Cell. Dr. Nishizuka's studies helped explain the intricate molecular signals that lead to the development of cancer within a cell. He discovered protein kinase C (PKC), a substance in cells that translates incoming chemical signals into instructions for the cell and that plays a critical role in growth control. Several oncogenes distort this translation process, so that PKC gives the command to keep growing. Researchers now are interested in developing ways to keep PKC under control.

Mammography Screening. Professor Shapiro and Dr. Strax received their prize for their groundbreaking breast cancer screening/mammography study begun during the 1960s for the Health Insurance Plan of Greater New York. The study proved that mammography could detect breast cancer at a very early and more curable stage and that regular mammograms could reduce breast cancer mortality by 38 percent. These results led to a number of other major mammography studies and stimulated the development of the mammography equipment in use today, which employs low-dose radiation. Recent statistics showing an increased incidence in breast cancer underline the importance of mammography screening.

Some researchers had disputed the cost-effectiveness of mammography for women under the age of 50, but recent reanalysis of data from the Health Insurance Plan study, using a follow-up period of at least 18 years, found 24 percent fewer breast cancer deaths among women who were screened at ages 40 to 49 than in women who were not screened. The weight of evidence in favor of beginning regular mammography screening at age 40 has reinforced the NCI's recommendations that women get a mammogram every one or two years from age 40 to 49 and annually after age 50. (The American Cancer Society also recommends a baseline mammogram between the ages of 35 and 39.) Many states are legislating mandated insurance coverage for mammography screening, so that cost does not remain a barrier. Despite the benefits of mammography, only 15 to 20 percent of women have ever had a mammogram.

See also the Spotlight on Health article DETECTING CANCER EARLY. PAUL F. ENGSTROM, M.D.
SHARON WATKINS DAVIS

Diabetes

Transplant Drug Offers Hope • Marker for Type I Diabetes • Preventing Kidney Damage • Doctor-Patient "Therapeutic Alliance"

New Drug Treatment?

The drug cyclosporine, widely used following transplant operations, is now being used experimentally to treat one type of diabetes. The drug suppresses the body's immune system (and therefore helps prevent rejection of transplanted organs). It is being tried against what is known as Type I diabetes, in which the body stops producing the hormone insulin, needed by body cells so that they can properly utilize glucose (sugar) circulating in the blood. Type I diabetes is known to be an autoimmune disease, or one in which the body's defenses attack its own tissues—in this case, the beta cells in the pancreas that produce insulin. It is well known that there may be a "honeymoon period" right after the diagnosis of Type I diabetes, during which the need for insulin injections decreases sharply, possibly because those beta cells that have not yet been destroyed increase their production of the hormone. The goal of cyclosporine treatment is to suppress the immune system's attack on these cells and prolong the honeymoon period.

In one recent study conducted in Paris, cyclosporine was given to 40 children, aged 7 to 15, who had shown initial symptoms of Type I diabetes over the previous three months. Within six weeks of starting to take cyclosporine, two-thirds of the children had improved to the point where they could totally discontinue insulin injections; in half of the children, the diabetes was still in remission after one year on the drug. In similar studies involving teenagers or adults, remission rates of up to 25 percent have been achieved, and remission has persisted, in some cases, for a year or more. It should be noted, though, that insulin dependence frequently returns within a few weeks if cyclosporine treatment is discontinued.

Moreover, the use of cyclosporine carries some risks, because suppressing the immune system reduces the body's overall ability to fight infection and perhaps to prevent the growth of tumors. There is also evidence that the drug may damage the kidneys. However, techniques are being developed to control the side effects of cyclosporine, and research into less toxic alternate drugs is continuing.

Predicting Diabetes

The effort to find a reliable "marker" that could identify people who will develop Type I diabetes in the future has recently met with success. The marker is a substance called 64K autoantibody, which attacks a protein (64K) that seems to occur only in the insulin-making cells of the pancreas. In previous studies 64K autoantibody had been found in the blood in 95 percent of those just developing the disease. In research reported in 1988, the autoantibody was found in blood samples taken from people three months to seven years before diabetes was diagnosed; all those in the 1988 study who developed diabetes had the autoantibody in their blood months or years earlier. This discovery could provide physicians with a vital tool to identify people who might be candidates for preventive cyclosporine or other immuno-suppressive therapy. It may also be possible to develop a drug that would prevent the onset of Type I diabetes by destroying the 64K autoantibodies (without harming other body cells).

So far, no definite marker has been found for Type II diabetes. In this much more common form of the disease, which mainly occurs in older people, the body continues to produce but cannot make use of insulin. It is already known, however, that those who have a family history of this type of diabetes and who are overweight and not physically active are very much at risk. For such people, a change to a more active life-style, coupled with weight loss and a balanced diet, may prevent the onset of the disease.

Preventing Kidney Failure

A useful test for kidney damage, a possible complication of diabetes, is now widely available. In general, people with diabetes are vulnerable to damage to the capillaries, the body's smallest blood vessels. When the capillaries in the kidneys are affected, eventually kidney failure may result. Since treatment for kidney damage is most effective when started early, people

with diabetes should have the new test once a year.

The test measures the amount of protein in urine samples collected from the patient over a 24-hour period. (When the kidneys are not functioning properly, protein "leaks" into the urine.) A class of drugs called angiotensin-converting enzyme (ACE) inhibitors, used in treating some types of high blood pressure, have been found effective in slowing the progression of kidney damage.

Update on Pancreas Transplants

Although pancreas transplants have been performed for 20 years as a treatment for Type I diabetes, serious problems remain. They include rejection of the foreign tissue and destruction of the new insulin-producing beta cells by the same process that initially caused the diabetes. Cyclosporine is used to try to prevent these reactions, but as noted, it can have serious side effects. Therefore, transplants of the whole pancreas have generally been reserved for those with advanced kidney failure who require a kidney transplant as well (and therefore would be receiving cyclosporine in any event). But as techniques improve, earlier transplantation may be indicated in certain carefully selected cases.

An alternative procedure currently being studied is the transplantation of fetal pancreatic tissue. In general, fetal tissue is less likely than other foreign tissue to be rejected by the body's immune system. The tissue used in the transplants are the islets of Langerhans, the tiny clusters of pancreatic cells in which the insulin-producing beta cells are located. To date, more than 600 fetal islet transplants have been performed outside the United States—with widely varying degrees of success.

Controlling Blood Glucose

A long-term research project funded by the U.S. National Institutes of Health (NIH) is under way, to study the relationship between blood glucose control in Type I diabetes and the development of various complications. Because, in people with diabetes, body cells have difficulty utilizing glucose, sugar tends to accumulate in excessive amounts in the blood; this buildup of glucose has been linked to many of the complications of the disease (including, for example, capillary damage). Keeping blood glucose levels as near normal as possible may minimize the risk of complications, and the NIH study is attempting to assess just how close the relationship between glucose level and complications in fact is.

In any event, for someone with Type I diabetes, tight control of blood glucose levels is, unfortunately, no easy task. People with diabetes have to walk a tightrope in attempting to manage their disease without unduly restricting their lives.

The current study has shed light on the value—and limitations—of insulin pumps as an alternative to regular injections to control blood glucose. With an insulin pump, a needle that remains under the skin continuously delivers insulin (generally from a reservoir worn on the belt) according to a set program. When the study was started, these pumps were popular, and they have since been improved, particularly through the development of a "soft needle" that can remain in place even during strenuous exercise. Nevertheless, experience has shown that the pumps are ideal only for a limited number of highly motivated people—who are willing to cope with the constant presence of the device and to accept the risk that its use will sometimes cause low blood sugar. It has been found that most people who want to carefully control their blood glucose levels prefer to give themselves multiple daily injections of insulin, guided by frequent checks of their own blood sugar to determine when an injection is needed.

Nasal Insulin

Press reports about the value of insulin taken in the form of a nasal spray have proved to be premature. Only short-acting insulin (effective for a comparatively short period of time) can be absorbed through the nasal tissues. Therefore, whenever longer-acting insulin is required for blood glucose control between meals or overnight, it still has to be injected. Moreover, the detergents used in the nasal insulin preparations may irritate nasal tissue or make it susceptible to infection. However, researchers are continuing efforts to improve the products, and nasal insulin may eventually be useful as an additional resource for controlling Type II diabetes, besides diet, exercise, and sometimes oral medication.

The "Therapeutic Alliance"

Controlling diabetes places restrictions on the way people live and reduces their freedom of action, both at work and at home. And even the most conscientious efforts cannot guarantee that the long-term effects of the disease will be entirely avoided. Many health professionals are now becoming aware of the extent to which both the restraints and the uncertainties affect the daily life of those with diabetes and make it difficult for many to adhere to their treatment plan. Moreover, diabetes affects the ability to respond to the challenges and problems that come with each stage of life, including adolescence, career choice,

marriage, pregnancy and parenting, and aging. At the same time, people with diabetes are taking a more active part in their own treatment; in particular, those who test their own blood glucose levels daily know how effective their treatment is. For all these reasons, many physicians and health educators are trying to build a partnership—or therapeutic alliance—with people who have diabetes and their families, rather than merely prescribing treatment for them. Such a relationship emphasizes cooperation and negotiation between patients and healthcare providers. For the partnership to work, people with diabetes need to feel assured that their healthcare providers are aware of the latest developments in treatment and honest about the limitations of therapy, and that they care about the welfare of each individual patient. Healthcare providers, for their part, need to trust their patients to be open about the problems they encounter in living with diabetes—and to be willing to learn and change. If such mutual respect and openness are present, realistic goals of therapy can be agreed upon and modified as necessary. In this way, the individual can strike the best possible bargain between leading a satisfying normal life and keeping diabetes under control.

ETHAN A. H. SIMS, M.D.
DOROTHEA F. SIMS

Digestive System

Heredity and Colorectal Cancer •
Salmonella-Infected Grade A Eggs •
Dangers of Eating Raw Fish

Heredity and Colorectal Cancer

The majority of people who develop colorectal polyps and cancers may have inherited a susceptibility to such abnormal growths in the large intestine, according to a recent study of Utah families. The new research adds an important dimension to earlier evidence that environmental factors, particularly a diet high in fat and low in fiber, play a major role in the development of most colorectal polyps and cancers: environmental factors may help determine which genetically susceptible people eventually develop cancer.

Colorectal cancer is the second leading cause of cancer deaths in the United States and Canada, resulting in some 61,300 U.S. and 5,900 Canadian deaths each year. Early detection and removal of precancerous growths and early cancers is critical to curing the disease. However, colorectal cancer produces few symptoms in its early stages. Thus, the new evidence may encourage wider screening among those whose close relatives had polyps or cancers.

Most colorectal cancers appear to arise from adenomatous polyps—benign, mushroom-like growths on the lining of the wall of the intestine. If not removed, about 5 percent of all adenomatous polyps develop into cancers. The role of genetics in the development of colorectal cancer has been established in some relatively rare conditions, such as familial colonic polyposis and Gardner's syndrome, in which individuals may have dozens of polyps in their colons and are at an extremely high risk for developing colorectal cancer. Both conditions have definite patterns of inheritance, but little information was available until now on the role of genetics in cases of colorectal cancer not associated with those diseases.

In the Utah study, which involved 670 people from 34 family groups, the researchers began by assuming that people who developed adenomatous polyps or colorectal cancers had inherited a gene or genes that made them susceptible to the growths. The scientists selected as subjects individuals who had an adenomatous polyp or who had a cluster of relatives with colon cancers; none of the cases involved the rare inherited disorders of familial colonic polyposis or Gardner's syndrome. The researchers then screened

the blood relatives of their subjects, as well as spouses. The spouses served as "controls" in the study, because they shared the same life-style and environment as the subjects but had different genetic makeups. Adenomatous polyps were found in 19 percent of the blood relatives of the subjects with colon abnormalities but in only 12 percent of the spouses.

The scientists believe that almost a third of white Americans may carry one or more genes that predispose them to developing adenomatous polyps and colorectal cancer. The researchers believe that there is an interaction between the gene or genes and the environment. While genetic factors determine relative susceptibility, environmental factors determine which genetically susceptible people develop cancers. The scientists emphasized that the results from their study were obtained from white subjects only, who were primarily of British and Northern European descent.

Results of a smaller study in California, involving approximately 150 close relatives of people with colon cancer, did not find evidence of a clear family link in the development of colorectal polyps and cancers. Nevertheless, both groups of researchers emphasize the need for close relatives of people with colorectal polyps or cancers to have regular screening tests to detect these conditions.

The American Cancer Society recommends that

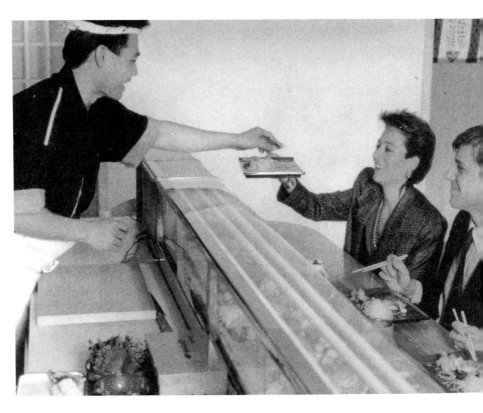

With the growing popularity of sushi bars in the United States, there has been an increase in intestinal parasitic infections caused by eating contaminated raw seafood.

everyone, regardless of family history, be screened for possible colon cancer starting at the age of 40. The society recommends an annual digital rectal examination beginning at age 40 and an annual stool blood test beginning at age 50. The society also recommends that people over 50 be examined with a proctosigmoidoscope, a lighted tube that allows the doctor to view the rectum and lower colon. This examination should be done annually at first, with later tests done at intervals of three to five years following two consecutive normal exams.

Grade A Eggs and *Salmonella*

Clean, disinfected grade A eggs have been linked to sometimes severe infections of the gastrointestinal tract. Prompted by a sixfold increase in infections caused by the bacterium *Salmonella enteritidis* in the northeastern United States between 1976 and 1986, researchers at the U.S. Centers for Disease Control (CDC) investigated all *S. enteritidis* outbreaks in eight northeastern states over a 2½-year period. They traced the source of the infections to grade A eggs or foods containing the eggs.

Salmonella, a bacterium that can cause abdominal cramps, fever, and diarrhea, is especially dangerous to the very young, the elderly, or people with impaired immune systems. *Salmonella* infections associated with eggs have been known for many years, but past infections were associated with the use of bulk egg products and ungraded or noncommercial eggs thought to have been contaminated by bacteria from chicken feces that got inside through cracks in the shell. To control this form of contamination, the U.S. government adopted policies in the 1970s requiring the pasteurization of bulk egg products and inspection and grading of eggs in the shells.

In the more recent northeastern infections, the CDC researchers investigated 65 outbreaks occurring between January 1985 and May 1987, involving over 2,000 people and resulting in 257 hospitalizations and 11 deaths. Food was identified as the vehicle by which the bacteria were transmitted in 35 of the outbreaks, and grade A eggs or foods containing such eggs were responsible for 77 percent of the food incidents. In most cases the eggs either were eaten raw or were inadequately cooked in such foods as hollandaise sauce, homemade eggnog, or Caesar salad dressing. The identification of grade A eggs as an important source of infection was unexpected since unbroken, unsoiled grade A eggs usually are not considered to be a source of infection. The researchers suspect that the bacteria might have contaminated the hens' ovaries and infected the egg yolks before they were surrounded by the shells.

There are many strains of *Salmonella*, and another type, *S. typhimurium*, was implicated in a California outbreak of food poisoning among people who attended a potluck birthday dinner in August 1988. The illness was traced to raw eggs used in the preparation of homemade strawberry ice cream. The eggs had apparently been handled and stored correctly.

To prevent *Salmonella* infection, individuals should use relatively fresh eggs that have been refrigerated and have no cracks. Adequate cooking is the most important means of prevention. To kill *Salmonella*, eggs should be boiled for seven minutes, poached for five minutes, or fried on each side for three minutes. People might also consider avoiding foods made with raw or undercooked eggs until more information is available on the association of grade A eggs with this type of infection.

Intestinal Infections and Sushi

Intestinal parasitic infections caused by eating raw or inadequately cooked fish are increasing worldwide, according to researchers from the U.S. Food and Drug Administration. Anisakiasis, an infection of the human intestinal tract caused by a fish parasite, was uncommon in the United States until recently. Researchers attribute much of the recent increase to changes in dietary habits, particularly the recent popularity of raw fish dishes, such as sushi and sashimi, and the trend toward undercooking seafood. The U.S. cases have all been caused by one of two roundworms—*Anisakis simplex* or *Pseudoterranova decipiens*. Pacific rockfish (also called Pacific red snapper) and Pacific salmon have most commonly been linked to the disease in the United States.

An increase in the number of human infections in the western United States (including Alaska and Hawaii) may well be related to the burgeoning populations of marine mammals found along the West Coast, such as California sea lions, elephant seals, and harbor seals. The worms can infest the stomachs of these mammals. Then, in their stool the mammals can pass worms in the form of larvae (a developmental stage in the worm life cycle). The larvae can then infect several species of fish that are closely associated with the mammals. The infection is transmitted to humans who eat raw fish containing the larvae.

Although the larvae of both *Anisakis simplex* and *Pseudoterranova decipiens* cause infections, *Pseudoterranova* infections are rarely serious from a medical standpoint since the larvae usually do not invade the wall of the stomach or intestines, and the worms eventually pass out of the body. Nevertheless, *Pseudoterranova* infestations can be frightening. Victims often cough up a live worm within 48 hours of eating infected fish, and they can sometimes feel the worm crawling around in the back of the throat.

However, *Anisakis* infections are much more serious since the larvae can penetrate the wall of the stomach, small intestine, and colon, producing marked inflammation resulting in abdominal pain, fever, diarrhea, nausea, or vomiting. These symptoms can occur within a few hours of eating infected fish. In some instances the symptoms are similar to and may be mistaken for acute appendicitis, a stomach ulcer, or some other gastrointestinal problem, making diagnosis of anisakiasis difficult. The diagnosis is made even more difficult because the presence of the parasite cannot be detected in the victim's feces.

About 50 cases of anisakiasis have been reported in the United States, but researchers believe that figure does not represent the true extent of the problem. Anisakiasis is currently not required to be reported to public health authorities, and accurate diagnostic tests are not available. The disease may be prevented by killing the parasites by cooking or freezing fish. Fish should be stored at -4°F for 60 hours or cooked to a temperature of at least 140°F for 10 minutes.

There is no effective drug to treat anisakiasis. However, the disease usually subsides on its own with conservative treatment of the symptoms (which can include providing fluids and giving antibiotics and possibly steroid drugs). Some people with intestinal anisakiasis undergo surgery because another condition is suspected. In these instances, removal of the diseased segment of the intestine represents definitive treatment for the condition.

See also the Spotlight on Health article HEMORRHOIDS.
DANIEL PELOT, M.D.

Drug Abuse

Addicts and AIDS • New Treatments for Cocaine Addiction • New Strategies for Prevention and Law Enforcement

AIDS

As more information becomes available about the spread of AIDS among drug users, researchers have found that the virus that causes the syndrome has infected different groups of abusers at different rates. The differences exist not only between geographically separate regions (New York City has much higher

rates of infection than Albany), but also between different parts of the same city (Chicago's west side has higher rates than the north and south sides). It is not yet clear what causes the differences, but many complex factors are probably involved, including the population within which the virus was first introduced and the behavior of individual drug users.

Several other important findings have also emerged from recent studies. One is that the proportion of intravenous (IV) drug users in New York City and San Francisco who are infected seems either to have leveled off or to be rising much more slowly now than in the late 1970s and early 1980s. It is uncertain whether this apparent slowing of the rate of infection is real or if it represents changes in how data are collected and analyzed or changes in the addict population (as some die, others quit, former addicts relapse, and new addicts enter the ranks). Nevertheless, these latest data present a slightly more optimistic picture than was seen in the recent past, when the rate of infection was rising sharply. It also appears that the AIDS virus is not spreading from drug users into the general population as rapidly as many had feared.

Another optimistic development is that many drug users have reduced their participation in activities that place them at risk for getting infected with the AIDS virus. This change is probably due, at least in part, to the public health educational programs that have been aimed at drug users. Needle-sharing and other unsterile practices for injecting drugs have been reduced more than high-risk sexual behavior; apparently, it is easier for drug abusers to change the way they use drugs than to change their sexual practices.

A related finding is that cocaine users are at particularly high risk for acquiring the AIDS virus. This discovery is especially important because cocaine is often used in ways that do not require injection, such as snorting, smoking (in the form of crack), or inhaling. Interviews with cocaine users have found that many exchange sex for drugs. Such transactions are particularly common among crack users who frequent so-called crack houses (usually apartments, where the drug can be both bought and smoked). During hours—and sometimes days—spent in crack houses, some users engage in sex with dozens of partners. As over one-third of the customers in crack houses have previously used IV drugs, and many of them are infected with the AIDS virus, the chances of infection being passed along are high.

For those who inject cocaine, the risks are also high. According to studies in New York and San Francisco, the AIDS virus is now spreading faster among people who inject cocaine than among those who use heroin, because cocaine users on a binge inject the drug several times in an hour. (Heroin's effects last longer, so the

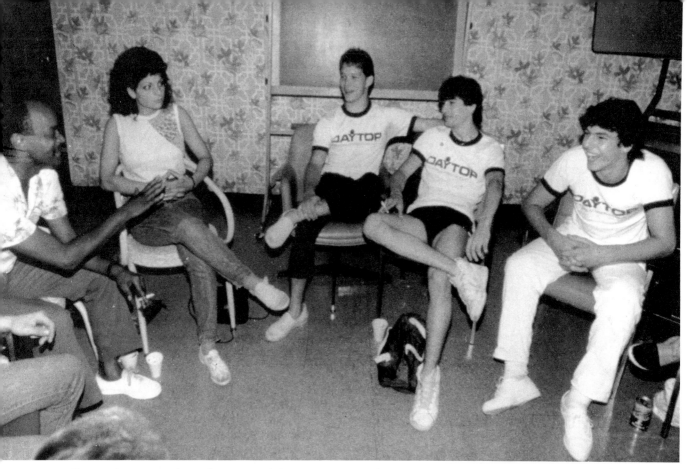

Recovering young drug abusers participate in a group therapy session at a Daytop Village drug rehabilitation center in Far Rockaway, N.Y.

typical heroin user injects it much less frequently.) Furthermore, regular cocaine users are more likely than other drug users to frequent so-called shooting galleries, where needle-sharing is common.

Overall, then, the AIDS epidemic continues to present a largely pessimistic prospect. A large wave of infected drug users who will eventually develop AIDS has not yet hit the healthcare system, and recent surveys indicate that hospitals in areas with high rates of infection, such as New York City, will be overwhelmed by AIDS cases unless drastic increases in resources are available. Among the most tragic victims of the epidemic are the infants who are infected with the AIDS virus during birth to mothers who acquired the virus themselves either through drug use or through sex with an infected addict.

See also the Spotlight on Health article CHILDREN WITH AIDS *and the Health and Medical News article* AIDS.

Cocaine Treatment

In the face of an epidemic of cocaine use, much work is being done to find effective treatments. Whereas heroin addicts can be given methadone, a synthetic drug that is taken by mouth and relieves the craving

for heroin as long as it continues to be taken, there is no such drug that can be given as a maintenance treatment for cocaine. Thus, all treatments for cocaine addiction aim at total abstinence.

Several studies have examined drugs that may help the addict stop using cocaine. Some of these have shown that desipramine, a commonly used antidepressant also sold under the brand names Norpramin and Pertofrane, can reduce cocaine use in people who are well motivated and attend regular drug counseling or psychotherapy sessions. Desipramine treatment, however, is not a "magic bullet" for cocaine addiction and is best seen as potentially helpful as the addict tries to become abstinent during the early stages of treatment. It probably must be supplemented by intensive psychosocial rehabilitation if long-term abstinence is to be achieved. People who respond to desipramine treatment usually do not stop cocaine use immediately, but only after being on the drug for two or three weeks.

Considerable attention has also been given to conditioned responses and the role they play in leading former cocaine users to start using the drug again. Conditioned responses are powerful feelings of craving for cocaine that are often accompanied by physical reactions, such as sweating or increased heart rate.

They occur frequently when the cocaine abuser is exposed to cues—situations, people, or even objects (such as white powder, pipes, or mirrors) that were previously associated with taking the drug. Studies now being done should lead to a better understanding of how much conditioned responses contribute to cocaine use and how an addict's chances of avoiding a relapse might be improved by extinguishing them. Extinguishing conditioned responses is a long-term process that aims to reverse the conditioning so that eventually cues lose their power to arouse craving for the drug. It is most often done in a setting of long-term psychotherapy.

A relatively new treatment method called relapse prevention is also being used in many drug treatment programs. Like the conditioning-extinction treatment, it emphasizes identifying cues that may cause an addict to relapse. However, while extinction treatment focuses on decreasing the arousal produced by such cues, relapse prevention goes beyond this, encouraging abusers to develop alternatives (such as new interests and new, drug-free friendships) that will substitute for cocaine use or keep them out of situations that may lead to cocaine use. This treatment is also being evaluated for its effectiveness.

Many programs treating cocaine abusers have found that for treatment to be effective, it must be intensive, with abusers visiting a hospital or treatment center daily or as inpatients. In addition to the techniques already mentioned, these programs use many of the same principles that have been developed to treat alcoholism, including self-help components that follow the Twelve Steps of Alcoholics Anonymous. (The Twelve Steps call on alcoholics to admit that they are powerless in the face of alcohol and need help from a greater "Power"; to admit their past mistakes and to try to make up for them; and to share their recovery experiences with others who need help.) After they have ended formal treatment, addicts are urged to attend a self-help group such as Cocaine Anonymous that will assist their effort to stay away from the drug.

A New Emphasis in Public Policy

The interconnected problems of AIDS and drug abuse, combined with the difficulties in controlling the latter by law enforcement alone, have led to a new emphasis in public policy on reducing the demand for drugs through prevention and treatment of drug abuse. This shift in emphasis is best reflected in the Anti-Drug Abuse Act of 1988, which authorized the spending of $2 billion and for the first time targeted more money (about 55 percent of the total) for prevention and treatment than for law enforcement. (However, only $500 million was actually allocated for fiscal 1989.)

AIDS prevention work among drug users focuses on educating users about how to avoid becoming infected. It is being carried out through increased amounts of AIDS counseling in drug treatment centers, through public service announcements on radio and television, and through the use of ex-addicts to explain AIDS prevention techniques to drug abusers who are not in treatment. Efforts to get addicts to swap their used needles for clean ones have, however, become bogged down in controversy. Other radio and TV advertisements, often using sports and entertainment personalities, aim to discourage drug use itself.

Under a new AIDS prevention strategy proposed by the U.S. government in March 1989, methadone would be made available to thousands more heroin addicts than ever before. More than 50 percent of IV drug users who seek methadone treatment are infected with the AIDS virus. Federal officials hoped that making methadone more widely available would reduce the number of infected addicts sharing needles and thus reduce the spread of the virus. Methadone has been available only to addicts enrolled in treatment programs with a full range of counseling and rehabilitative services, but such programs have long waiting lists. Under the new proposal, all addicts seeking treatment could get methadone, with the only counseling being AIDS counseling.

Another prevention strategy is urine testing to identify workers who are using illicit drugs. The most controversial form of urine testing—random, unannounced tests on employees who show no signs of drug use—has been done in the military (with great success) and in certain industries, such as nuclear power. However, efforts by the federal government to implement random urine testing among certain segments of its civilian work force have been contested in the courts on the grounds that they are an unconstitutional invasion of privacy. In March 1989 the U.S. Supreme Court, ruling for the first time on the constitutionality of such drug testing programs, upheld the federal government's testing programs involving railroad industry employees and most employees of the U.S. Customs Service. The Court upheld testing of railroad employees because their work involves public safety and of Customs Service employees because they safeguard the borders, are often involved in drug interdiction efforts, and may carry firearms.

Under a provision of the Anti-Drug Abuse Act, a civil penalty of up to $10,000 can be imposed for possession of illicit drugs, even if they were intended solely for personal use. Another new strategy is the confiscation of money and personal property from convicted drug dealers—police in some areas have confiscated millions of dollars in cash or possessions in this way. The cash and the proceeds from the sale of the confiscated property are then turned over to law enforcement and drug treatment agencies. It is too early to tell if these programs will reduce drug use and distribution, but more information should be available within one or two years.

It is also too early to tell what kind of impact the U.S. government's new "drug czar," William Bennett, will have on the drug problem. As head of the Office of National Drug Control Policy, an agency authorized by the Anti-Drug Abuse Act, the drug czar has responsibility for coordinating the work of more than 30 federal agencies involved in drug-related law enforcement, education, and treatment efforts.

GEORGE E. WOODY, M.D.
A. THOMAS McLELLAN, PH.D.
CHARLES P. O'BRIEN, M.D., PH.D.

Ears, Nose, and Throat

Technology Aids Those With Hearing Loss • Treating Head and Neck Cancers

Help for the Hearing Impaired

Hearing loss is one of the most prevalent disabilities in the United States, affecting an estimated 18 million to 20 million people. A small percentage of individuals with hearing impairment can undergo surgery to have their hearing restored. Researchers continue to develop and test new and improved devices to assist the remaining 15 million to 16 million Americans who are not candidates for surgery.

Conventional hearing aids are useful for many people with impaired hearing. A hearing aid usually consists of a microphone, amplifier, and loudspeaker which electronically amplify and transmit the incoming sound. The drawback to this conventional device is that *all* incoming sounds are amplified. In noisy environments, amplification of background noise often makes it difficult for the hearing aid wearer to perceive the desired sound, such as the speech of another person.

Newer models of hearing aids incorporate automatic signal processors that filter out background noise. Most such noise is low-frequency sound. In the newer hearing aids, this type of sound is selectively canceled, and only sounds in the higher frequencies, such as speech sounds, are enhanced. The benefit of such signal processing is improved speech understanding for wearers of the devices. Newer hearing aids also tend to have better volume control and to be smaller and less conspicuous than older models.

Aids for the Theater. Despite the improvements in hearing aids, some hearing-impaired persons continue to experience difficulty with speech perception. Two communication systems that can benefit such people are available. One system, which can be owned by individuals or installed in theaters, churches, courtrooms, and other large meeting places, uses what is called the assistive listening device (ALD). A microphone is placed close to the speaking source. This microphone is attached to an amplifier/transmitter (the ALD), and the desired sound is sent from the transmitter to a receiver worn by the listener. Since the ALD transmits only the sound closest to the microphone, background noise is not transmitted and does not interfere with listening.

Infrared listening systems can also make large indoor spaces more accessible to the hearing impaired. In this system, the original sound—made, say, by the actors on stage—is picked up by a microphone or mixing board that feeds it into an infrared transmitter. The transmitter modulates the sound waves into infrared light that is then broadcast throughout the room by emitter panels. (Infrared light is not within the visible light spectrum, so no one in the audience sees it.) The infrared signals are picked up by special headsets, worn by members of the audience, that demodulate the light waves back to the original sound signal. Users report that the sound is crystal clear. Even theatergoers with normal hearing sometimes rent the headphones to enjoy the undistorted sound.

Surgical Implants. Surgically implanted devices are now an option for some individuals who cannot wear or do not benefit from conventional hearing aids. An implantable bone conduction hearing aid may help people in whom the tiny bones in the middle ear are damaged (these bones normally conduct sound vibrations to the inner ear). The implant consists of a small disk that is surgically inserted into the skull behind the ear. The device, which is stimulated by a small external sound processor, transmits vibrations through the surrounding bone to the inner ear. One of the principal benefits of this implantable aid is the relative absence of feedback and distortion, which are common with conventional hearing aids.

Researchers continue to improve and miniaturize cochlear implants, electrical devices that are helpful in some cases of profound hearing loss. Use of these devices in appropriately selected patients was endorsed by a panel of experts convened by the U.S.

National Institutes of Health in May 1988. Cochlear implants can be beneficial for the small percentage of the hearing impaired who have suffered damage to the hair cells in the cochlea (a snail-shaped organ in the inner ear), which convert sound vibrations to electrical impulses for transmission to the brain via the auditory nerve. A device is surgically implanted in the bone behind the ear, and it receives electrical signals from a sound receiver. These signals are then transmitted into the cochlea. The auditory nerve is directly stimulated, bypassing the damaged hair cells.

Although normal hearing is not restored by the device, a sense of sound is perceived. Many cochlear implant patients gain great improvement in lip reading skills and speech comprehension. Some individuals who receive the type of implant called a multichannel device can understand speech without lip reading and may successfully use a telephone. Such results are confined to adults who developed speech and language skills prior to the onset of hearing loss. The value of cochlear implants in congenitally deaf children remains a topic of debate, although an estimated 300 children throughout the world have been fitted with the devices.

Head and Neck Tumors

Improving the diagnosis and treatment of head and neck tumors continues to be a goal of doctors who treat ear, nose, and throat disorders. By examining the genetic material of cells, researchers are trying to find out what causes a normal cell to become cancerous. Other recently developed laboratory techniques are being used to try to characterize the patterns of growth and spread of certain cancers.

The refinement of older surgical procedures and the development of new techniques are helping head and neck surgeons to remove tumors from difficult to reach areas such as the base of the skull. Despite improvements, surgery for head or neck cancer may leave the patient with disabilities such as impaired speech and difficulty in swallowing (dysphagia). Improved techniques in reconstructive surgery are enabling physicians to remedy many of these disabilities, and several medical institutions in the United States have set up special "swallowing centers" to help those suffering from dysphagia.

Radiation therapy continues to be an important form of treatment for head and neck cancer. Such therapy is curative in many early forms of cancer, and it is useful in preventing recurrences after surgery in advanced cases. Like many other types of treatment, radiation therapy has some undesirable side effects, including extreme dry mouth, loss of taste, and difficulty swallowing. These side effects can be treated symptomatically.

The results of chemotherapy for head and neck tumors are somewhat disappointing so far; the drugs have been ineffective in providing long-term control of head and neck cancer. There are, however, a few exceptions. The combined use of certain drugs (such as cis-platinum and 5-fluorouracil) shows promise in treating some cases of advanced head and neck cancer.

DAVID L. CALLENDER, M.D.

Environment and Health

The Long Hot Summer • Increased Concern Over the Greenhouse Effect • Health Hazards From Nuclear Weapons Plants • Lead and Children's Health

Summer Heat and Drought

An extended heat wave that enveloped much of the United States and Canada during the summer of 1988 was accompanied by the worst drought since the Dust Bowl days of the 1930s. The hot, dry weather brought illness and death to vulnerable population groups, along with health-threatening pollution.

The incidences of heat-related deaths and illnesses were noticeably higher than usual in Chicago, Boston, New York, and a large part of the Midwest. In Chicago, for example, which experienced its hottest recorded summer, the actual number of people who died of heat-related causes—46—may not appear large, but they were the most visible sign of a need for extraordinary public health measures. These ranged from providing people with electric fans to flooding the roofs of nursing homes for emergency cooling. Most of Chicago's deaths were from heatstroke, and they occurred overwhelmingly among people in their 70s, 80s, and 90s. The danger was greatest among older people who had sealed their homes tightly for security or to prevent loss of heat during the winter.

The intense heat and drought led to an increase in both water and air pollution. Heat and drought left the Mississippi, Missouri, and other rivers far below their expected levels. Many set records for low flow.

In coastal Louisiana, saltwater moved far up the Mississippi River channel, contaminating drinking water sources. In some areas the water was too low to dilute sewage properly, creating a potential health hazard. Dredging to keep navigation channels open increased the risk of releasing toxic substances buried in the river bottom.

Stagnant air prevented the dispersion of air pollutants generated by cars, electricity generating plants, and other sources. As a result, ozone pollution in the lower atmosphere was the worst since the 1970s. Contributing to pollution in many areas was the haze from large forest fires in the western United States—the worst in decades. The abnormal dryness contributed to causing fires affecting over 4 million acres.

A combination of climatic conditions caused the excessive heat and drought and their complications. One was a drier than usual winter of 1987-1988, so that water levels were low even before the heat arrived. In addition, the jet stream (the main high-altitude west-to-east air current) remained unusually far north, blocking the flow of cool air from Canada. This allowed a large mass of hot air to stagnate over the Midwest for most of the summer. Both the dry winter and the jet stream behavior were probably triggered by El Niño, an abnormally strong warming that occurs every few years in the eastern Pacific Ocean near the equator.

The Greenhouse Effect

The unusual size and persistence of the summer's weather pattern led some scientists to speculate that it was the first clear sign of the long-anticipated greenhouse effect—a global warming trend caused by air pollutants that trap the sun's heat near the surface of the earth. The greenhouse effect probably didn't cause the 1988 heat wave, since global temperatures fluctuate in both short-term and long-term patterns that are not yet fully understood. But the drought and heat wave did give everyone a taste of what rapid climatic change could mean for health, the environment, and the economy. Just as important, they strongly pointed up the interrelated causes of global warming, smog, acid rain, and damage to the stratospheric (upper atmosphere) ozone layer.

What Causes It? Carbon dioxide is a trace gas—a gas naturally found in small amounts in the environment. It is the key to greenhouse warming. Trees and other plants require large amounts of the gas in order to live, incorporating it through photosynthesis into their tissues. It also prevents the escape of heat into outer space, and in the past there has been just enough excess carbon dioxide to provide a thermal

"blanket" for the earth that has permitted the evolution of the present mixture of plant and animal life.

Since fossil fuels—coal, oil, and natural gas—are made of plant material, they give off carbon dioxide when burned. Rapid industrialization during the past century has meant that ever larger amounts of fossil fuels are burned and ever larger amounts of carbon dioxide are released, so that its concentration in the atmosphere today is 25 percent greater than it was a century ago. Thus, more heat is retained near the earth.

Other trace gases also play a role in greenhouse warming. These include methane, which is given off by various natural processes; sulfates and oxides of nitrogen, which are waste gases from industry and automobiles that are responsible for smog and acid rain; and manufactured gases known as chlorofluorocarbons (CFCs), which are used in refrigerators, aerosol spray cans, air conditioners, and plastic foams. Scientists consider CFCs to be responsible for the thinning of the stratospheric ozone layer, which protects the earth from harmful levels of the sun's ultraviolet radiation. Additional factors that contribute to the greenhouse effect include water vapor in the atmosphere, natural pollution from volcanic eruptions and desert dust storms, and ocean warming.

Three major studies of global warming published in 1988, all based on computer simulations of future climatic conditions derived from current trends in gas

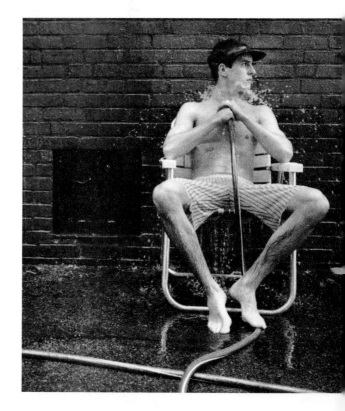

emissions and temperature patterns, found that the amount of carbon dioxide in the environment is increasing and that an unprecedented increase in global temperature is possible within the next 50 years. These studies suggest that trace gases already emitted into the atmosphere probably have begun the process of greenhouse heating, so that even if emissions are cut back, such heating will take place. The studies also indicate that the temperature increases expected in the future will be greater and more rapid than any experienced in the past; that human health, agriculture, the natural environment, engineered structures, and life-styles will all be affected; and that action should be taken now to ensure that the changes are as slow and moderate as possible.

Health Effects. Among the major health-related effects anticipated from rapid global warming are those involving water. As in the 1988 heat wave, higher temperatures increase the rate of evaporation, diminishing water supplies. Decreased rates of river flow may mean increased health hazards from undiluted sanitary and toxic wastes. Dredging of waterways to keep navigation channels open could recycle settled toxic metals and other pollutants into the environment. The increased agricultural use of chemical fertilizers and pesticides in the greenhouse-warmed Great Plains could additionally threaten groundwater quality and human health.

Another effect of greenhouse warming will be a rise in sea levels, resulting from melting of polar ice. (The melting ice will also result in a decrease in reflected sunlight and other solar radiation, which could have as yet unknown climatic effects.) Encroaching saltwater could contaminate rivers and groundwater, threatening drinking water supplies. Whatever the effect of rising sea levels in North America, it could be far more drastic in parts of the world where most people live in low-lying areas, such as Bangladesh, the nations of the Caribbean and the East Indies, China, and some Arctic regions.

Heat-caused changes in wind speed and direction, precipitation patterns, cloud cover, atmospheric water vapor, and global air circulation patterns all affect air quality and would contribute to air pollution from unexpected sources. For example, Arctic soils are rich in organic material; as they dry in the warmer climate, they could release additional carbon dioxide and methane into the atmosphere.

Also, according to the U.S. Environmental Protection Agency (EPA), global warming will increase the demand for electricity in the United States over the increase that would occur without such warming. Depending on the fuels used, the generation of more electricity would mean the release of more carbon dioxide, sulfates, nitrates, and ozone and an increase in acid rain.

Heat Wave

A suffocating heat wave covered much of North America in the summer of 1988, causing a number of heat-related deaths and raising water and air pollution levels. Among the people who took extraordinary measures to keep cool: at left, a Boston resident hoses himself down; right, two library users in Des Moines read in comparative comfort.

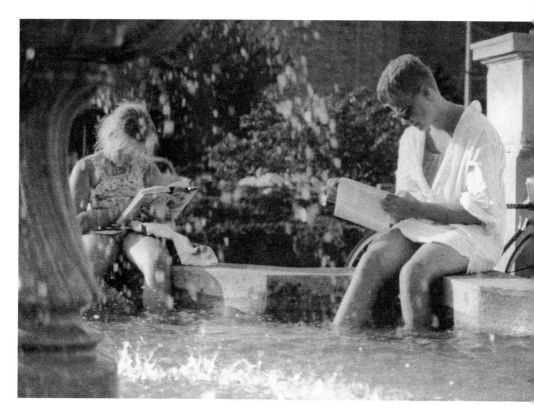

Increased temperature also magnifies the effects of existing pollution. As an example, ozone pollution (in the lower atmosphere) in the San Francisco area already exceeds the limits set by the EPA. A 4°C temperature increase could raise ozone concentrations by 20 percent and double the amount by which the area exceeds EPA limits, even if the actual level of discharged pollutants remained the same. Also, the area of greatest pollution would widen eastward to Sacramento. Smaller changes of this type could be expected in other regions of the United States.

As temperatures and air pollution increase, rates of illness and death from such diseases as influenza, pneumonia, emphysema, and asthma will rise among the elderly and those who are already very ill. In the North, the increases in physical stress, illness, and deaths caused by hotter summers would probably more than offset the decreases during the expected milder winters, although the exact relationship is as yet unknown. Increases in temperature and changes in rainfall patterns could also affect the life cycles and habitats of mosquitoes, fleas, ticks, and other arthropods, the EPA says. Larger numbers of these creatures resulting from such changes could increase people's risk of acquiring diseases transmitted by them, such as dengue, malaria, and Rocky Mountain spotted fever. Changes in climate may also change the incidence of skin diseases caused by organisms that thrive in warmer conditions, diseases such as ringworm, candidiasis, and scabies.

Combating Warming Trends. The trace gases mentioned above do not yet determine global temperatures, which are also influenced by various natural phenomena. For instance, the sun's radiation decreased between 1979 and 1985, essentially canceling the effect of trace gases. But that radiation fluctuates, possibly in 11-year or 22-year cycles, and so will increase again. El Niño ended in 1988, removing a source of added heat for the next several years, but it reappears at unpredictable intervals. In addition, major volcanic eruptions and desert dust storms could occur at any time.

One of the 1988 studies recommended attempting to hold global warming to 0.1°C per decade by cutting the increase in carbon dioxide releases by two thirds. This could be done by drastically slowing deforestation and increasing reforestation, using fossil fuels more efficiently, substituting other energy sources for fossil fuels, shifting from fossil fuels that contain high amounts of carbon dioxide to those with low amounts of it (for example, from coal to natural gas), and disposing of carbon dioxide deep in the ocean. The report also recommended measures to cut the release of other gases, including those that deplete the stratospheric ozone layer.

Reforestation can remove significant amounts of carbon dioxide from the air. According to one expert, replanting forests on about 500,000 acres would store 1 billion tons of carbon dioxide a year for half a century, as the trees grow to maturity. One power plant operator is planting 52 million trees on 250,000 acres in the tropics to offset carbon dioxide emissions from its new coal-fired power plant in Connecticut. Scientists are also studying ways to slow the burning of tropical forests to clear land for agriculture and are embarking on a major study of the effects of the oceans on climate.

In related actions, the United States has joined over 20 nations in limiting the amount of nitrogen oxides emitted into the atmosphere by the mid-1990s. The United States, the largest producer of nitrogen oxides, will restrict its emissions to the level of 1978. The limitation will help in controlling smog and acid rain as well as global temperature increases.

If, as some expect, greenhouse warming takes effect in the next few years, action to combat it will become more critical. For example, a smaller water supply will need to be carefully allocated for drinking, industrial, agricultural, and other needs. People may have to adjust priorities and adopt new, more efficient ways of using water. In general, greenhouse warming will require wide-ranging adaptations by individuals, as well as governments, institutions, and societies.

Understanding Air Pollution

The high levels of smog and ozone during the hot summer of 1988 and the expected arrival of greenhouse warming gave added urgency to the need to understand the sources of air pollution, the way pollution works in the environment and in the human body, and effective methods of controlling it. In 1988 a scientist at the University of California, Irvine, found that ozone pollution is far more damaging to human lungs when combined with other pollutants, such as oxides of sulfur (sulfates) and nitrogen oxides. In effect, the sulfates and nitrogen oxides become health hazards themselves in the presence of ozone.

Scientists at the EPA have found a major but previously neglected source of hydrocarbon emissions from cars—gasoline that, during hot weather, becomes overheated while being recycled from the fuel injection system to the fuel tank. The car's pollution control system is unable to process it, and it evaporates. The researchers believe this evaporation is the reason that cities have been unable to meet EPA ozone limits.

In Los Angeles, where ozone and smog are pervasive, the EPA has forbidden the construction of large new pollution sources (large industrial plants such as electric utilities, steel production plants, and petroleum refineries) in an attempt to lower pollution levels. However, smaller polluters are not included in the ban. Moreover, the EPA decided not to regulate brief surges of sulfur dioxide emissions from coal-fired power plants and other sources. Environmentalists had requested such a ban to limit the harmful health effects (especially to asthmatics) that could result. Current regulations set limits on average emissions during 24-hour periods; the proposed standard would have specified limits for 1-hour periods.

Hazards From Nuclear Weapons Plants

In 1988 the U.S. Department of Energy (DOE) acknowledged that it and its predecessor agencies had improperly stored radioactive and other toxic and cancer-causing wastes at the 16 nuclear weapons plants it operates. The resulting health hazards for workers and the general public living near those plants are unknown. Equipment failures and improper handling of materials at the plants have created additional health hazards.

DOE's admission of problems at the plants came both in congressional testimony and in the closing of several of the facilities. Production reactors at the Savannah River plant in South Carolina were removed from service indefinitely because of leaks of plutonium and other radioactive materials and cracks in their cooling systems. Similar problems at the Hanford, Wash., plant forced DOE to announce the permanent shutdown of the facility's last operating reactor. (The other eight reactors at Hanford had already closed.) Plutonium processing was stopped at the Rocky Flats plant, near Boulder, Colo., because of fires, the inability to store wastes properly, and other hazards. In addition, DOE officials admitted that large-scale radioactive releases from the Feed Materials Production Center near Fernald, Ohio, had occurred over several decades.

DOE was also forced to postpone the opening of the first permanent U.S. repository for military and civilian nuclear wastes. Operation of the Waste Isolation Pilot Plant in Nevada is problematic because of uncertainty about its ability to completely prevent leakage into the environment of wastes that remain dangerous for centuries.

Some actions have been taken or are planned to rectify these situations. The federal government consented to a court order to pay the state of Ohio for violations of state and federal pollution laws at Fernald and to obey state and federal pollution laws in the future. And in 1989 all 16 facilities were put under stronger regulatory control by the newly created Defense Nuclear Facilities Safety Board.

Environmental Survey of Weapons Facilities. In the first environmental survey at the 16 plants, the DOE found 155 instances of contamination that it considers existing or suspected health hazards, 40 percent of which are significant. Among the contaminants cited were volatile organic compounds, solvents, heavy metals, radioactive substances, and polychlorinated biphenyls (PCBs). An additional 46 areas were found to contain potential hazards. The DOE did not make public the amount of hazardous material involved.

The most serious existing health threat involves large amounts of volatile, cancer-causing organic compounds that have leaked from inactive waste sites at the Rocky Flats plant and into shallow groundwater (water that supplies wells and springs). From the groundwater the chemicals can quickly migrate to surface water, becoming part of the supply of drinking water and of irrigation water for crops and grazing. Another serious problem is the possible leakage of solvents from an unlined waste pit at the Pantex facility, near Amarillo, Texas. The pit received wastes from 1954 to 1980, and the contents are believed to be seeping into an underground aquifer that serves as a water supply for the plant and surrounding communities.

Remedying the Situation. Unlike private nuclear reactors, DOE's facilities have not been subject to independent regulation, nor have they obeyed various environmental laws. Past government policy apparently emphasized production of weapons at the expense of the safe operation of the facilities and the health of workers and the public. Dealing with the resulting problems will cost billions of dollars and will mean balancing health and safety considerations against the need for the materials produced by the plants and the realities of the already overburdened federal budget.

Costly waste cleanup, repair and replacement of equipment, and improved operating and handling procedures will be needed to reduce the health risks. The first priority is to collect more complete information and perform thorough investigations of the extent of the hazards. Independent studies of the health of the 300,000 workers at the weapons facilities have been impossible because DOE has denied access to the records; however, the department gave some indication that this policy may change. Also, the Centers for Disease Control (CDC) in Atlanta began studies of the health of people who live near the Hanford plant, and similar investigations at other facilities may be performed. DOE planned to complete its environmental survey in 1989; the survey will form the basis for the department's cleanup plan, which could cost over $90 billion.

The Effects of Lead on Children

In 1980, 4 percent of children under the age of five in the United States had what were considered toxic levels of lead in their systems. That year, the U.S. Public Health Service set a goal of reducing this incidence to 0.5 percent by 1990. Since then a major source of lead in the environment, leaded gasoline, has been largely eliminated. Screening programs have been established in many city neighborhoods to detect and treat children with high lead levels. Some of the more obvious signs of lead poisoning—such as anemia and kidney, cardiovascular, and neurological damage—have been greatly diminished. But the goal for 1990 won't be met.

Rather than being reduced, in fact, estimates of the extent of lead poisoning actually increased dramatically after 1980, because of new evidence that lead in the body is toxic at much lower levels than previously thought. Using today's standard for the maximum level of lead in the body that health authorities (including the CDC) commonly recognize as safe—25 micrograms of lead per deciliter of blood—not 4 but 9 percent of children in 1980 suffered from lead poisoning. And even this definition may be inadequate. Research shows that concentrations as low as 15 micrograms per deciliter impair a child's physical and mental development.

New Evidence of Low-Level Effects. Additional evidence of the harmful effects of relatively low levels of lead came from an Australian study published in 1988, which showed that 6 to 21 micrograms per deciliter of blood in children's bodies during their first four years of life can impair cognitive, verbal, and physical development. The harm comes from exposure over the long term, and the effect is cumulative. The higher the level of lead, the lower the children's scores on standard developmental tests.

The study covered over 500 children born between 1979 and 1983 in and around a community located near a lead smelter. Their mothers' blood lead levels were measured during pregnancy; the children's blood lead concentrations were measured at birth and regularly thereafter.

A child's development also depends on a variety of home factors, including the parents' health, intelligence, educational level, and emotional responsiveness. Other influences include the child's own health before and during birth, the child's play activities, and the variety of stimulation within the home. The scientists found that about half of the developmental deficits could be attributed to the lead concentrations; however, they said this was a conservative estimate.

Sources and Remedies. Two of the major unregulated sources of lead in the environment are house paint in old buildings and drinking water. Lead paint was used extensively in housing for decades into the 1970s and remains exposed in an estimated 37 million houses and apartments in the United States. The oldest paint is the greatest hazard. Children who chew on painted surfaces, such as window sills, or eat paint chips that flake from walls are potential victims of lead poisoning. So are those who inhale or eat lead-contaminated house dust. Lead from paint that has been carelessly disposed of, flaking paint, smelting, and auto emissions mixes with soil, providing another means of exposure to the body, especially for children using contaminated backyards, fields, and playgrounds.

The EPA estimates that drinking water accounts for about 20 percent of the average U.S. child's lead exposure. Tap water can be contaminated with lead from two sources. One is the water supply itself, but the more important source is water piping. The EPA estimates that about 25 percent of public water suppliers have some lead water mains. In the home, water may flow through lead fittings and pipes, as well as lead-soldered sections of copper piping. Corrosive substances in the water leach lead from all of these. Generally, the more acidic the water the more corrosive it is. Chlorine, minerals, and oxygen also make water corrosive. A ban on lead solder was contained in the Safe Drinking Water Act, passed in 1986, but the lead can leach out for at least five years, both because of corrosive water and through the electrochemical reaction of lead and copper.

In any water supply, the amount of lead reaching the user varies from building to building and with the time of day. Water that has been standing in the pipes for a long time (such as overnight) has higher levels of lead than free-flowing water. And the levels are often higher in hot water than in cold.

Lead is one of dozens of contaminants to be regulated by the EPA under the 1986 amendments to the Clean Water Act. But regulation will not begin until 1990 at the earliest, and accurate information on the extent of lead in drinking water is just being collected.

The United States has several pressing needs if it is to come anywhere near the 1990 goal, the Public Health Service says. One is improved local and state housing codes to eliminate the threat caused by lead paint. If this is not removed, the paint will continue to be a hazard for decades. The lead in drinking water must be adequately regulated. Also needed are continuing efforts to educate the public about lead's dangers and sources. Finally, there must be a nationwide clearinghouse of information on the incidence of lead poisoning and the measures being taken to treat it and to eliminate its sources.

ELLEN THRO

Eyes

Freezing Technique Reduces Eye Damage in Newborns • Drug Treatment for Squint and Eyelid Spasms • Progress on "Living Contact Lenses"

Freezing Saves Infants' Vision

A tremendous breakthrough was reported in 1988 in the treatment of an eye disease that sometimes strikes extremely premature infants. Preliminary results from a study involving 23 U.S. medical centers showed that freezing certain parts of the eye with a supercooled probe halved the risk of severe damage to the retina, the light-sensitive tissue lining the eyeball.

The disease, called retinopathy of prematurity or ROP, involves excessive growth of blood vessels in the retina, potentially leading to bleeding, scarring, and detachment of the retina. ROP was first identified in the late 1940s. After much study it was shown in 1952 to be due to exposure to excessive amounts of oxygen in incubators. Doctors began keeping close track of oxygen concentration, and the disease virtually disappeared for the next two decades. But then came a resurgence, as the 1970s and 1980s saw great advances in medical science's ability to keep alive infants born with a very low weight. Babies nearly four months premature and weighing only 500-700 grams (about 18-25 ounces) were now surviving, and some of them developed ROP. Most such low-birth-weight babies need oxygen for longer periods of time, and are far sicker, than the premature children of the 1950s.

The infants most at risk for developing the most severe cases of ROP weigh under 1,000 grams (2.2 pounds) at birth. Of these babies, 10-20 percent in recent years could be expected to become legally blind. Blindness from ROP has been occurring in approximately 1,000 infants annually in the United States, with numerous others left with partially reduced vision. Many of the children affected by ROP have additional handicaps (often involving the nervous system) that are caused by prematurity, and the vision problems augment the developmental difficulty faced by the premature child. No completely effective means of preventing retinopathy of prematurity has yet been discovered.

The new breakthrough in treatment originated in reports by physicians in Japan, Israel, and the United States, who found that they could reduce the severity of eye damage by freezing a portion of the infants' eyes. Other doctors were not convinced that this approach, known as cryotherapy, was effective, and they also voiced concern that the treatment might injure the eye. A major study was mounted under the direction of Dr. Earl A. Palmer of the Oregon Health Sciences University to determine whether cryotherapy did reduce the number of cases, and the severity, of blindness produced by ROP. Between 1986 and 1988 over 100 investigators at medical centers across the United States took part in the effort with the close cooperation of officials from the National Eye Institute.

The scientists hypothesized that the treatment retards the development of the abnormal blood vessels, which grow along the line separating the front part of the retina, where there are no blood vessels, from the vesseled back part. The treatment is carried out with the baby asleep or under anesthesia. The cold probe is applied to the white, or sclera, of the eye at about 50 spots around the eyeball, just to the front of

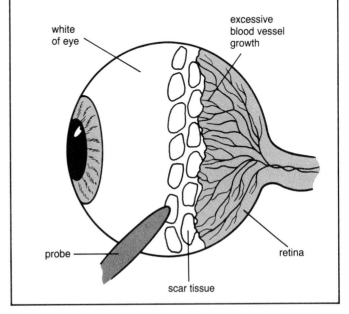

Averting Blindness With Cold

Some premature babies suffer from excessive growth of blood vessels in the retina, which can lead to blindness. Applying a supercooled probe to the white of the eye creates a ring of scar tissue that slows or stops the abnormal growth.

white of eye

excessive blood vessel growth

probe

retina

scar tissue

the line on the retina. The result is a ring of scar tissue in front of the abnormal area that slows or stops the abnormal growth.

Not all babies, however, are helped by the new procedure: for the infants in the study, 22 percent of the eyes treated with cryotherapy got worse. For this reason, doctors continue trying to determine which babies should have cryotherapy, whether one or both eyes should be treated, and at what stage in the disease's development the procedure should be done. Other avenues of research being followed include supplementing babies' diets with vitamins E and A, reducing the levels of lighting in hospital nurseries, and developing more sophisticated microsurgical techniques for repairing damaged retinas.

Over the next few years ophthalmologists plan to reexamine the cryo-treated patients to learn what variations in vision development the children may experience as they grow. Children with ROP are at higher than normal risk for amblyopia (reduced vision), crossed eyes, nearsightedness, and glaucoma, as well as retinal detachment. Only many years of follow-up study will tell ophthalmologists and pediatricians whether the new treatment has truly improved the ability to see.

Drug for Squint and Eyelid Spasms

Researchers have reported good results from the use of a bacteria-produced chemical called botulinum toxin (Oculinum) in the treatment of strabismus and blepharospasm. In strabismus, also known as squint, the eyes fail to align properly, with the result that they do not both look at the same target. Cross-eye and walleye are forms of strabismus. In addition to being a potential source of embarrassment, the problem may lead to double vision, loss of depth perception, or even loss of vision in children. Blepharospasm is a constant spasmodic condition of the muscles of the face around the eyes that produces constant eyelid closure, leading in effect to blindness. Both strabismus and blepharospasm have been treated in the past with surgery. Although the operation has frequently been effective, more than one-third of patients need repeat surgery. This led scientists to search for a nonsurgical alternative.

Botulinum toxin is made by the bacterium *Clostridium botulinum*. It is the same substance that, when ingested with improperly prepared food, causes the form of food poisoning called botulism. The toxin chemically disconnects muscles from their controlling nerves, rendering the muscles functionless. When used as a drug, botulinum toxin is administered in minute fractions of the toxic dose. No adverse effects have been reported from its use. The drug is injected through a fine needle into the muscle the physician wishes to weaken.

The best-established use of botulinum toxin is for the treatment of blepharospasm. Well over 7,000 patients have been injected across the United States; more than 90 percent received relief of their symptoms and were able to return to near-normal activity. Prior to treatment, many patients were so debilitated by the constant eyelid closure that they could not drive; a considerable number could not even leave their homes and were functionally blind. They achieved a remarkable restoration of function.

As to strabismus, researchers have used the drug in both adults and children. Excellent results have been reported for patients with temporary eye misalignments, which may occur after a serious head injury, a mild stroke, or neurosurgery. Since the drug can be administered at any age, it may also be a useful adjunct to eye muscle surgery in infants. If it is given immediately after the onset of misalignment, it may realign the eyes. This may help preserve normal vision until the child is old enough to undergo general anesthesia and surgery. Much more research remains to be done to determine exactly which patients will benefit from the treatment. A major drawback of the drug is that its effects last only two to four months in the majority of patients. Then the injection must be repeated. Researchers are looking for a longer-acting drug that might make the changes permanent. Meanwhile, the U.S. Food and Drug Administration was expected to approve Oculinum for use in treating both strabismus and blepharospasm.

Eye Injuries

Injuries to the eye are a major cause of impaired vision. They account for 8 to 10 percent of all visual impairment, including 5 percent of all severe cases, in the United States. Researchers from New England, Israel, and Brazil in 1988 released a number of studies evaluating the risk factors for eye injuries in adults and children.

Children under 18 were found to have as many injuries as all adults. This means that children were more often victims of eye injuries. Not only were children more at risk, but the data showed that they more often sustained injuries to both eyes, and had more severe injuries, than did adults. Of all segments of the population, children up to five years of age, boys and girls alike, were at the greatest risk. Among people over five years old, males were more frequently affected than females.

Eye injuries occurred most frequently at home, notably among children. Children were injured most often when playing without adequate adult supervision. The Brazilian study found that active supervision of play produced a marked reduction in the number of accidents. The home was followed closely by the workplace in frequency of eye accidents. Young male adults were injured most frequently at work, usually when not observing safety guidelines.

Since eye injuries constitute a significant portion of potentially treatable visual impairment, educational efforts to prevent them need to be stepped up. These should be directed particularly toward safeguarding young adult males in the workplace, where the use of sufficient eye protection should be encouraged or required, and toward protecting children at home and at play through the provision of active adult supervision. Any person who has only one good eye should be sure to wear the appropriate protective spectacles at all times.

"Living Lens" Update

During 1988 further refinements were made in the procedure known as epikeratophakia, in which a "contact lens" is made from a frozen piece of a deceased person's cornea (the transparent membrane at the front of the eye). Because of the way the lens is produced, there is no risk that it will carry an infectious disease. The lens is sewn, or grafted, onto the patient's cornea and becomes a permanent part of the eye in a few months. Such lenses, which are now commercially available in a freeze-dried state, can be used to correct nearsightedness and farsightedness, especially in patients who undergo cataract surgery. They have also found use as a structural reinforcement for patients with thin diseased corneas.

The procedure can be effective and is relatively safe, although complications such as scarring or rejection of the transplanted lens have been reported in some cases. Also, care must be taken that the lens used is of the correct power. Much more accurate power-prediction formulas, coupled with increased experience with the procedure, have improved doctors' ability to graft the correct lens. With children it is still difficult to predict what power the lens should have. This problem has led physicians to avoid the procedure in children under two years of age. Advantages of epikeratophakia include the relative technical ease of the surgical procedure and the convenience for the patient of not having to cope with the day-to-day care problems presented by normal plastic contact lenses. The procedure has been simplified so that no corneal tissue needs to be removed from the recipient. At present, epikeratophakia is used only for patients who cannot wear an ordinary contact lens or who are poor candidates for implantation of an artificial lens. MICHAEL X. REPKA, M.D.

Family Planning

New Options Available • Ongoing Controversy Over Abortion Pill • Injectable and Implantable Contraceptives

More Options for Birth Control

A copper intrauterine device and a cervical cap became available in the United States in 1988.

New IUD. An intrauterine device (IUD) called ParaGard Copper T 380A went on the market in June 1988 and was the first new IUD made available to American women since most IUDs were removed from the U.S. market in the mid-1980s. The new IUD was developed by the nonprofit Population Council of New York and was actually approved by the U.S. Food and Drug Administration (FDA) in 1984. However, even though it was widely used in other countries, including Canada, its introduction in the United States was delayed in part because of the unfavorable publicity about IUDs in the mid-1980s and because the Population Council was negotiating a licensing agreement for distribution with a New Jersey firm, GynoPharma.

A cloud of suspicion has hung over IUDs since the 1970s, when women who used an IUD called the Dalkon Shield began developing serious problems, including pelvic infections, miscarriages, and infertility. (The Dalkon Shield was manufactured by the A. H. Robins Company, which took the product off the market and in 1985 filed for protection under federal bankruptcy laws because of the number of claims filed by women who used the device. In 1988 the American Home Products Corporation offered to buy Robins and set up a $2.5 billion fund to compensate women claiming injury from the Dalkon Shield, but that plan was being challenged in court.) The publicity led many women to believe that the risks of IUDs were much greater and the benefits much smaller than they actually are. When IUDs made by other companies were withdrawn from the market in the mid-1980s, those actions fueled the belief that IUDs were unsafe. In fact, the companies stopped selling the devices not because they were unsafe but for economic reasons, in particular because of the financial risks posed by lawsuits. Until ParaGard became available, the only IUD on the U.S. market since 1986 was Progestasert, a hormone-releasing IUD.

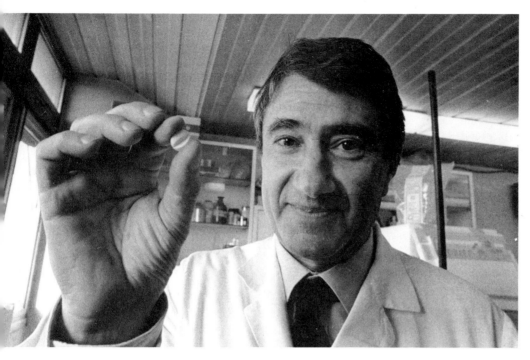

French chemist Etienne-Emile Baulieu displays RU 486, the controversial abortion pill he developed, approved for use in France. The drug is effective for inducing abortion during very early pregnancy.

ParaGard, the new IUD, is a T-shaped polyethylene device about 1½ inches long and 1¼ inches wide with an exposed surface area of copper. It is most effective in women over 25 and is designed to be effective for four years after insertion. International trials have shown ParaGard to be one of the most effective methods of contraception ever developed, with pregnancy rates of less than 1 in 100 women. Although there is an increased risk of pelvic inflammatory disease (PID, a potentially serious infection of the uterus and fallopian tubes), that risk is largely limited to the first four months after insertion; women who are not monogamous and are exposed to sexually transmitted diseases are at greatest risk.

Not all women should use IUDs, so careful screening is necessary. Women with multiple sex partners should choose another birth control method because of the risk of sexually transmitted diseases (the bacteria responsible for some of those diseases are the leading cause of PID). IUDs are also unsuitable for women with a history of PID or ectopic pregnancy (outside the uterus), for women with genital bleeding of unknown cause, or for women with known or suspected uterine or cervical cancer, including an abnormal Pap test. (Pap tests indicate cancer and precancerous conditions in the cervix and occasionally infections.)

Cervical Cap. The FDA approved the Prentif Cavity-Rim Cervical Cap in May 1988. It is a barrier contraceptive smaller than but somewhat similar to the diaphragm. The cap is a latex, dome-shaped device to which the user applies a small amount of spermicide. The cap is then inserted into the vagina, where it fits snugly over the cervix, blocking the passage of sperm. The cap is about 1½ inches long with a firm flexible rim at the open end. It has a narrow groove along the inner surface of the rim that creates a seal when it is placed over the cervix. Like the diaphragm, it is a prescription device that must initially be fitted by a physician.

The modern rubber cervical cap was invented in the 19th century and has been used in Europe for years. Cervical covers made of various materials were one of the earliest family planning methods, dating back over 2,500 years.

At the request of the FDA, the National Institutes of Health funded a study on the effectiveness of the cervical cap, involving more than 1,000 women at eight California clinics. The study found that the cap was approximately 83 percent effective—about as effective as the diaphragm in preventing pregnancy. As with the diaphragm, most unanticipated pregnancies can be traced to improper use of the cap, including incorrect placement, inconsistent use, or failure to use spermicide with it.

The advantages of the cap are that it can be left in place for up to 48 hours and requires only one application of spermicide. The diaphragm, in contrast, should not be left in place for more than 24 hours and requires reapplication of spermicide before each act of intercourse. Cap users may not suffer the urinary tract infections that are associated with diaphragm use. The cap also has fewer and less serious side effects than the pill and IUDs and is not associated with an increased risk of pelvic infections or toxic shock syndrome, a serious bacterial infection.

The disadvantages of the cap are that it can be more difficult to insert and remove than the diaphragm and that it can be dislodged from the cervix during sex. With practice, most women find they can insert the cap quickly and effectively, but they are advised to use a backup method of contraception until they are sure they can insert the cap correctly.

About 10 percent of women should not use the cervical cap, including those whose cervix is an unusual shape or length. It should also not be used by women with cervicitis, vaginal infections, a history of cervical lacerations or scarring, or abnormal Pap tests. Of the women who used the cap in the California trials, 4 percent had an abnormal Pap test after three months of using the device, as compared with 1.7 percent of diaphragm users. After six months, the rates of abnormal Pap tests were about the same for both methods. The FDA advises that cap users have Pap tests after using the device for three months and discontinue use if the results are abnormal.

Abortion Pill

An oral drug that induces abortion very early in pregnancy is now available in some countries, but it may never be marketed in the United States. The drug—RU 486—is manufactured by the French firm Groupe Roussel Uclaf. It works by blocking the action of the hormone progesterone, causing the lining of the uterus—and the embryo implanted there—to slough off, in effect bringing on a menstrual period and thus ending the pregnancy. RU 486 is approved in France to induce abortions in women up to seven weeks pregnant. Its main advantages are that it is considerably cheaper than a surgical abortion and possibly safer, since the woman avoids the risks of an operation. A woman should be medically supervised over the several days in which the drug works. It can be used only early in pregnancy and is about 90 percent effective. (If it does not work, the woman can have a surgical abortion.) Antiabortion groups in the United States fear use of the drug will make abortion easier and say that many women who might otherwise continue their pregnancies will decide to have abortions with RU 486.

In September 1988, China and France became the first nations to approve the use of RU 486. But in October, Roussel announced it would withdraw the drug from the world market in response to threats of boycotts of other company products and because of personal harassment of company executives by anti-abortion groups. However, two days later the French health minister ordered Roussel to continue distribution of the drug in the interests of public health.

Besides inducing abortion, RU 486 holds promise in treating breast cancer, preventing conception, making labor easier to induce, and treating endometriosis (the growth of uterine tissue in the pelvic cavity and outside the uterus, which can cause pain and infertility). There has been no attempt to seek approval for its distribution in the United States for two main reasons—the political activity of antiabortion groups and the national product liability insurance crisis, which has already had an impact on birth control options for U.S. women.

Hormonal Contraceptives

Several long-acting hormonal contraceptives have been developed and could be available in the United States in coming years. The precursors of the new preparations are the long-acting injectable contraceptives that have been available in many countries for years: Depo-Provera, which prevents pregnancy for three months, and Noristerat, which prevents pregnancy for two months. Neither is available for contraception in the United States or Canada, although Depo-Provera is available in the United States for other uses and its manufacturer, the Upjohn Company, may in the future apply to the FDA for approval to market the drug as a contraceptive. All the hormonal preparations contain the synthetic female sex hormone progestin. They appear to be effective, convenient, and long-acting, but to varying degrees all change or disrupt menstrual patterns.

Norplant implants, not yet available in the United States and Canada, are widely used in other parts of the world. Six tubes are surgically placed just under the skin on the inside of a woman's arm where they release progestin at a slow, steady rate and prevent nearly all pregnancies for five years before they must be replaced. There are also biodegradable implants, which are placed under the skin and dissolve and eventually disappear. These implants prevent pregnancy for at least 18 months. A new type of injectable contraceptive—still investigational—contains microspheres and microcapsules suspended in a solution. Once injected, these particles provide a constant dose of medication that prevents pregnancy for up to six months. Monthly injectable contraceptives containing female hormones are being used in China and Latin America. The last of the new hormonal contraceptives is the vaginal ring, which is worn in the vagina and gradually releases hormone over a three-month period, after which it is removed.

VIRGINIA COWART

279

Genetics and Genetic Engineering

Genes That Prevent Cancer • Hormone Affects Women's Skills • Advances in Genetic Testing • Understanding Garbled DNA

Genes and Cancer

In the short time since the discovery of anticancer genes that serve as sentinels against the development of tumors, scientists have made enormous progress in understanding these genes and their potential use in therapy.

Eye Tumors. In December 1988 it was reported that researchers had for the first time succeeded in causing cancer cells growing in the laboratory to revert to normal by replacing a defective gene with a healthy one. The gene involved is named Rb. When it is defective, retinoblastoma can develop. This is a rare form of eye disease that strikes about 1 in 20,000 children annually in the United States. The Rb gene, discovered in October 1986 by researchers at the Massachusetts Eye and Ear Infirmary in Boston, was the first of the anticancer genes to be found. These genes—known as anti-oncogenes—apparently protect against cancer by preventing adult cells from proliferating.

Normally, an individual receives two Rb genes at conception, one from the father and one from the mother. If each of the two received is healthy, a tumor can arise later on only if both genes in one cell are disabled by a chemical or virus—which rarely happens. But if a child inherits one defective Rb gene, only the one healthy gene must be disabled for cancer to occur—a more common event. Many children who inherit the defective gene, in fact, suffer from multiple eye tumors.

Early in 1988 the Boston researchers announced that they had developed a test for the defective Rb gene that would allow them to identify children who are predisposed to retinoblastoma. Those children could then be monitored closely for the first signs of tumor formation. Treatment at that stage can destroy the tumor and save the child's vision. When tumors are found at later stages, the child's eye may have to be removed.

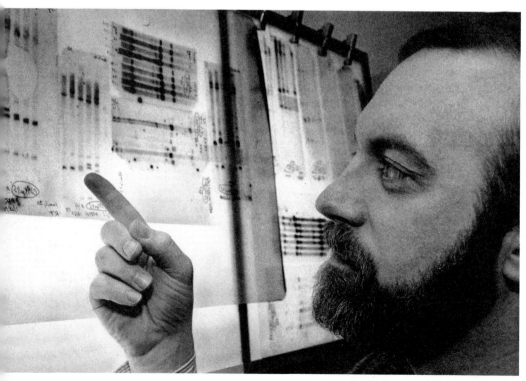

A scientist examines patterns in a patient's genetic material for signs of the defect that causes Huntington's disease, a progressive, degenerative nervous system disorder. Several Canadian and U.S. medical centers now offer to screen individuals who have relatives with Huntington's, to determine if they have inherited the defect.

Three groups of researchers reported at midyear that a defective Rb gene is also present in cells from about 20 percent of breast tumors, more than half of small-cell lung cancers, and most bone tumors.

The successful conversion of cancerous cells into normal ones that was reported in December was carried out by scientists at the University of California at San Diego. They used a specially engineered virus to insert the healthy Rb gene into retinoblastoma and bone cancer cells. Once the gene had been inserted into the cells, the cells immediately stopped proliferating. When the engineered cells were then injected into special laboratory mice that have no immune system (and thus cannot reject transplanted tumors), no tumors formed, indicating that the cells were no longer malignant. The researchers predicted that the technique could be tested in humans within five years and might be useful in treating genetically linked conditions such as some cancers and Alzheimer's disease.

Colon Tumors. In 1987 scientists discovered that many individuals with colon cancer had a defective gene that, like the Rb gene, seems to protect against cancer when it is healthy; this gene was located on chromosome 5. In 1988, Japanese and American research groups independently found evidence that victims of colon or rectal cancer had defective genes on at least six other chromosomes. Some victims had only one genetic defect, while others had as many as five. Biologists now believe that colorectal cancer (which strikes over 165,000 people in the United States and Canada each year) is an unusually complex form of cancer in which both inherited defects and poor diet must interact to form a tumor.

Meanwhile, a study found that as many as a third of white Americans have a genetic predisposition to colorectal cancer and that more than half of all colorectal tumors are associated with such a genetic predisposition. The researchers, at the University of Utah Medical Center in Salt Lake City, did not identify specific genes associated with the disease but rather determined from physical examinations the incidence of cancer in groups of blood relatives. The study was the first to give evidence of the wide prevalence of a genetic predisposition to the disease.

Leukemia and Lymphoma. A team of researchers reported in mid-1988 that some types of leukemia and lymphoma—cancers of the blood and the lymph nodes—might be caused by a genetic defect that prevents cells from manufacturing alpha-interferon and beta-interferon, which are naturally occurring proteins that the body produces to fight tumors and viruses. In the late 1970s interferons had been hailed as potentially powerful antitumor drugs, but scientists have since found that they are active against only a few forms of

cancer. The new results suggest that the interferons may be useful only in treating those types of tumors in which the body is not able to manufacture the proteins itself.

Sex-Linked Differences

Researchers from the University of Western Ontario reported finding the first scientific evidence that thought processes and certain physical abilities of women are related to hormone levels in the blood. Studies of three separate groups of women showed that their success on tests involving precise muscle control and verbal skills increased by as much as 10 percent during parts of the month immediately before ovulation and during the ten days before menstruation, when blood levels of the female hormone estrogen were high. At those same times the women's ability on tests involving spatial reasoning, such as discovering hidden figures in complex designs, dropped by about the same amount.

On average, women are generally believed to be better than men at tasks involving fine muscle control and verbal skills, while men are thought to be better at spatial reasoning. The new results suggest that those differences may partly arise from hormonal differences. Similar testing on men has not yet been conducted, according to the researchers.

Signposts to Genetic Defects

Geneticists made new progress in deciphering the molecular bases of inherited diseases and developing screening tests.

Friedreich's Ataxia. One recent discovery was the approximate location of the defective gene that causes Friedreich's ataxia. This crippling degenerative disease, which can lead to reduced muscle coordination, speech difficulties, and an irregular gait, strikes several thousand people in the United States each year. The finding was reported in mid-1988 by researchers in Great Britain, Sweden, and the United States. The scientists studied 22 families, each of which had three or more affected siblings, and found that the gene lies in a small region of chromosome 9. The team is now developing a test to screen for predisposition to the disease.

Drug Reactions. Another 1988 discovery was that as many as 10 percent of whites in North America and Europe are genetically unable to metabolize some drugs properly, a problem that causes toxic reactions in their bodies when they take the drugs. The multinational research team responsible for the finding studied the blood pressure drug debrisoquine, which had been withdrawn from the market in the United

States and some European countries because of toxic, but nonfatal reactions among some users. The team found that the individuals who suffered adverse reactions were missing a normal liver enzyme that helps detoxify the drug. The missing enzyme also prevents the body from processing at least 20 other commonly prescribed drugs, including antidepressants, antiarrhythmics (to smooth out irregular heartbeats), and the cough suppressant dextromethorphan (found in preparations marketed under such names as Triaminic-DM Cough Formula, Tylenol Cold Medication, and Naldecon DX). The study was conducted only in whites; preliminary evidence suggests that blacks share the genetic defect, while Orientals do not.

At the present time doctors cannot predict which patients will suffer adverse reactions to drugs; they can only halt a dosage if a patient demonstrates such a reaction. The new findings may lead to a test to detect people with an inability to metabolize certain drugs.

Huntington's Disease. In August 1988, Canadian scientists announced that 14 medical centers across the country would offer screening for individuals who are susceptible to Huntington's disease, a devastating, usually fatal brain disease that strikes people without warning in their mid-30s and mid-40s. Only a handful of research centers in other countries test for the disease, offering screening to individuals with a relative who has Huntington's or has died from it. Canadian medical experts estimated that there are 3,000 Huntington's victims in the country and another 20,000 people at risk of developing the disease.

In the United States there are 25,000 Huntington's patients and more than 100,000 at risk. Integrated Genetics, Inc., of Framingham, Mass., has made available a newly developed test for the disease. The test costs about $2,750. The company said that because of the extraordinary impact a positive test has on an individual, it is processing tests only from medical centers that also offer extensive psychological counseling. Previous studies have shown that individuals who know that they are susceptible to Huntington's disease have a high suicide rate.

Down's Syndrome. British and American researchers developed a simple test of a pregnant woman's blood that can tell if her fetus is at high risk of developing Down's syndrome. Children born with the condition, once known as mongolism, are mentally retarded. The syndrome, which affects as many as 2 babies in every 100 live births, can be positively identified by amniocentesis or chorionic villus sampling, both of which require removing cells from the amniotic sac in which the fetus is carried. These tests carry a small, but definite risk for the fetus. The researchers said that their blood test could be used to screen out fetuses at low risk of developing the syndrome, so that the riskier procedures of amniocentesis or chorionic villus sampling could be reserved for those most likely to have the syndrome. The testing could be widely available in two years, the researchers predicted.

Linking Alcohol With Cancer

A possible way in which alcohol may cause cancer has been identified by researchers at the University of California at Berkeley. They reported in mid-1988 that alcohol and a major product of the body's processing of alcohol called acetaldehyde may react directly with DNA (deoxyribonucleic acid) in the cells of mammals to produce changes known to be associated with the onset of cancer. In the past, the only evidence that alcohol may cause cancer came from statistical epidemiological studies, which suggested a higher incidence of breast, liver, rectal, and oral cancer in drinkers.

Garbled DNA

A surprising deviation from a fundamental assumption of genetics was reported in mid-1988 by researchers from the University of California at Los Angeles and the University of Washington. Scientists had believed that all genetic information in living organisms (aside from some viruses) is found in DNA and that this information is copied in the production of proteins and other components of cells. But the researchers found that in a family of parasitic organisms called kinetoplastids, which cause a variety of widespread tropical diseases, the DNA information for at least five separate proteins is garbled and unusable. Somehow the kinetoplastid cells alter the information content of these genes, in two cases by 60 percent, so that useful proteins can be produced. The ultimate source of the genetic information used to repair the genes is unknown.

The discovery could lead to new ways to treat the diseases caused by the parasites, such as sleeping sickness and Chagas' disease. The latter, a chronic wasting disease that causes high fever and enlargement of the liver, spleen, and lymph nodes, affects more than 30 million people worldwide. There are no drugs to treat it. But the discovery has potentially greater ramifications. Many organisms, including humans, have what are known as pseudogenes: long stretches of DNA that somewhat resemble genes but lack key segments necessary for genes to function. Such pseudogenes might, the researchers said, be genuine genes that must first be processed by cells before the products they code for can be produced.

Phenylketonuria

Mental retardation due to phenylketonuria (PKU)—an inherited inability of the body to process the amino acid phenylalanine, which is found in foods—has been largely eliminated, thanks to routine screening of newborn infants in hospitals and the use of special diets for babies found to suffer the defect. But women who are born with PKU run the risk of bearing brain-damaged children themselves, according to researchers from West Penn Hospital in Pittsburgh. If a phenylketonuric woman becomes pregnant while not adhering to a diet containing very low amounts of phenylalanine, the amino acid and its by-products can cross the placenta and damage the heart and nervous system of the fetus. Between 60 and 70 percent of such fetuses carried to term have small heads and underdeveloped brains; 25 percent have congenital heart disease. The researchers said that the risk can be reduced to between 0 and 20 percent if a woman stays on a PKU diet before conceiving.

THOMAS H. MAUGH II, PH.D.

Government Policies and Programs

UNITED STATES

Improvements in Medicare • AIDS Bill Passed • Surgeon General Speaks Out

Catastrophic Coverage Act

In 1988 the U.S. Congress approved and President Ronald Reagan signed into law the most significant liberalization of the Medicare program, which provides health insurance for millions of elderly or disabled Americans, since its creation in 1965. The Medicare Catastrophic Coverage Act of 1988 provided, for the first time, protection to elderly and disabled Americans against prolonged acute healthcare expenses associated with a major illness or serious injury. The legislation also placed an upper limit on the financial liability of Medicare participants for services covered by Medicare and established a program to ease the financial burden of prescription drug purchases. To control costs, the increased protection will be phased in over a period of several years. In 1989 only the hospital insurance component of Medicare (known as Part A) was affected.

Hospital Insurance Component. Under the new law, once a Medicare beneficiary meets the annual deductible (set at $564 for 1989), Medicare coverage for acute care in hospitals will be unlimited. This is a major change from the previous law, which had imposed a limit on the number of days of hospitalization covered. Previously, Medicare paid for only 90 hospital days per illness, along with a lifetime reserve of 60 additional days to draw upon if a hospital stay exceeded 90 days. Another change is that once the annual deductible has been met, beneficiaries will no longer be required to share the costs of hospitalization (called co-insurance or copayments). Under previous law, beneficiaries had to pay a deductible for each separate hospital stay, and they also were required to make co-insurance payments if the stay exceeded 60 days. Now Medicare will cover all the costs of unlimited hospitalization, beyond the patient's once-a-year deductible.

Benefits for nursing home care were also liberalized. (Most nursing home patients need custodial care, not "skilled" nursing; Medicare covers only the latter type.) The limit on Medicare coverage for each spell of illness in a skilled nursing facility was increased, effective January 1989, from 100 to 150 days. In addition, beneficiaries can stay in such a facility without a prior three-day hospital stay, as required before enactment of the new law. Beneficiaries are now liable for co-insurance payments of the cost of a skilled nursing facility for only the first eight days each year; after that, Medicare pays the full cost. Prior to the act, co-insurance payments were required after the 20th day of residence. Also, the new co-insurance amounts are lower than under previous law. The amount, based on the national average daily rate for care in a skilled nursing facility, is estimated to be $20.50 in 1989; in contrast, the daily co-insurance amount in 1988 was $67.50.

The third hospital insurance component of the act that becomes effective in 1989 is a major liberalization in coverage for hospice care. A hospice is a facility that keeps a terminally ill patient as comfortable as possible rather than attempt heroic efforts to prolong the patient's life. Beginning in 1989, the new act eliminates the 210-day limit for hospice care and contributes up to $68 a day for it. Small co-insurance requirements for drug and in-home respite expenses associated with terminal illness will continue. The latter is the use of temporary in-home assistance for the relief of relatives who care for homebound Medicare recipients.

The Catastrophic Coverage Act will also expand benefits for skilled nursing care provided in the home. Previously, the frequency of home health benefits was limited to no more than 5 days a week, for up to three consecutive weeks. Starting in 1990, the act will allow up to 38 consecutive days of care. For people who required home healthcare for less than 5 days a week, the previous law provided unlimited coverage. In contrast, the new law provides unlimited coverage for those who require home healthcare services 6 or fewer times a week.

Supplementary Insurance. Starting in 1990, significant changes will take effect in the second component of the Medicare program—the supplementary medical insurance program, or Part B, which covers services provided by physicians, outpatient clinics, and clinical laboratories. Under previous law, for such services beneficiaries had to pay an annual deductible of $75 and copayments of 20 percent of reasonable charges above the deductible (Medicare paid 80 percent). There was no limit on the liability for copayments. Starting in 1990, though, a beneficiary's total annual Part B liability for copayments and the deductible will be limited to $1,370. This amount will be adjusted each year to ensure that at least 7 percent of enrollees will have copayment liabilities that reach the limit.

Medicare coverage will also be expanded in 1990 to include periodic mammograms for women. These will be subject to the usual 20 percent copayment requirement.

Effective in 1990, a new catastrophic drug insurance program will be phased in. Currently, Medicare pays only for prescription drugs administered while a beneficiary is hospitalized, as well as paying for limited use of immunosuppressive drugs, which are administered following an organ transplant to prevent rejection by the body's immune system. Under the new program, in 1990 coverage will be provided for prescription drugs administered intravenously at home; these will be subject to an annual $550 deductible and 20 percent copayment. In addition, immunosuppressive drugs will get expanded coverage. Under current law, Medicare covers 80 percent of the cost of such drugs in the first year following an organ transplant. Beginning in 1990, the beneficiary's copayment will rise to 50 percent and there will be a $550 deductible, but the costs of immunosuppressive drugs will be covered as long as they are needed.

The drug insurance program will be further expanded in 1991. Subject to a deductible and copayment, Medicare coverage will be provided for insulin and all prescription drugs, including immunosuppressive drugs and intravenous drugs administered at home. The deductible will be $600 in 1991 and $652

in 1992; it will be adjusted in subsequent years to ensure that at least 16.8 percent of the enrollees reach the full deductible. The co-insurance amounts beneficiaries pay will be on a sliding scale, moving from 50 percent of reasonable charges above the deductible in 1991, to 40 percent in 1992 and 20 percent in 1993 and thereafter.

Financing the New Coverage. The added catastrophic protection will be financed completely by individuals enrolled in Medicare. Prior to 1989, the hospital insurance component (Part A) was financed solely through a Social Security payroll tax. The supplementary medical insurance component (Part B) has been financed by general funds from the U.S. Treasury as well as monthly premiums paid by people enrolled in Part B.

Money from two sources will pay for the increased Medicare benefits. First, the monthly Part B premium is being increased. The initial increase in 1989 is $4.80 a month, so that people will pay $31.90 a month compared with $27.10 a month under previous law. The premium will continue to rise so that by 1993, the total monthly payment will be $43.60.

The second source of financing for the new catastrophic protection is a supplemental premium that beneficiaries will pay through a surtax in their federal tax return. The surtax will be applied to all people eligible for Medicare (whether or not they have applied for or received Medicare benefits) who owe more than $150 in federal income tax. The maximum liability for this surtax will be limited by a ceiling, which will be $800 per beneficiary in 1989 and rise to $1,050 by 1993.

By the end of 1988, a political backlash began among the elderly against the increased costs they would incur to finance the new catastrophic protection. Sentiment was building in Congress to roll back the premium increases. Those opposed to the costs noted that unlike other government aid programs that are financed by charging all segments of society, only one group—the elderly—would pay for the new coverage. Texas Representative Bill Archer, the ranking Republican on the House Ways and Means Committee, introduced legislation to postpone the increases. On the other side, supporters of the act argued that because of Social Security and Medicare, the elderly were now better off than they were 20 years ago and had poverty rates dramatically below the rates of families with children. Thus, they argued, it was fair to expect the elderly to pay for the expanded protection. The federal budget deficit was also cited by those supporting the premium increases. The chairman of the House Ways and Means Committee, Illinois Democrat Dan Rostenkowski, and the chairman of the Senate Finance Committee, Texas Democrat Lloyd

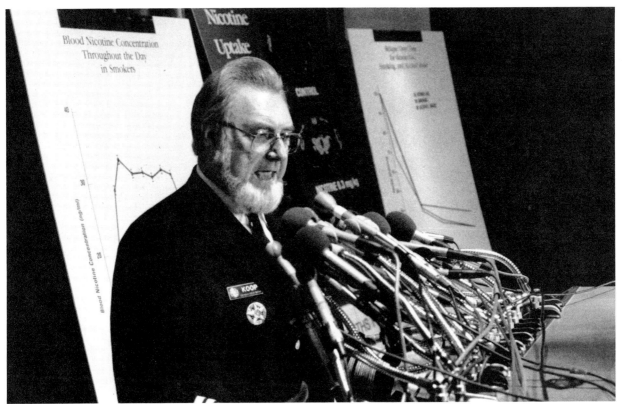

Dr. C. Everett Koop, the outspoken U.S. surgeon general, speaks publicly about the addictive nature of nicotine. He maintained a high profile throughout 1988, addressing the issues of AIDS, smoking, and nutrition.

Bentsen, both opposed changes in the financing of the Catastrophic Coverage Act.

There was no question that the taxes and premiums paid by the elderly to finance the new protection would be significant. Still, the Congressional Budget Office estimated that overall, the average Medicare enrollee would come out ahead when both the increased benefits and increased liabilities were taken into account.

AIDS Issues

In October 1988, Congress passed its first major AIDS legislation. The measure, signed into law in November, provided $900 million over three years for AIDS research and $400 million over two years for home healthcare for AIDS patients, counseling, and anonymous blood testing. The question of privacy was a major issue in the legislative battle. In September 1988 the House had overwhelmingly approved a three-year, $1.2 billion program to fight AIDS. One important provision of the House plan was a confidentiality requirement for AIDS test results, with penalties for their unauthorized disclosure. The opposition of Sen-

ate conservatives to this provision forced a House-Senate compromise that omitted the requirement.

The civil liberties problem of the AIDS crisis also figured prominently in two reports issued in June 1988. The first report, a National Academy of Sciences update of its 1986 report "Confronting AIDS," criticized federal policy in the AIDS war as inadequate. It also called for a law banning discrimination against persons infected with the virus. The second report was produced by the Presidential Commission on the Human Immunodefiency Virus Epidemic, a 13-member panel chaired by retired Admiral James D. Watkins. The key recommendation of the panel was the enactment of a federal antidiscrimination law to protect AIDS victims, as a way to encourage people to be tested and treated for AIDS. The Reagan administration, however, opposed the idea, deeming it unnecessary and a matter best left to the individual states for action.

Late in the spring of 1988, a brochure on AIDS, produced by the U.S. Public Health Service and the Centers for Disease Control, was sent to every household in the United States. The brochure contained an explicit description of the ways in which the AIDS

285

virus is transmitted. It included a discussion of the risk of anal sex and recommended which kinds of condoms to use to minimize the risk of spreading the disease. The distribution of the brochure had been ordered by Congress after the White House rejected a similar pamphlet in 1987 on the grounds that a mass mailing would cost too much money and that distributing a brochure was an inefficient way to reach persons most at risk of AIDS. To prevent censorship or suppression of the 1988 brochure, Congress took the unusual step of specifying that it would not require White House clearance.

Surgeon General Weighs In

In 1988 the surgeon general of the United States, Dr. C. Everett Koop, took controversial positions on some of the most sensitive health policy issues facing the country. In addition to his public statements on dealing with the AIDS crisis, Koop addressed the issues of nutrition and abortion. The highly visible chief medical officer of the United States became, to many, America's personal physician.

Report on Diet. In July 1988 the surgeon general released a comprehensive report on the American diet that had taken four years to prepare. In releasing the report, Koop stated, "If you are among the two out of three Americans who do not smoke or drink excessively, your choice of diet can influence your long-term health prospects more than any other action you might take." A startling statistic in the report was that of the 2.1 million deaths occurring in the United States in 1987, two-thirds were the result of conditions influenced by dietary factors.

Effect of Abortion. After meeting with right-to-life advocates, President Reagan in 1987 requested Dr. Koop to prepare a report on the physical and emotional impact of abortion on women. It had been expected that the surgeon general, who personally opposes abortion, would prepare a report supporting the right-to-life position that abortion is traumatic for women, both physically and emotionally. Instead, Koop submitted a letter to Reagan early in 1989 stating that he could not complete the assignment because existing studies of the issue did not "provide conclusive data about the health effects of abortion on women." Koop was criticized by both abortion supporters and opponents. Each side argued that existing studies, while not without flaws, contained enough data to support their respective positions. Proponents of abortion contend that abortions have few physical or psychological consequences.

See also the Spotlight on Health article How Drugs Are Approved.

JAMES A. ROTHERHAM

CANADA

Abortion Debate • Tougher Antitobacco Laws • Policy on AIDS Drugs • New Efforts to Rein in Ontario Healthcare Costs

Abortion Policy Controversy

A legislative vacuum surrounded the abortion issue for more than a year after a January 1988 decision by the Supreme Court of Canada that the country's existing abortion law was unconstitutional. (The court said the 1969 law, which required that abortions be performed only in accredited hospitals and only after approval by a committee of doctors, interfered with a woman's right to control her body and thus violated the constitution's Charter of Rights and Freedoms.) For two days at the end of July 1988, members of Parliament debated the issue hotly without coming to any agreement. The MPs were responding to a motion by the Progressive Conservative government proposing that abortions in the early stages of pregnancy be allowed after consultation between a woman and her doctor but that those to be performed at a later stage—exactly when was not specified—require two medical opinions agreeing that the mother's life or health was seriously threatened. Crossing party lines, groups of MPs including members of all three political parties—the Progressive Conservative Party and the opposition Liberal and New Democratic parties—drew up five different amendments to the motion. On July 28, however, the two pro-choice and three pro-life amendments, as well as the government's motion, were all defeated.

The government had introduced the motion (instead of a bill) in order to provide an opportunity for an open debate on the issue, and its rejection indicated how difficult it would be to reach a consensus and pass abortion legislation. In fact, the amendment with the most support called for a total ban on abortion unless the mother's life was at stake. It was narrowly rejected, by a vote of 118 to 105. The government's motion was defeated 147 to 76.

Meanwhile, provincial governments filled the legal vacuum with various temporary measures. The Alberta and New Brunswick governments required a woman seeking an abortion to get two medical opinions that the procedure was necessary, a position that Saskatchewan doctors followed in the absence of provincial government policy. (Medical necessity was being very broadly defined by many doctors.) British Columbia's original interim policy, declared by Premier Bill Vander Zalm early in 1988, stated that his

Social Credit government would not pay for abortion through public health insurance (which every Canadian has) unless the mother's life was endangered. But Vander Zalm was forced to adopt a more moderate policy—similar to Alberta's—when the provincial Supreme Court ruled that his position was illegal. Ontario left the decision on abortion up to a woman and her doctor.

While the government efforts to settle the issue were going on, the Supreme Court of Canada was facing a case brought by Joe Borowski, a former Manitoba cabinet minister and ardent antiabortionist. Borowski asked the court to rule that a fetus has the constitutional right to life, liberty, and security of the person, as well as equal protection under the law. However, in March 1989 the court refused to rule on the question of fetal rights. Issuing a 25-page statement, the justices unanimously maintained, 7-0, that in the absence of a federal abortion law, the court had no jurisdiction to decide the matter. For his part, Prime Minister Brian Mulroney had said in 1988 that his government would wait until after the Supreme Court ruling in the Borowski case before proposing any new abortion legislation.

New Curbs on Tobacco

Two stiff antitobacco laws were passed June 28, 1988, giving Canada some of the toughest legislation on this subject adopted by any tobacco-producing country. One of the laws guarantees a smoke-free work environment, if desired, to all federal employees and to employees who work under federal jurisdiction (for example, in banks and Crown corporations); employers who set up smoking rooms are required to make "reasonable efforts" to have them ventilated. The law also requires planes, ships, trains, and buses that come under federal jurisdiction to be smoke-free except in designated areas. Penalties under the law, which comes into effect when the cabinet proclaims it, include fines of $1,000 for the first offense and $10,000 for the second offense for companies failing to comply and fines of $50 for the first offense and $100 for the second offense for smokers who light up where they are not supposed to. (Canadian dollars used throughout.)

The other law, which is going into effect in stages beginning January 1, 1989, requires tobacco packages to include detailed health warnings and bans all forms

During a province-wide illegal strike for higher wages, these picketing nurses in Calgary, Alberta, pause for a coffee break. The 19-day walkout, which caused temporary nursing shortages at hospitals, was settled after a negotiated wage increase.

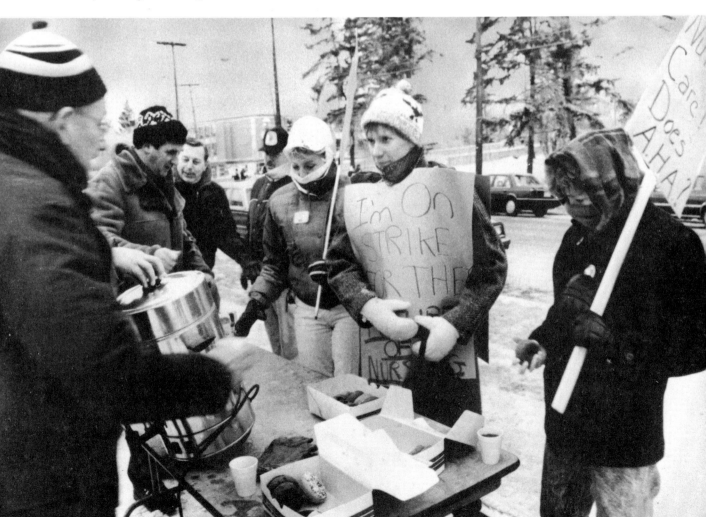

of tobacco advertising in Canada. Exceptions to the ban include television or radio broadcasts that originate outside Canada, as well as imported magazines and newspapers. Penalties for violating the law include fines ranging from $2,000 to $300,000 and maximum prison terms of six months to two years.

AIDS Drug Policy

Early in 1989 the Canadian government notified all Canadian doctors that it was speeding up the approval process for drugs to prevent and treat AIDS. The government also drew the doctors' attention to an emergency program that allows patients with life-threatening diseases, including AIDS, to get any drugs that pharmaceutical companies will sell, even if the drugs are still experimental and have not been approved by any nation for general use. The program has existed for several years, but it had become clear that few doctors and federal health officials knew about it.

Under the program, a doctor must apply for government permission to use an experimental drug on a critically ill patient. Permission can be refused if health officials feel that the doctor does not properly understand the drug. If permission is granted, the doctor must keep officials informed of the patient's progress. According to the government notice, several drug companies had already agreed to sell some experimental AIDS drugs on an emergency basis. But it was not immediately clear how many others would become available. Manufacturers might be reluctant to provide drugs out of concerns about legal liability and about how they could test their drugs in controlled scientific studies if they were already in wide use.

There was also some concern among federal officials that the healthcare system might be overburdened if AIDS patients from the United States tried to use the program to gain access, through Canadian doctors, to experimental drugs.

Ontario Healthcare Costs

The Ontario government undertook a major reorganization of its Health Ministry in May 1988 and initiated several broad inquiries—including one into the use, misuse, and cost of prescription drugs—as part of efforts to control the escalating cost of its healthcare system, which amounted to $12.7 billion in the 1988-1989 fiscal year. The system is one of the most expensive in the world on a per capita basis.

In April 1988, Health Minister Elinor Caplan ordered the province's 222 hospitals (all government-financed) to cut costs and submit balanced budgets for the 1988-1989 fiscal year. Although 105 of them did so, 117

facilities predicted deficits totaling $124 million, saying they had no fat left to trim. In May the minister imposed a freeze on all new or expanded hospital programs in order to curtail the deficits. Later, the government offered $42 million to bail out those hospitals whose shortfalls were unavoidable.

Ontario's 19,000 doctors, who are paid on a fee-for-service basis by the provincial government, were also affected by the government's cost-control efforts. After ten months of negotiations with the Ontario Medical Association, the government unilaterally imposed a 1.75 percent fee increase in December 1988. The hike, which the government had said four months earlier was its final offer, had been rejected by the OMA in October. Caplan said the increase in doctors' income would turn out to be closer to 9 percent after number of patient visits and other factors were taken into account. In 1987 doctors had received a 4.8 percent fee increase.

Caplan also said she wanted doctors to get more involved in discussing health policy issues. In June 1988 she made a plea for help at the OMA's annual conference, challenging members to be creative in finding ways to control government healthcare spending, which comprises a third of the provincial budget.

The government also raised the possibility of limiting the number of doctors allowed to practice in the province. Premier David Peterson said in early June that this option could not be ruled out. In recent years the number of doctors in Ontario has been rising by 5 percent annually, five times the rate of the population increase.

Alberta Nurses Strike

Alberta's 11,400 nurses went on strike illegally for 19 days in early 1988, and their union was charged a total of $400,000 in contempt of court fines as a result. In defiance of a 1983 law that bans strikes by nurses because they are considered essential employees, the members of the United Nurses of Alberta walked off the job January 24, demanding a wage increase of $1.50 an hour by October 1. Nurses were earning between $14.25 and $16.47 per hour, for an average yearly salary of about $30,000. The strike left almost all of the province's 104 hospitals without nursing assistance for nonemergency surgery and caused a temporary closure of Alberta's only abortion clinic. The union and the Alberta Hospital Association finally reached a tentative agreement February 11, ending the walkout. The settlement included a wage hike of 8 percent over 27 months, with an additional 2.9 percent for nurses who had worked for more than six years. The increase gave nurses from $1.16 to $1.82 per hour in additional wages.

Ruling on Billing Numbers

The British Columbia Court of Appeal ruled in August 1988 that the province's government was depriving doctors of their constitutional rights by denying them billing numbers, needed to collect fees under Canada's national health system. The decision was a triumph for a group of physicians who had taken the government to court in 1983 over its policy of restricting billing numbers, which the government argued was necessary to control healthcare costs. British Columbia was the only Canadian province restricting billing numbers for doctors. The court found the government's rules on assigning billing numbers "procedurally flawed and . . . manifestly unfair in substance."

LYNNE COHEN

Heart and Circulatory System

Type A's After a Heart Attack • Another Look at Balloon Therapy • Combining Aspirin With Clot-Busting Drugs • Preventing Sudden Death • Hypertension: Which Drug First?

The "Cardiac-Prone" Personality

Over the past three decades several scientific studies have suggested that people with Type A personalities—aggressive, hard-driving, fiercely competitive individuals—are more likely to develop premature coronary artery disease (hardening of the arteries supplying the heart muscle) than their more easygoing counterparts (Type B's). Coronary artery disease puts one at high risk for a heart attack. Although the hypothesis has had widespread popular appeal, it has not been completely accepted by the medical community because of conflicting scientific evidence.

Now researchers at the University of California at Berkeley have examined the effect of personality on survival *after* a heart attack. Their study, published in 1988, came up with surprising results. The researchers followed a group of men for more than 12 years after hospital discharge and found that those with Type A personalities were 58 percent less likely

than Type B's to die of a second heart attack. Seeking to explain this finding, some experts have suggested that people with Type A personalities may be more motivated than Type B's to take action to lower the risks of a second heart attack, for example, giving up cigarette smoking, lowering blood cholesterol levels through diet changes, and taking prescribed medications. Type A's also may be more likely to seek medical care when new symptoms arise.

Balloon Therapy

Angioplasty Update. Researchers continue to look for ways to reduce the incidence of reblockage of narrowed coronary arteries dilated by balloon angioplasty. In this procedure a deflated balloon attached to a catheter is snaked through the bloodstream to the spot where severe narrowing has occurred; the balloon is then inflated, widening the artery. Unfortunately, in about one-third of cases, the artery becomes narrowed again within a matter of months. A recent study found fish oil pills to be surprisingly successful in reducing the likelihood of reblockage (or restenosis). In patients who were given approximately 3 grams daily of eicosapentaenoic acid (a fatty acid found in fish oil), the incidence of restenosis within four months was 16 percent. In a control group treated with aspirin, restenosis occurred more than twice as often—in 36 percent of the cases. Since only 82 patients were studied, further investigation of the effect of fish oil is indicated.

Another recent study, this one involving nearly 400 patients, also found that aspirin did not reduce the rate of restenosis. Six months after successful angioplasty, both the patients treated with aspirin and those given a placebo had a 38 percent incidence of reblockage.

Opening Heart Valves. The use of balloons to open up narrowed heart valves continues to increase. This relatively new procedure, similar to angioplasty, is known as balloon valvuloplasty. It is often performed on the aortic valve, through which blood leaves the heart. In some people the valve narrows as they age. When this happens, the heart cannot empty properly, resulting in chest pain and possibly heart failure and sudden death. Surgical replacement of the valve has been the standard method of correcting this problem.

Although balloon valvuloplasty has now been used in place of surgery in many patients, until recently the success rate of the procedure has not been well documented, and the risks have not been well defined. In 1988 investigators in Boston reported on the results of over 170 valvuloplasties performed on elderly patients (average age, 77) who were considered poor candidates for cardiac surgery or who refused surgery

LET'S TAKE A WALK

Even if jogging sounds like too much work, you don't have to turn into a total couch potato. Regular brisk walking is good for the cardiovascular system, easier on the joints than running, and growing in popularity. Like all good aerobic exercise, it can lower the risk of heart disease.

There are an estimated 25 million walking enthusiasts in the United States, with a wide variety of life-styles. No special facilities, training, or equipment is required, aside from comfortable clothing and footgear. For those wishing to walk in high fashion, however, special walking shoes (at prices that can go well over $100) and chic walking outfits are available.

Many people take brisk walks every day, but a schedule of three or four walks a week can be enough for significant cardiovascular benefit. Walkers should set a pace of 4 to 4½ miles an hour and keep it up for about 60 minutes. (Besides helping your heart, that will burn up about 500 calories.)

For those who want a higher level of fitness, there's race walking, with its faster speeds and distinctive hip-rolling stride. Even that peculiar gait is becoming a more common neighborhood sight. To race walk properly, the heel of the front foot must touch the ground before the toe of the back foot leaves the ground, and the knee of the front leg must be straight as the body passes over it. The arms move diagonally across the body, in sync with the legs. Mastering this stride, as well as mustering the courage to perform it in public, may take some time. Top race walkers achieve speeds of 7 miles an hour, faster than most people can run.

More important than speed, however, is consistency. Walking regularly, alone or with company, is a healthful, relaxing habit that can be enjoyed for a lifetime.

as the initial choice. Only 3.4 percent of the patients died while still in the hospital. However, the mortality rate dramatically increased—to 26 percent—when the patients were followed for one year. Additionally, 50 percent of the patients developed valve restenosis (renarrowing of the valve), requiring either a second valvuloplasty or else surgery.

These results indicate that although aortic valvuloplasty shows some promise, it also carries significant risks; more information is required before the technique's advisability can be weighed against that of surgery. It already seems clear from the incidence of restenosis, however, that valvuloplasty should not be considered a cure.

Treating Heart Attacks

Dissolving Blood Clots. The "clot-busting" drugs streptokinase and tissue plasminogen activator (TPA) are now used extensively in emergency rooms throughout the United States to treat heart attack victims. These drugs dissolve clots in coronary arteries that cut off the blood supply to part of the heart muscle, precipitating a heart attack. If given in the first hours after a heart attack, they can save lives and reduce the damage to heart tissue.

A major study from Europe has further demonstrated the power of streptokinase to save the lives of heart attack victims, particularly when given in combination with aspirin. In the largest such study ever performed, more than 17,000 patients were given streptokinase, aspirin, both, or neither within 24 hours of the onset of chest pain—with striking results.

There were 23 percent fewer deaths in the group treated with aspirin, and 25 percent fewer in the group treated with streptokinase, as compared with the group that was not given any drug. However, the combination of both drugs reduced mortality by an amazing 42 percent, showing aspirin had an additive benefit when given with a clot-busting drug.

Immediate Angioplasty. Even after streptokinase or TPA has dissolved a blood clot, there is almost always an underlying buildup of cholesterol and fat in the artery wall (atherosclerotic plaque) that narrows the artery and impairs blood flow. Some doctors have suggested that using balloon angioplasty to dilate the coronary artery shortly after the administration of a clot-busting drug might lessen the severity of heart damage and hence improve the chances of survival. But the results of a study sponsored by the U.S. National Heart, Lung, and Blood Institute suggest that such an aggressive approach is unnecessary.

In the study, 3,200 heart attack patients who had been given TPA were divided into two groups. One group received angioplasty 18 to 48 hours after the TPA; the other received noninvasive medical care. A year later, the complications and death rate were the same for both groups, suggesting that angioplasty is not mandatory immediately after clot-dissolving therapy. Although 20 percent of those assigned to noninvasive care did develop recurrent chest pain within six weeks and thus required balloon angioplasty, the majority did very well without immediate post-heart attack balloon treatment.

Combating Sudden Death

Of the more than half a million people who die of heart attacks each year in the United States, the majority suffer sudden death, that is, death within minutes of the attack. Those who are fortunate enough to survive cardiac arrest often do so because a bystander, police officer, or fire fighter administers cardiopulmonary resuscitation (CPR) until trained medical support becomes available. Two recent experiments in Seattle (a city whose 20-year-old emergency medical system has long been a model for others) attempted, with the help of new technology, to speed delivery of treatment to heart attack victims and thereby save more lives.

In one experiment, fire fighters—often the first on the scene of a medical emergency—were trained to use an automatic electric defibrillator on heart attack victims. Paramedics, who generally arrive later, frequently use a defibrillator, a machine that administers an electric shock to the heart, often restoring normal cardiac function and saving the patient's life. Medical training is required to identify the proper situations for use of the standard defibrillator. But the new, automatic one used in Seattle can itself analyze the patient's cardiac rhythm and then deliver an electric shock if this is indicated. Of 276 patients who were initially treated by fire fighters using the automatic defibrillator, 84 (30 percent) survived long enough to be discharged from the hospital. In comparison, only 44 of 228 patients (19 percent) survived when the fire fighters delivered just basic CPR. For this latter group of patients, the first electric defibrillation was performed only after the arrival of the paramedic team. Use of the new automatic defibrillator improved survival rates by more than 50 percent, indicating this device may prove to be an important part of treatment for out-of-hospital cardiac arrest.

In another Seattle experiment to reduce the incidence of sudden death, every paramedic team has been equipped with a newly developed portable electrocardiogram machine in which a cellular phone is incorporated. The very complete and detailed data this machine provides (it can produce a complete cardiogram) are transmitted by the cellular phone to a hospital, where they are reviewed by a cardiologist. The doctor then decides whether the paramedic team should administer a clot-dissolving drug. (Previously, patients who would benefit from such a drug did not receive it until they reached the hospital.) A long-term study will evaluate the results of this new approach. New York City is also experimenting with a new portable electrocardiogram machine, but on a much more limited basis.

Silent Ischemia

Greater efforts are being made to treat patients with the condition known as silent ischemia, and more is being learned about the situations in which it occurs.

Ischemia is the term for chemical and physiological changes in the heart muscle resulting from an insufficient supply of blood. It often occurs when a person with coronary artery disease performs intense physical activity. Normal arteries supply more than enough blood to satisfy the needs of the working heart muscle, but those narrowed by coronary artery disease limit blood flow and impede cardiac functioning. Episodes of cardiac ischemia can be identified by changes in the individual's electrocardiogram (ECG), and until recently it was thought that these changes were typically accompanied by angina—pain or discomfort in the chest, arm, or throat. Recent evidence suggests, however, that the ECG changes can also occur without symptoms—this is silent ischemia.

Investigators have now discovered that in patients with coronary artery disease, emotional stress and

Seattle fire department paramedics use a portable electrocardiogram machine with a cellular phone to speed data on a heart attack victim to a hospital. A physician can then decide whether drugs should be administered even before the patient reaches the hospital.

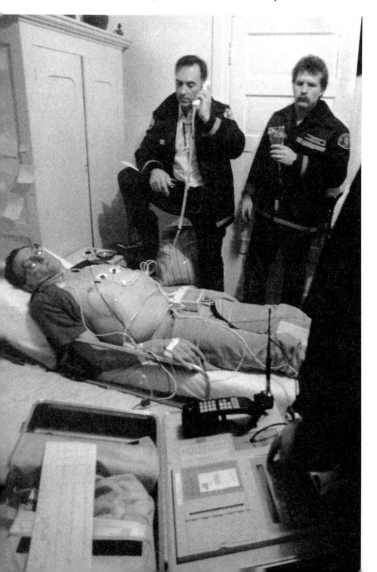

mental as well as physical exertion may lead to silent ischemia. A study showed that performing mathematical calculations, undergoing psychological testing, and delivering a speech all induced abnormal changes in subjects' electrocardiograms and in the functioning of their heart muscle. These episodes occurred in the absence of chest discomfort or other symptoms—the patients were totally unaware that their hearts were in a stressed state. Scientists have further discovered that silent episodes occur more commonly than episodes accompanied by symptoms, even in patients who also have angina attacks.

Although it is not yet clear whether these silent episodes are dangerous, they have caused concern both in patients and doctors, who had previously assumed that in the absence of chest discomfort the heart was working normally. It was further assumed that drug therapy for angina was successful if the patient's symptoms disappeared; doctors now know this may not be the case. As a result, some patients taking medication for coronary artery disease are being advised by cardiologists to wear 24-hour ambulatory electrocardiogram machines and undergo exercise stress tests to ensure that their medication is adequate to prevent silent ischemia.

Alcohol and the Heart

Research has shown that moderate alcohol consumption reduces the risk of coronary heart disease in men. The most plausible explanation of alcohol's protective effect is that it elevates levels of high-density lipoprotein (HDL) cholesterol, the "good" cholesterol that helps remove excess cholesterol from the blood.

A major study published in 1988 also found a relationship between alcohol consumption and the risk of heart attack in women. More than 87,000 female nurses between 34 and 59 years of age completed a dietary questionnaire that assessed their alcohol consumption. The nurses were then followed for four years. Adjusting for other risk factors, the study found that women who consumed from three to nine drinks a week were 40 percent less likely to have a heart attack than women who did not drink at all. Having more than nine drinks a week did not offer any greater protection.

Although the results were statistically impressive, the absolute number of heart attacks prevented by alcohol was not very large. To prevent one heart attack, 500 women had to drink moderately for four years; 499 of them therefore received no benefit. It is also worth noting that although mild to moderate alcohol consumption may help reduce the risk of coronary heart disease, excessive drinking is responsible for many significant medical and social problems.

A Head Start in Fighting Heart Disease

Heart disease, the number one killer of adults in the United States, often begins in childhood. Cholesterol and fat begin to deposit in the arteries of the heart in children as young as 10 to 15 years of age. It has therefore been suggested that changing children's eating patterns and certain other habits could help lower their cholesterol levels and possibly reduce their risk of heart disease later in life.

A five-year experiment in the New York City area, which involved more than 3,000 children in the fourth through eighth grades in 37 different schools, was conducted to examine the effectiveness of education in lowering cholesterol levels. The children were exposed to an intensive curriculum focusing on the importance of proper diet and physical activity and on the risks of cigarette smoking. The result was a modest decrease in total cholesterol levels over the five-year period. On average the cholesterol levels of participating students went down from 169 to 159. (The numbers refer to milligrams of cholesterol per deciliter of blood.) Nonparticipating students saw virtually no change in their cholesterol levels.

Although the program did not produce dramatic improvement, the results do suggest that children can respond to health education. And since there are some 45 million youngsters from 5 to 18 years of age enrolled in U.S. schools, the potential to improve the health habits of the next generation is considerable.

Heart Attacks and the Pill

It is well established that current use of oral contraceptives (birth control pills) increases the user's risk of heart attack. This is especially true for older women and cigarette smokers. It has not been clear, however, whether past use of the pill adds to the risk of heart attack. A study published in 1988 provided conclusive evidence on the latter question. The study, which followed more than 119,000 women for eight years, found that those who had used the pill in the past— even for prolonged periods of time—were not at greater risk for heart disease once they stopped using it. However, active users were found to be twice as likely to have a heart attack as those not on the pill (although their risk was still quite low, especially if they were nonsmokers).

Hypertension: Which Drug First?

Better understanding of the effectiveness of different types of medication promises improved treatment for high blood pressure (hypertension). It is estimated that there are more than 30 million adults with hypertension in the United States, and the condition is the most common reason for visits to the doctor's office. Although high blood pressure rarely has any symptoms, it often leads to stroke, kidney failure, heart attack, and premature death. In many cases, drugs are prescribed to control patients' hypertension and reduce the likelihood of these complications.

Many medications are effective in treating hypertension. In 1972 a government-sponsored panel recommended a diuretic as the best first drug if weight loss and a low-salt diet failed to reduce blood pressure. (Diuretics, or water pills, promote elimination of sodium and water from the body.) The panel also recommended adding a beta blocker to the diuretic if blood pressure was still unacceptably elevated, and in some cases a third or even a fourth medication. (Beta blockers are a class of drugs that, by occupying so-called beta receptors in the heart and kidneys, reduce the heart's workload.) This sequential use of medication, starting with a diuretic, is known as stepped care and has been widely used in the United States. However, recent scientific information has raised doubts about the validity of the approach.

A study conducted in Europe and published in 1988 examined the effects of different drug therapies on more than 3,200 men, aged 40 to 64, with mild to moderate hypertension. Half of the men were first prescribed a diuretic (as in typical stepped care) while the other half were given a beta blocker called metoprolol as the initial medication. The two drugs proved equally effective in controlling blood pressure. However, after four years of continued therapy, the death rate in the group of men treated with metoprolol was found to be 48 percent lower than in the group of men treated with the diuretic. This finding suggests that a diuretic may be the wrong first-choice drug in treating hypertension.

In recent years, new classes of medications have become available for the treatment of hypertension. In guidelines published in 1988, the same government-sponsored panel, which had been reconvened, recommended that the choice of medication as first therapy should be based on individual factors, such as the type of hypertension and how high a particular patient's blood pressure is. Thus, the concept of stepped care as the standard approach has been virtually discarded.

Artificial Heart Update

In 1988 the U.S. government seemed to be of two minds about funding artificial heart research—first stopping, then reinstating such funding. In May the National Institutes of Health announced that beginning in the next fiscal year, it would no longer finance artificial heart research and instead would concentrate its limited resources on a simpler mechanism, the left ventricular assist device. (This device is essentially a blood pump that would help one chamber of the heart, the left ventricle, send oxygen-rich blood out to the body.) In announcing the funding cutoff, NIH officials cited the complications suffered by the five individuals who had received the Jarvik-7 artificial heart, the most commonly used model, as a permanent replacement for a diseased heart. These complications included infections, blood clots, and strokes. All five men died within two years of receiving their hearts, some within just a few months. Proponents of the artificial heart point to its current value as a stopgap measure, to keep a potential transplant recipient alive until another human heart becomes available (dozens of Jarvik-7's have been used this way); they also see a successful permanent artificial heart as an attainable goal.

Less than two months after its initial decision, the NIH, under pressure from Congress, backtracked and announced it would continue artificial heart funding. Current research is focusing on the development of a new generation of artificial hearts that would be completely implantable, in contrast to present devices, which must be tethered to a power source outside the body. The project is an ambitious one, and testing in humans of an implantable artificial heart is perhaps a decade away. An implantable left ventricular assist device, on the other hand, could be ready for testing in humans within three years.

BRUCE D. CHARASH, M.D.
JEFFREY FISHER, M.D.

Liver

Hepatitis Virus Discovered • Advance in Liver Transplants • Treating Gallstones

Non-A, Non-B Hepatitis

In the United States the form of hepatitis most commonly transmitted by blood transfusions is the type called long-incubation non-A, non-B hepatitis. Although it is usually a mild illness, it can cause chronic liver disease, including cirrhosis (in which the liver develops excess scar tissue, leaving it unable to function properly), and possibly cancer. In 1988 researchers at a California biotechnology company announced that, after 5½ years of trying, they had isolated proteins of a virus responsible for the disease (although other viruses, not yet discovered, may also cause it). The virus appears to be unrelated to any virus already known.

Isolation of the proteins has already led to the development of a screening test to identify donated blood that may contain the virus. The test detects the presence of antibodies to the virus in the blood of people who have been infected. (Up to 70 percent of people who have had non-A, non-B hepatitis may become lifelong carriers of the virus.) If approved by the Food and Drug Administration, the test could be in use in the United States by the end of 1989, and it is expected to detect at least 80 percent of donated blood units that could transmit non-A, non-B hepatitis. Over the longer term, isolation of the virus may lead to development of a vaccine.

Treating Alcoholic Hepatitis

Several recent studies have provided new hope for those suffering from alcoholic hepatitis, a severe form of liver disease that develops in 15 to 20 percent of chronic alcoholics. In half of those who get it, cirrhosis follows. For those most severely ill from alcoholic hepatitis, the mortality rate is up to 40 percent. There is no cure for alcoholic hepatitis other than stopping alcohol consumption. But a number of drugs may improve patients' health. Cortisone-like drugs may help selected patients, especially women and those who go into a coma from brain dysfunction or whose blood clots too slowly because of their liver disease. Anabolic steroids similar to those utilized by body builders may also be effective. In a large Veterans Administration study, an anabolic steroid appeared to decrease long-term mortality.

A drug used to treat overactive thyroid glands may also help patients with alcoholic hepatitis. In a Canadian study, the drug propylthiouracil increased the survival rate of patients with alcoholic hepatitis and other forms of severe alcoholic liver disease. Studies are underway to confirm these findings.

Colchicine, a drug used to treat gout, may slow the growth of scar tissue in the liver, impeding the development of cirrhosis in patients who are chronic alcoholics. Some patients even appear to lose scar tissue while taking the drug.

For those who develop the life-threatening complications of alcoholic cirrhosis, a liver transplant may be the only means of prolonging life. According to one recent report, few of the patients studied returned to alcohol following a transplant operation. It has been feared that alcoholics receiving such transplants might continue to drink and thus destroy their new livers. Further studies of the effectiveness of transplants for alcoholic cirrhosis are underway.

Liver Transplants

Early in 1989 it was reported that a new chemical solution developed at the University of Wisconsin had kept human livers viable outside the body for up to 34 hours, more than three times as long as the solution traditionally used. The Wisconsin solution may revolutionize the field of liver transplantation. With more time to get a donated liver into a dying patient, doctors are no longer limited to looking for donors in the same geographic area—donor livers stored in the new solution have even been transported across the Atlantic. Doctors also have more time to examine a donor liver before deciding to go ahead with a transplant and more time to spend on the transplant procedure itself. During clinical trials it was found that transplants using livers preserved in the new solution for up to 24 hours had a higher success rate than transplants using livers preserved in the old solution for up to 9½ hours, success being measured by whether the new liver functioned properly. The U.S. Food and Drug Administration has been asked to approve the Wisconsin solution for general use.

Dissolving Gallstones

An experimental therapy that dissolves cholesterol gallstones seems promising. Gallstones are small solid lumps that form in the gallbladder, a small sac on the underside of the liver in which bile is stored and concentrated. Bile, which plays an important role in the digestive system, is made in the liver. It contains cholesterol, as well as various other substances. Sometimes, when the balance of these substances is upset, small particles of cholesterol may gather in the gallbladder and stones develop around them; these cholesterol stones are the most common kind of gallstone.

Researchers have discovered that cholesterol stones bathed in methyl tert-butyl ether may dissolve completely in a matter of hours. The solvent can be delivered through a small catheter placed through the skin into the gallbladder. The catheter can even be incorporated into a pump controlled by a microprocessor, so that less continuous, hands-on medical attention is needed. The new technique appears promising for patients who are not good candidates for surgery to remove the gallbladder but whose symptoms are so severe that immediate treatment is needed. ROWEN K. ZETTERMAN, M.D.

Medical Technology

Blood Plasma Filter • New Type of Pacemaker • Laser Probe for Blocked Blood Vessels

Helping the Immune System

A device to improve the functioning of the immune system in patients with a particular autoimmune disorder was approved by the U.S. Food and Drug Administration (FDA) in December 1987. Called the Prosorba Immunoadsorption Treatment Column, the device essentially acts as filter, removing specific substances from the blood plasma (the liquid part of blood). The Prosorba Column was approved for use in treating the condition known as idiopathic thrombocytopenic purpura, or ITP. The device is manufactured by the Imré Corporation of Seattle.

ITP is an autoimmune disease, that is, one in which the immune system attacks the body's own tissues. In the case of ITP, platelets (cell fragments in the blood that assist in clotting) are destroyed. As their platelet counts drop, patients develop purplish blotches caused by hemorrhaging into the skin. ITP is most common in children, in whom it typically begins following a viral infection. When it occurs in adults, there is often no apparent reason for the onset of ITP. Patients may experience abrupt or acute bleeding from the mucous membranes, and tests may show changes in the bone marrow. In most patients, the disease goes into remission without treatment in two to six weeks, but a small percentage will develop chronic ITP. Standard treatment usually begins with large doses of oral steroid medications. In some patients removal of the spleen is an effective cure, since significant numbers of antibodies directed against platelets are produced in the spleen. However, some patients (especially those over 45 years of age) are not sufficiently helped by either form of therapy.

When the Prosorba Column is used, blood is removed from the patient, the plasma is separated out, and the red blood cells are returned to the patient. The plasma is passed through the column, which filters out substances called immunoglobulin G (IgG) and IgG-containing circulating immune complexes (CIC). The plasma then is also returned to the patient.

Although beneficial effects have been seen in patients when as little as one unit (pint) of blood was treated, at least two units were treated in most patients in tests of the products.

The Prosorba Column appears to produce a greater benefit than can be attributed to the amounts of IgG and CIC it removes. The makers of the column believe it also produces changes in the composition of CIC and stimulates the body to remove additional CIC.

In one study of the effectiveness of the Prosorba Column, 11 of 16 patients (69 percent) had increases in platelet count following treatment. One patient who had undergone extensive prior therapy had a complete remission that lasted for more than six months. The most commonly reported side effects of therapy with the Prosorba Column are pain, fever, chills, and nausea.

New laser technology allows surgeons to remove fatty deposits from blocked blood vessels in the legs more quickly and cheaply than with conventional vascular surgery.

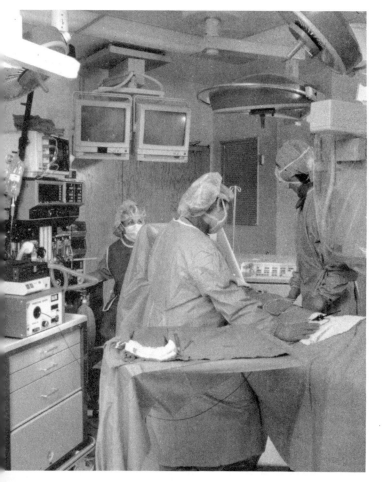

Decreased platelet counts sometimes occur following infection with human immunodeficiency virus (HIV), the virus that causes AIDS. In a study involving 29 patients with ITP as a complication of HIV infection, 16 (55 percent) showed significant platelet count increases after four to eight treatments with the Prosorba Column.

Although the Prosorba Column has been approved only for the treatment of ITP, it may well have future applications in treating other autoimmune diseases.

Heat-Sensitive Pacemaker

In April 1988 the FDA approved a new type of pacemaker, the Kelvin 500, that is expected to improve the quality of life for some pacemaker users by allowing them to engage in a broader range of activities. It is manufactured by the Cook Pacemaker Corporation of Leechburg, Pa.

More than 350,000 people in the United States have pacemakers to regulate their heartbeats, and more than 100,000 pacemakers (including replacements) are implanted each year. One of the problems with conventional pacemakers is that they operate at a fixed rate, usually about 70 beats per minute, that does not vary when the wearer exercises or is under some type of stress—conditions that would normally cause the heart to pump faster in order to deliver more oxygen and nutrients to body cells. With no way of increasing blood flow or oxygen delivery, patients with fixed-rate pacemakers are limited in the extent to which they can engage in physical activity. Just walking up a flight of stairs might be more vigorous exercise than someone with a fixed-rate pacemaker can tolerate.

In recent years, a great deal of research has gone into producing "rate responsive" pacemakers, which increase the number of heartbeats per minute during stress and exercise. The Kelvin 500 is the first device to use temperature as the signal for the pacemaker to implement a change in the patient's heart rate.

At the beginning of exercise, a person's blood temperature normally drops. Then, as exercise continues, it steadily rises. The Kelvin 500 responds to the initial decrease in temperature by increasing the heart rate to an intermediate level. If blood temperature then rises, confirming that physical activity is taking place, the pacemaker further increases the heart rate to a preprogrammed upper rate. When the patient finishes exercising, blood temperature starts dropping, and the pacemaker detects that decrease and reduces the heart rate. Each pacemaker is custom-programmed according to the recipient's normal temperature changes during activity. Programming is a relatively simple procedure that can be done in a

DOWN THE HATCH

The familiar mercury-filled thermometer is being replaced—at least in some special cases—by a new battery-powered device that people swallow. Called CorTemp, the device provides constant readings of the body's internal temperature for the one to two days it takes to move through the digestive tract and be passed out of the body. Developed at the Applied Physics Laboratory at the Johns Hopkins University and approved by the U.S. Food and Drug Administration in November 1988, CorTemp is the size of a vitamin pill and consists of a silicone shell enclosing a quartz crystal whose vibration frequency depends on its temperature. Vibrations are transmitted to a receiver wired to a personal computer or to a calculator-sized unit worn on the belt.

Accurate to within 0.01°C, CorTemp has many uses. It can help doctors monitor treatment for hypothermia, in which body temperature drops dangerously low; treatment involves warming the body at a slow, steady rate. It can also be used for monitoring heart transplant patients after surgery, since the slightest rise in temperature can be a sign of infection. And it can aid women trying to become pregnant, since body temperature rises about a degree just before a woman ovulates. (CorTemp does have to be prescribed by a doctor, and currently each capsule costs about $75 and can be used only once.)

Johns Hopkins veterinary labs are investigating possible uses for CorTemp in animals. Larger animals, such as horses, often awake from anesthesia confused and hostile and frequently kick or bite veterinarians who get too close. With CorTemp, vets can take temperature readings from a safe distance. Certain industries have expressed interest as well. The canning industry suspects CorTemp, placed in newly canned goods, could allow packers to ensure that food temperatures remain at safe levels to prevent the growth of dangerous bacteria. The photography industry could similarly use CorTemp to check the temperature of packaged film, as an aid in preventing film spoilage.

---

doctor's office. In addition to exercise, the pacemaker can respond to body or skin temperature changes—such as those caused by a fever or by using a sauna—that would normally cause an increase in heart rate. Unlike some rate-modulating pacemakers, the Kelvin 500 is not affected by medications the patient may be taking.

Like other pacemakers, the Kelvin 500 is small and made of a biologically compatible material (titanium), so that it can be implanted under the skin of the upper chest. A thin tube containing the heat-sensing probe extends from the device into the right ventricle of the heart.

Unblocking Blood Vessels

A device for opening blocked blood vessels—called the Spectraprobe-PLR Catheter and manufactured by Trimedyne, Inc., of Santa Ana, Calif.—was approved by the FDA in June 1988. It is used in conjunction with a laser to remove fatty deposits clogging a vein or artery in a limb, most often one of the legs. The Spectraprobe-PLR differs from a previously approved laser probe in that it emits a small amount of laser energy directly onto the blood vessel wall, vaporizing some of the fatty material. The rest of the laser energy heats the metallic tip of the probe, and the heated tip also vaporizes fatty material. (The previous probe works solely by heating the tip.) In addition, use of the Spectraprobe-PLR does not always require followup with balloon angioplasty—a therapy in which an uninflated balloon is threaded into a partially clogged area of a blood vessel, then inflated to enlarge the passageway through which blood flows.

A blocked vessel in the leg can cause pain, as well as weakness in the affected leg when a person walks, so that the individual becomes lame. A patient may develop sores that do not heal and that sometimes lead to gangrene, forcing doctors to consider amputation. Laser treatment is preferable to conventional surgery to open such vessels because it requires a shorter hospital stay, costs less, and is a less invasive procedure.

The removal of a blockage with the Spectraprobe-PLR can be performed under either local or general anesthesia. An incision is made, and the probe is inserted into the blood vessel and guided to the obstruction. Then, 10-12 watts of laser energy are delivered. As the fatty deposits are vaporized, the probe is slowly advanced through the blocked area;

doctors track its path on a screen. The probe usually is passed through the blocked channel two or three times to maximize the width of the opening.

Doctors in the United States and England tested the device by performing some 250 procedures in over 200 patients. Some of the patients had had previous surgery on their leg vessels, and a few had undergone amputation because of vessel blockage; the average age of the patients was 64 years. In some cases Spectraprobe-PLR was used as the sole therapeutic device. In others it was combined with balloon dilation or some type of vascular surgery or both.

The Spectraprobe-PLR was able to open a channel through the entire length of the obstruction in most of the patients, both when used as the sole therapy and when combined with other treatment methods. Long-term follow-up revealed that most of the treated blood vessels remained open for at least 9 to 12 months.

Adverse reactions, including leg spasms, infection, and perforation of the blood vessel being treated, occurred in a small percentage of cases.

VIRGINIA COWART

Medications and Drugs

New Infection Fighters • Preventing Pneumonia in AIDS Patients • New Uses for Alpha-Interferon • More Drugs for High Blood Pressure

Drugs That Fight Infection

Under a new Food and Drug Administration (FDA) regulation, two kinds of products became available in the United States for use in some infections caused by a virus called cytomegalovirus (CMV). Intended primarily to speed promising drugs to AIDS patients, the regulation allows the distribution of what are called treatment investigational new drugs (treatment INDs) to doctors treating patients with various life-threatening or disabling diseases. (*See also the Spotlight on Health article* HOW DRUGS ARE APPROVED.)

The usually harmless CMV can cause serious illness in patients whose immune systems are impaired by AIDS or deliberately suppressed by drugs given to prevent rejection of organ transplants (immunosuppressive drugs). One of the new CMV treatments is

a biological product called cytomegalovirus immune globulin (CMVIG). The other, ganciclovir (Cytovene), is a drug for treating AIDS-related complications caused by CMV.

CMVIG has proved effective in preventing infections in patients whose donated kidney was thought to have carried the cytomegalovirus. Patients treated with CMVIG suffered CMV infections only one-third as often as untreated kidney recipients, and their symptoms were milder. The transplants were more often successful in those who got CMVIG along with an immunosuppressive drug than in patients treated with an immunosuppressive drug only.

Ganciclovir, a drug already available in Europe, has been shown to prevent blindness in AIDS patients with long-standing CMV infections of the retina—the eye structure most important for sight. Given by intravenous injection, ganciclovir seems to stop the spread of infection in the inner part of the retina.

A genetically engineered form of an antiviral and antitumor protein called alpha-interferon (brand names, Intron A and Roferon) produced naturally by cells of the human immune system was previously approved only for treating one rare form of leukemia. Alpha-interferon is now also approved in both the United States and Canada for treating a cancer associated with AIDS (see Treating Leukemia and Cancer, below) and in the United States only (in the form of Intron A) for treating genital warts—growths that appear on the penis, vagina, anus, and elsewhere. Genital warts are now the fourth most frequently diagnosed sexually transmitted infection in the United States.

To remove genital warts by eliminating their cause—the human papilloma virus—alpha-interferon is injected into the base of each wart three times weekly for up to three weeks. In close to half the cases all warts clear up completely and in most other cases the size of the remaining warts is reduced. This new treatment seems more effective than the many other measures employed to rid infected areas of genital warts. However, as happens with all other treatments, warts often recur after interferon therapy.

Pentamidine (Pentam 300), a drug previously approved for use by injection to treat a form of pneumonia called *Pneumocystis carinii*, was made available in aerosol form on a treatment IND basis in the United States and on a similar basis (called emergency drug release) in Canada. More than 50 percent of AIDS patients get this form of pneumonia, the most common fatal complication of the disease. Preliminary tests indicate that aerosol pentamidine, when inhaled once a month by AIDS patients who have had one or more attacks of *Pneumocystis carinii*, can prevent further attacks. The drug is also being made available to those infected with AIDS whose immune systems are seriously weakened, in the hope that it can ward off a first attack.

A new improved version of a vaccine for preventing infections caused by *Haemophilus influenzae* type b (Hib) bacteria became available in the United States and Canada in 1988. Called Haemophilus b conjugate vaccine and marketed as ProHIBiT and Hib TITER, it is made by linking noninfective parts of Hib bacteria with diphtheria toxoid, a very strong immune system stimulant. A single injection of this combination produces much higher and longer-lasting levels of antibodies than the previously approved vaccine. The earlier vaccine was not recommended for use on youngsters under two years of age, but the new one stimulates the immature immune systems of children as young as 18 months old to produce the antibodies needed to attack and kill invading Hib bacteria, thus protecting them from serious Hib infections. These include bacterial meningitis—an inflammation of brain and spinal cord membranes that is still a killer and can leave survivors deaf, partially blind, or mentally retarded—pneumonia, and epiglottitis, an inflammation and swelling of soft tissues in the throat that can cause sudden suffocation by closing the opening to the trachea, or windpipe. The new vaccine, which is being tested in infants as young as two months, is said to have few side effects.

Cefuroxime axetil, a new oral form of a cephalosporin antibiotic approved earlier for injection only, was marketed in the United States as Ceftin, an easy-to-swallow tablet that need be taken only twice a day. The new antibiotic is especially useful for treating acute respiratory infections such as strep throat, bronchitis, and middle ear infections in children, and it causes few side effects. One difficulty, however, is that it is not available in a flavored liquid form for children too young to swallow a tablet. Since the crushed tablet has a bitter taste even when mixed with applesauce or ice cream, toddlers may refuse to take it.

A new antibiotic called mupirocin (brand name, Bactroban), was made available as an ointment and approved for use in treating impetigo, a skin infection that is seen mainly in children. Impetigo is marked by small blisters that break and release a fluid that forms thick yellow crusts as it dries. Parents of young children should first wash the crusts away with warm soapy water. They should then spread the antibiotic ointment directly on the child's underlying reddened skin.

When mupirocin is applied three times daily (and covered with a gauze dressing if desired), most cases of impetigo clear up within a week. This treatment is said to be at least as effective as taking other antibiotics by mouth. A high local concentration of mupirocin builds up without risk of the serious adverse effects that sometimes occur with oral antibiotics. Use of this ointment has caused only occasional complaints of a mild stinging or burning sensation and, rarely, itching.

The first of a new chemical class of antifungal agents was approved by the FDA for use in treating vaginal infections caused by the yeast *Candida albicans*. Terconazole is available in two forms: a suppository called Terazol 3 that is inserted into the vagina at bedtime on three consecutive days and a cream called Terazol 7 that is applied at bedtime to the vagina and the nearby female genital areas (the vulva) for seven consecutive days. Both products act rapidly to eradicate the yeastlike fungi responsible for candidal vulvovaginitis. Many women report complete relief of itching, redness, and discharge in as few as three days. (*See also the Spotlight on Health article* YEAST INFECTIONS.)

A new antifungal agent, naftifine, was approved by the FDA for use as a cream and marketed as Naftin. Applied daily to the skin, the cream rapidly relieves the typical itchy red rashes of ringworm infections. Although its use seems safe, some patients complain of stinging, burning, redness, and dryness of the skin when applying the cream.

Metronidazole, long available for use orally or intravenously against many kinds of infections, was recently approved by the FDA for application to the skin in a gel form (Metro Gel). When applied on the face by patients with rosacea whose condition has not been helped by oral antibiotics, this product markedly reduces the number of unsightly blemishes. (Rosacea is a chronic inflammatory condition that resembles acne.) Local application of metronidazole seems safe as well as effective when used daily for two months or more. However, because it cannot reduce the size of dilated blood vessels on the faces of people with rosacea, it cannot cure this potentially disfiguring disease.

Treating Leukemia and Cancer

Mitoxantrone (marketed as Novantrone), the first new chemotherapeutic drug developed during the past decade for treating leukemia, was approved for use in the United States in one relatively uncommon kind of blood cell cancer, acute nonlymphocytic leukemia. However, some U.S. doctors are also using it to treat some other types of leukemia and some lymphomas (lymph tissue tumors) and even prescribing it for women with widespread breast cancer. (In Canada, where the drug has been approved for a number of years, it is prescribed for breast cancer, lymphoma, and liver cancer.)

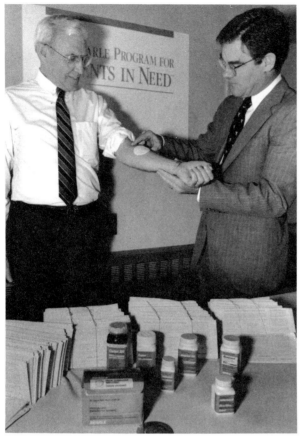

At Boston City Hospital, the G. D. Searle Company demonstrates the application of a nitroglycerin patch for angina sufferers—one of the cardiovascular products that the drug company is distributing free to medically indigent patients nationwide.

Two alpha-interferon products, Intron A and Roferon, previously approved for treating hairy cell leukemia, received FDA approval in 1988 for use in another kind of cancer, AIDS-associated Kaposi's sarcoma. Roferon was approved for the same use in Canada. Kaposi's sarcoma was once a rare and relatively slow-growing tumor confined mainly to the skin; in AIDS patients, however, it grows aggressively and rapidly invades various internal organs. This form of the disease is fatal, and those who have it live, on the average, for less than two years.

Interferon therapy works best when given in the early stages of AIDS to patients whose immune systems are still functioning fairly well. In such patients, injections of the drug three times a week often lead to long periods of improvement, marked by partial to complete disappearance of tumors from the skin, lungs, and abdominal organs. Patients who respond

to interferon live about a year longer than those who do not respond and require radiation or chemotherapy.

Interferon is also safer than the standard treatments, which can do further damage to the already weakened immune defenses of AIDS patients. The drug causes frequent but less serious side effects—mainly flu-like symptoms such as chills and fever, fatigue, headache, and muscle pain. Such symptoms can usually be controlled by acetaminophen (Tylenol and other brand names).

A synthetic drug called octreotide, which acts like the natural hormone somatostatin, was recently marketed in the United States as Sandostatin after it was approved for use in treating certain rare cancers of the intestine and pancreas. These are malignant tumors containing cells that secrete excessive amounts of chemicals capable of adversely affecting gastrointestinal, heart, and blood vessel functions. Patients suffer from frequent, disabling bouts of watery diarrhea, facial flushing, wheezing, and cardiac rhythm irregularities or even heart failure.

Octreotide does not cure the digestive system cancers, which are best removed surgically before they have spread to the liver, or treated with chemotherapy when they have become inoperable. However, the drug improves patients' quality of life by quickly controlling their disabling diarrhea and life-threatening cardiac conditions. This synthetic relative of somatostatin is more useful than the natural hormone because its effects last for hours rather than only minutes.

Cardiovascular Drugs

Lowering Blood Pressure. A long-acting drug that reduces mild to moderate high blood pressure by widening the patient's arterioles, or smallest arteries, was recently approved in both the United States and Canada. Taken in a single daily morning dose, terazosin (brand name, Hytrin) exerts a pressure-lowering effect that lasts until the following morning. Its effectiveness does not appear to decrease after several years of steady use.

Some doctors advocate beginning treatment for high blood pressure with terazosin instead of with a diuretic or a beta blocker, the two types of medication most commonly prescribed as initial treatment. This is because the new drug is said to be safer, especially for patients who have other conditions that can worsen when they take the standard drugs for hypertension. However, while terazosin is well tolerated by most patients, some may suffer a fainting spell after taking their first dose. Patients are therefore warned to get up slowly from a sitting or lying position so as to avoid injury from falls. Because dizziness and drowsiness may also occur at first, patients are also advised to avoid driving during the period when their initially low doses are being gradually adjusted upward.

Lisinopril (available as Prinivil and Zestril) received FDA approval for treatment of mild, moderate, and severe degrees of hypertension. The product acts like two previously approved drugs of the same class, captopril and enalapril. Drugs of this class, called angiotensin-converting enzyme (ACE) inhibitors, act by blocking the action of an enzyme that converts angiotensin I, an inactive circulating substance, into angiotensin II, a powerful pressure-raising hormone. Because lisinopril's effects last longer than those of the earlier drugs, it is recommended for administration only once daily.

A single daily dose of lisinopril lowers high blood pressure to normal levels in more than half the patients taking it. For some reason, blacks do not respond as readily as nonblacks; but when blacks—as well as others with mild to moderate hypertension who do not respond adequately to lisinopril alone—are given a diuretic, the combined therapy is effective in almost every case.

Lisinopril's most common side effects—dizziness, headache, diarrhea, and fatigue—are well tolerated by most patients. However, some patients react with a persistent hacking cough and may have to discontinue this drug. As with all ACE inhibitors, a rare but serious reaction marked by sudden swelling of the face, tongue, and throat tissues requires immediate lifesaving measures and, of course, discontinuance of the drug. So far, no severe reduction in the white blood cell count—a potentially dangerous adverse reaction to the earlier ACE inhibitors—has been reported in the case of lisinopril.

Another drug to control blood pressure, a diuretic called metolazone, which has been available for close to 15 years in high-dose tablet form, was marketed in the United States in 1988 in a new low-dose formulation called Mykrox. A single daily dose is said to cause less loss of potassium than the earlier form while reducing high blood pressure equally well. However, about one of every five patients does develop a drop in serum potassium levels (hypokalemia).

Mykrox is claimed to be the best drug with which to begin treatment of hypertensive blacks who, as noted above, often do not benefit from initial treatment with other drugs such as beta blockers or ACE inhibitors. Combining Mykrox with these drugs helps make them more effective for such patients.

Preventing Clots. Dipyridamole (Persantine), a drug long available for preventing chest pains (angina pectoris) in patients with coronary artery disease, has received FDA approval for another purpose. It is given together with an oral anticoagulant drug such as warfarin to help prevent blood clots (thrombi) from forming on artificial heart valves after open-heart surgery to replace patients' diseased valves. Its use lessens the likelihood of a clot's breaking loose from a new valve and then traveling to the brain or elsewhere to block arterial blood flow. Such clots can cause strokes or other complications by cutting off part of the blood supply to the brain or other organs.

New Drugs for Mental and Neurologic Conditions

Fluoxetine (Prozac), an antidepressant drug that differs from other drugs of this class, was approved in the United States and Canada for treating patients suffering from mental depression. A single daily dose taken in the morning exerts its therapeutic effect for 24 hours. However, as with other antidepressants, it may take two weeks for the first benefits to be felt and up to a month for the full effects to develop.

This drug is as effective as all previous antidepressants for improving a patient's mental status, but without the adverse effects sometimes caused by the older drugs. No cases have been reported of patients dying from deliberate overdoses. The most common side effects of fluoxetine—nausea, nervousness, and insomnia—subside with continued treatment. Caution is required, however, in patients with a history of convulsive disorders, as they may suffer seizures when taking this medication. Moreover, the drug can accumulate to toxic levels in patients with poor liver or kidney function, so that if it is prescribed at all to such patients, it is given in lower doses, with longer intervals between doses. It should not be prescribed in combination with an antidepressant drug of the class called monoamine oxidase (MAO) inhibitors. (*See also the feature article* MANIA AND DEPRESSION.)

Clomipramine (Anafranil), another treatment IND, has been approved by the FDA for use by psychiatrists treating patients with severe symptoms of obsessive-compulsive disorder. Patients with this condition are plagued by persistent thoughts that they cannot get out of their minds (obsessions) and by behavioral patterns that they cannot control (compulsions). Clomipramine is more effective than earlier drugs in lessening such symptoms; patients often improve enough to function well in their daily activities. However, since the drug can set off seizures, patients are cautioned not to undertake tasks that could prove hazardous if they suffer a sudden lapse in consciousness.

Another treatment IND, selegiline (Eldepryl), improves the response of Parkinson's disease patients to the standard drug levodopa, which is converted into dopamine by the brain. (Parkinson's disease results from reduced levels in the brain of dopamine, a substance that sends signals from one nerve cell to another in a special nerve pathway that modifies body movement.) Over time, however, levodopa loses its effectiveness so that higher doses have to be given, and these higher doses have serious side effects. Selegiline works by inhibiting the activity of an enzyme that reduces the level of dopamine. Treatment with selegiline and low doses of levodopa has been shown to improve Parkinson's patients' mobility and keep levodopa's side effects under control.

Treating Digestive System Disorders

A new drug for dissolving gallstones received FDA approval after being available in some countries for close to ten years. Ursodiol (Actigall) works only on stones made up mainly of cholesterol, and then only when the cholesterol has not been hardened by calcium salts. The drug may be of greatest benefit to patients whose stones have not yet caused gallbladder damage, and who continue to take it daily for as long as one or two years.

Ursodiol dissolves stones completely in about one of every three patients. But since new stones tend to develop in half of them after treatment is discontinued, patients are checked periodically by ultrasound images to see if they need a second course of treatment. Fortunately, unlike a previously approved stone-dissolving drug called chenodiol (Chenix), ursodiol can be taken for long periods without affecting liver function or raising blood cholesterol levels.

Nizatidine (Axid), the fourth drug of the histamine 2 antagonist type to be approved for peptic ulcer treatment, is just as effective as the earlier ones and has some advantages over cimetidine (Tagamet), the first drug of this class to be marketed. A single dose taken at bedtime promptly reduces stomach acid secretions and relieves abdominal pain for a long period. Most patients' active ulcers heal within four weeks. Patients then continue on half the previous dose to prevent new ulcers from developing during the next six months or so.

Unlike cimetidine, this new drug does not interact with the anticoagulant warfarin (Coumadin, Panwarfin) or with diazepam (Valium) to make these drugs accumulate to toxic levels. Nor does it affect the level of the hormones testosterone and prolactin, as cimetidine does, so that reports of increased breast size or impotence in men are very rare. The few side effects that occur are not long-lasting or discomforting enough to make patients discontinue nizatidine therapy.

The drug mesalamine (Rowasa in the United States, Salofalk in Canada) was approved for treatment of a chronic inflammatory bowel disease called ulcerative colitis. A liquid suspension administered rectally once daily, preferably at bedtime, brings about improvement in most patients. It does so by reducing inflammation in the last segment of the large intestine, including the S-shaped sigmoid colon and the rectum. An oral form of mesalamine—a tablet coated to keep it from dissolving in the stomach and being absorbed from the small intestine before it can reach the colon—is available in other countries but not yet in the United States or Canada.

A Drug to Fight Baldness

The first drug for fighting baldness received FDA approval in 1988, two years after it became available in Canada. Applied directly to hairless scalp areas, a solution of minoxidil (marketed as Rogaine) helps hair to grow in varying degrees in about two out of five individuals. It works best in young men who are just beginning to lose hair on the crown, but does not prevent the forehead hairline from receding. Because the treatment is not a cure—the new growth falls out a few months after a person stops applying the solution—the drug must be used indefinitely to retain hair and increase new growth.

Minoxidil was first introduced for treating high blood pressure, and it can cause serious side effects when taken orally. However, no adverse effects have developed from application of the drug solution to the skin of a healthy scalp. Doctors must check, however, to see that the patient's scalp is free of cuts or inflamed areas through which the drug might be absorbed into the bloodstream.

Another Choice in Treating Arthritis

Diclofenac (Voltaren), a drug that reduces joint inflammation, received FDA approval for treating rheumatoid arthritis, osteoarthritis, and ankylosing spondylitis, a potentially crippling form of spinal arthritis. The drug, which has been available for many years in Canada and most other countries, is the first of a new chemical class of the large group of antiarthritic medications called nonsteroidal anti-inflammatory drugs (NSAIDs). One of the advantages claimed for diclofenac is that it diffuses quickly from the bloodstream into inflamed joints and stays in the surrounding fluid for up to 24 hours. Medical scientists are not sure, however, that this property makes diclofenac any more effective than other drugs in this group. And while its daily use is said to cause less fecal blood loss than aspirin, indomethacin (Indocin), and ibuprofen (Motrin, Advil, Nuprin, and other brand names), there is no proof that this will hold true during long-term treatment of chronic arthritis. Nevertheless, since arthritis patients vary widely in their responses to different NSAIDs, the drug offers physicians an alternative in treating patients who have not responded well to other drugs.

Help With Glaucoma

A new drug became available to treat complications that sometimes arise after laser surgery for acute glaucoma. Glaucoma is a disorder in which abnormally high pressure builds up within the eye and can cause optic nerve damage and blindness. In laser surgery, a beam is used to burn small holes in blocked eye structures in order to let out the excess fluid that causes the pressure. While this usually lessens pressure on the head of the optic nerve, some patients paradoxically experience a rise of pressure within the eye after surgery.

Instilling one drop of apraclonidine (marketed as Iopidine) solution into the eye an hour before laser surgery and another drop immediately after the procedure can prevent such sudden rises in pressure. This prevents further damage to the patient's already impaired optic nerve, which would lead to more loss of sight.   MORTON J. RODMAN, PH.D.

Mental Health

*Genetic Marker for Schizophrenia •
How Mental State Affects the
Immune System • New Approach to
Dealing With Drug Abuse*

Genetic Research

Schizophrenia. A study published in November 1988 reported the first concrete evidence that a specific gene defect plays a role in the development of schizophrenia. Afflicting perhaps 1 person in 100 throughout the world at some time in life, schizophrenia involves a loss of contact with reality and often bizarre behavior, delusions, and hallucinations.

Scientists have believed for several decades that major psychiatric illnesses such as schizophrenia are caused at least in part by a genetic vulnerability. Several studies involving twins have shown that schizophrenia is more likely to occur in both individuals when they are identical twins than when they are fraternal twins. (Identical twins have identical genetic material, whereas in fraternal twins only half the genetic material is the same.) Furthermore, major adoption studies have shown that the offspring of schizophrenic parents have a higher than average risk of themselves becoming schizophrenic, even when raised by nonschizophrenic adoptive parents. In general, however, the rates of disease in the offspring of schizophrenic parents are not as high as they would be in a classic genetic disorder. Only 7 percent of people who have one schizophrenic parent actually develop schizophrenia. This figure suggests some more complex interaction between a genetic vulnerability to the disease and environmental influences.

Recently, techniques that enable researchers to determine the structure of genetic material have been applied to the study of psychiatric illness. The goal is to isolate specific defective genes that might trigger certain disorders, or at least to identify such a gene's approximate location by finding a genetic marker—a section of genetic material that lies close to the defective gene and is inherited along with it. The November 1988 study reported finding a genetic marker for schizophrenia on chromosome 5, one of the 23 chromosomes that occur in pairs in humans and that contain a person's genetic material. The researchers studied genetic material of extended families, looking for portions of genetic material that were similar among those who had the illness—and different from the genetic material of those who did not.

It is too soon to say whether the definitive site of the genetic defect that predisposes one to schizophrenia has been determined, since another group of researchers reported at the same time that they did not find a link between the disease and chromosome 5. But the finding holds promise that one or more specific chromosomal sites will be clearly identified as being associated with the development of schizophrenia. This in turn might lead to the development of new treatments. At the least it provides further solid evidence that schizophrenia is not simply the result of poor parenting or adverse early life experiences, but is rather the product of some biological vulnerability that may in turn be affected by environmental influences.

Genetics of Personality. A researcher at the University of Minnesota recently conducted a large-scale study of personality traits in families and found that genetics played a strong role in determining personality. How socially outgoing, how perfectionistic or impulsive individuals are seems to be determined not simply by upbringing and life experience but by genes as well. Thus, when parents comment that two siblings seemed different from the day they were born, despite being raised similarly, they may well be right.

Brain Studies

Imaging. Research using new brain imaging techniques continues, in an attempt to understand more about the biology of serious psychiatric illness. Earlier studies of schizophrenic patients using positron emission tomography (PET scanning), which measures biochemical activity in different areas of the brain, indicated a relative deficit in activity in the front part of the brain. More recent research has found less activity in the cortex, or outer portion of the brain, compared to the structures deep inside the brain. All of these studies suggest some deficit in the functioning of certain portions of the brain responsible for initiating and planning activity.

Lesions and Depression. Researchers continue to look for specific sites in the brain that may be associated with major mental illness. One recent study found that patients suffering from depression had damage at two sites in the brain stem (the portion of the brain that connects it to the spinal cord)—the locus coeruleus and the substantia nigra. This damage, not found in patients who did not suffer from depression, was discovered at autopsy. These parts of the brain had previously been identified with other disorders: the locus coeruleus with anxiety disorders, and the substantia nigra with Parkinson's disease. They produce two important neurotransmitters (chemicals that are necessary for communication between nerve cells). One, norepinephrine, is important in regulating mood and sleep and is thought to be deficient in patients suffering from depression; the other, dopamine, is important in maintaining normal motor activity. Evidence of damage to these specific sites in the brain stem in patients with depression, while insufficient to explain the disease, is helpful in linking psychiatrists' understanding of the role of neurotransmitters in certain parts of the brain to severe disturbances of mood.

The Mind and the Immune System

A new field called psychoneuroimmunology has been growing rapidly in the past few years. It is the study of the effects of one's mental state and social environment on the functioning of the body's immune system (which combats disease-causing and other foreign microorganisms). Research has demonstrated that in rats decreased immune system activity can be conditioned. Rats given a certain kind of food along with a drug that suppresses the immune system eventually will have reduced immune system activity when given the food alone, without the drug. Hundreds of studies have been conducted in animals and humans to test the hypothesis that stress, depression, bereavement, social isolation, and other factors may adversely affect immune system. Some studies have found that individuals who have recently lost a spouse, parent, or other close relative or who are under acute stress do show some reduction in various measures of immune system activity. In general, animal research seems to show that acute stress reduces measures of immune

Researchers in the new field of psychoneuroimmunology believe mental processes may affect the immune system's ability to fight disease. Here, biologist Joan Borysenko (third from left) leads a group in a psychological technique called guided imagery, in which patients hope to improve their physical health by visualizing positive images. AIDS or cancer patients may, for example, imagine themselves as light energy in a river of light.

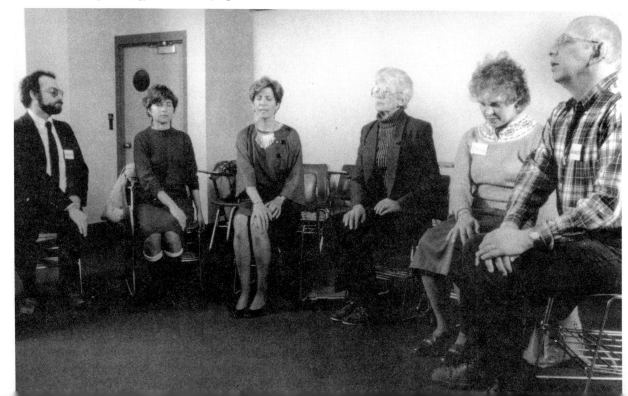

system functioning, but interestingly, chronic stress, if anything, increases them. Animals seem to adapt to chronic stress by mobilizing their immune systems.

Recently, there has also been interest in psychological techniques that may enhance immune system activity. One study found that children asked to imagine their body fighting off disease showed an increase in their production of immunoglobulins—proteins in the blood that fight infections.

Evidence from all such research is far from uniform. It is understandably difficult, although by no means impossible, to demonstrate a definite link between a particular mental state and level of immune system activity. Also, many of the measures of how the immune system is functioning are themselves not terribly reliable, involving as they do drawing blood samples, culturing immune system cells taken from the blood, and then testing the activity of these cells. Many factors can influence such cell activity once the cells are out of the body, so that what researchers measure in the laboratory is not necessarily a good indication of how the immune system is acting within a person or animal. Further research is needed to clearly document the nature of the connection between the brain and the activity of the immune system, and more work than that is needed to demonstrate that mental state can alter the way the immune system functions so as to affect the course of disease. Nonetheless, accumulating evidence suggests that the immune system is responsive to factors such as stress and relaxation.

Treating Drug Abuse

Recent research into the problem of how to treat drug abuse has focused on the continued craving for drugs and consequent high risk of relapse in individuals who have already gone through the physical symptoms of withdrawal and been drug free for a time. Many illicit drugs mimic or stimulate the release of naturally existing neurotransmitters in the brain that provide pleasure. Because of this effect, drug use is immediately and powerfully reinforced physiologically. As a result, people who have used drugs are strongly conditioned to want to repeat that behavior. (Studies with animals show that, given the opportunity to engage in behavior rewarded with drugs like cocaine or heroin, they will shun all other pleasures, including food and sex, even to the point of consuming the drug until they die from starvation.)

A related problem is that drug abuse tends to reduce other sources of positive reinforcement. Individuals using drugs often perform less well at school or work, they may resort to illegal and sometimes violent activities to obtain money for drugs, and they may exploit and antagonize family members. They often create a social environment in which their only positive reinforcement comes from drug use. Breaking this cycle is difficult. Those treating drug abusers, as well as family and friends, must find a way not to deny or collude with the drug-seeking behavior and at the same time provide positive reinforcement for change. But family and friends are often so disillusioned or frightened by drug abusers' deceit in obtaining money for drugs or their erratic behavior when under the influence of drugs that they discount a change in behavior as one more deception, thereby depriving drug users of what positive reinforcement they might get for initiating and maintaining change.

Although the actions of illicit drugs on the nervous system are now well understood and many medications can be helpful in getting addicts through the initial period of withdrawal without serious danger, for drug abusers trying to quit, an ability to combat their own cravings and to maintain their determination to abstain are the key factors influencing long-term success.

Long-Term Effects of Trauma

Recent research has been directed toward better understanding and treating the psychological aftereffects of physical and mental trauma. Two recent studies confirm that people who undergo what is called dissociation—a "disintegration of experience"—during and after a traumatic event are more likely to suffer later psychological problems.

Dissociation seems to occur in many people during physical trauma. Rape victims, for example, often experience the event as if they were floating above their own bodies feeling sorry for the person being assaulted below. Many people involved in combat or in natural disasters such as earthquakes have an acute sense of unreality about the situation. They may feel strangely distant from what is happening and for a period of time be relatively insensitive to pain. The traumatic experiences become mentally walled off, somehow separate from the rest of life. Yet, over time, they may exert an unwelcome and demoralizing influence on a person's ability to function—a condition known as posttraumatic stress disorder. Individuals who suffer from this disorder intensely relive the traumatic event. They find themselves strangely disconnected from friends, family, and experiences that previously gave them pleasure. They are hypersensitive to stimuli that remind them of the trauma, such as loud noises (for combat veterans) or a place reminiscent of the one where the assault took place (for a rape victim).

Confirmation of the connection between dissociation

during trauma and posttraumatic stress disorder has come from two recent studies which found that a measurable indicator of the capacity for dissociation—the ability to experience hypnosis—is significantly greater in patients with posttraumatic stress disorder than in other people. It is hoped that improved understanding of the condition will lead to better treatment of posttraumatic stress disorder. For example, techniques such as hypnosis, which can help individuals gain conscious access to dissociated mental states, should be helpful in treatment.

See also the feature article MANIA AND DEPRESSION.

DAVID SPIEGEL, M.D.

Nutrition and Diet

Government Recommendations • Campaign Against Palm and Coconut Oils • Very-Low-Calorie Diets • Yo-Yo Dieting • Apples and Cancer

Government Reports

The first nutrition report ever released by a U.S. surgeon general, published in July 1988, singled out overconsumption of fat, especially saturated fat, as the number one problem in the American diet. The report noted that five of the ten leading causes of death in the United States are associated with diet: coronary heart disease, stroke, certain cancers, diabetes, and atherosclerosis. While recognizing that diet is only one of many factors involved in the development of these diseases, the *Surgeon General's Report on Nutrition and Health* pointed out that it is now quite clear that modifying the diet in certain ways can reduce the risk for all of them.

Surgeon General C. Everett Koop's report broke no new ground. Intended primarily for nutritional policymakers, it drew on more than 2,500 scientific articles related to diet and chronic diseases to provide a scientific basis for nutrition and health programs and for legislation on related issues. It did not give specific guidelines about the ideal amounts of different foods that should be included in the diet, on the grounds that the scientific basis for such advice does not yet exist. (Some critics of the report disagreed with this assertion.) It did, however, offer common-sense recommendations, similar to those in other government and private studies, for people who want

to reduce their risk of various diseases. These range from cutting down on fat and salt to eating more complex carbohydrates and fiber-rich foods such as whole grains, fruits, and vegetables. (For more on the recommendations, see the box on page 309.)

In March 1989 a second national report on nutrition and health was issued, this one by the National Research Council, the research arm of the National Academy of Sciences. *Diet and Health* was based on a three-year review of published research. Like the surgeon general's report, it offered little new information, although it did provide specific guidelines on food quantities. The report recommended that Americans reduce their consumption of fat to 30 percent of total calories (less than 10 percent of which should be saturated fat) and of cholesterol to less than 300 milligrams a day. Americans should also eat less than 6 grams of salt a day and reduce consumption of alcohol. In addition, the daily diet should include five or more half-cup servings of fruits and vegetables and six or more servings of breads, cereals, and legumes (the six servings should comprise 55 percent of total daily calories). *Diet and Health* did not specifically recommend that people eat more fiber and recommended against the use of fiber supplements, as well as other dietary supplements.

Fat and Cholesterol

A More Healthful Saturated Fat? Saturated fat has had such a bad press in recent years that it was big news when a study published in 1988 announced that not all saturated fats were created equal. The study found that while one saturated fatty acid, palmitic acid, raises blood cholesterol levels, another one, stearic acid, does not. This was actually first demonstrated more than 20 years ago, but the new report captured media attention now because both beef and chocolate—shunned by cholesterol-conscious Americans—are high in the less damaging stearic acid.

Participants in the new study were fed liquid-formula diets high in stearic acid, palmitic acid, or a third type of fatty acid—oleic acid, which is mono-unsaturated and is found in olive oil. Investigators found that blood cholesterol levels were highest when people were on the palmitic-acid diet and lowest when they were on the stearic-acid diet. The authors pointed out that although stearic acid does not raise blood cholesterol levels, it will not lower blood cholesterol if it is simply added to a diet already high in palmitic acid. Thus, the study's results do not mean that people can eat as much beef or chocolate as they want because both foods contain large amounts of harmful palmitic acid in addition to stearic acid.

In fact, no food contains only stearic acid. About

half the fat in beef, for example, is saturated; 20 percent of that is stearic acid, but 50 percent is palmitic acid. In addition, because Americans eat a great deal of beef, it is a major source of total fat, saturated fat, and cholesterol, all of which contribute to high blood cholesterol levels.

Palm and Coconut Oils. The use in processed foods of palm and coconut oils came under increased public attention when consumer groups publicized the fact that the oils were potentially harmful to people's health. Meanwhile, major companies announced a phasing out of the oils from their products.

Palm and coconut oils are largely saturated fat. The amount of saturated fat in palm oil is about 50 percent; in palm kernel oil, 80 percent; and in coconut oil, 90 percent. The stearic acid content of these oils is very low. But economics rather than scientific evidence about saturated fat intake and heart disease has traditionally determined which oils manufacturers put into processed foods. Palm and coconut oils cost less than the unsaturated soybean, cottonseed, corn, and olive oils, and thus, many companies utilize large amounts of palm and coconut oils.

In congressional hearings, lobbying groups for the palm and coconut oil industries (which are important to the economies of Malaysia and the Philippines, respectively) claimed that neither of these oils raises blood cholesterol levels. Evidence cited to support these claims has been challenged by scientists. At present, there seems no good scientific basis on which to conclude that palm and coconut oils—unlike other saturated fats—do not raise blood cholesterol.

So far, consumer interest groups have not been able to persuade the U.S. Food and Drug Administration that product labels should declare exactly what oil is used. Labels often state that a product contains "one or more of the following" and then list, for example, both palm oil and cottonseed oil—leaving the consumer no basis on which to determine whether the product contains a saturated or an unsaturated oil. But success seems to have come on another front, following a campaign run by an organization called the National Heart Savers Association. This organization ran full-page ads in several prominent newspapers, picturing specific products and noting, "A large number of food processors use the most highly saturated fats—coconut and palm oil" although fully aware of "the negative health ramifications." Following the negative publicity, a number of major U.S. food processing companies, including General Mills, Pillsbury, and Pepperidge Farm, announced that they would replace the palm and coconut oils in their products with vegetable oils containing less saturated fat. At least one manufacturer also planned to stop using lard and beef fat, which are also saturated fats.

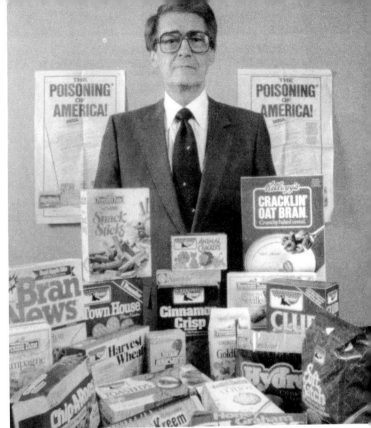

Irate about the presence of highly saturated fats in consumer food products, Philip Sokolof, an Omaha businessman who is head of the National Heart Savers Association, spent over $2 million on full-page newspaper ads excoriating manufacturers for using palm and coconut oils in popular brands of food. Here, Sokolof displays items in which the manufacturers are eliminating these tropical oils.

New Artificial Sweetener

In 1988 the U.S. Food and Drug Administration approved a new artificial sweetener with the brand name Sunette (technically acesulfame potassium), which is 200 times sweeter than sucrose (ordinary table sugar). Like the already marketed sweetener saccharin, it is noncaloric. Sunette is approved for use in processed dry food products such as chewing gum and nondairy creamers, as well as in dry mixes for beverages, instant coffee and tea, gelatins, and puddings. It is also approved for sale in powder or tablet form as a tabletop sweetener. Sunette is already on sale in some parts of the United States.

Dieting and Weight Control

Liquid Protein Diets. Talk show host Oprah Winfrey boosted public interest in 1988 in very-low-calorie (VLC) diets when she lost 67 pounds on such a diet and discussed it on her television show. But VLC diets were already big business. Several national chains offer VLC diet programs through hospitals and doctors' offices. Under the programs, participants eat no solid food, but instead drink a low-calorie liquid formula (400 to 800 calories per day) containing protein and carbohydrates, with vitamin and mineral supplements. The liquid is available by prescription only. Most programs tell patients to see the program's doctor weekly for a checkup and to attend a behavior-modification class, ostensibly to learn how to change food habits. Patients stay on the diet from three to six months at a cost of about $100 per week. Women may lose as much as three pounds per week and men, five pounds. This rapid weight loss is a great incentive for remaining on the diet, although 30 to 40 percent of patients do not finish the program.

In the 1970s similar low-calorie liquid protein diets resulted in several deaths because the diets were not nutritionally balanced. The new programs seem to have solved the safety problem, but there are still concerns about the advisability of using this method of weight control. First, the diet is so extreme that some experts would like patients to be at least 50 percent overweight to qualify. Most programs specify, however, that patients should be 15 to 30 percent over normal weight. And because the programs exist to make a profit, many people may be admitted who are less than 15 percent overweight. (In general, physicians consider people to be obese if they are 20 percent or more over normal weight.)

A major concern is that patients may not be able to maintain their weight loss, particularly since it has been rapid. They are apt to regain weight quickly, chiefly because it is difficult to learn new ways of eating while not eating. About 90 percent of women and 85 percent of men on all kinds of diets regain weight after they go off the special diet.

Before (left) and after: Talk show host Oprah Winfrey shows off her new, svelte figure, achieved by following a low-calorie liquid diet.

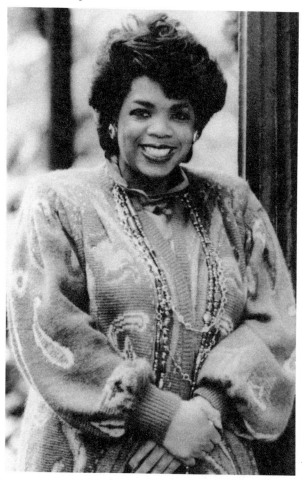

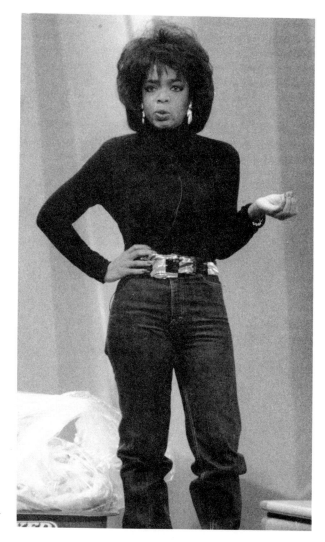

The Surgeon General's Dietary Recommendations

Issues for Most People:

● *Fats and cholesterol:* Reduce consumption of fat (especially saturated fat) and cholesterol. Choose foods relatively low in these substances, such as vegetables, fruits, whole grain foods, fish, poultry, lean meats, and low-fat dairy products. Use food preparation methods that add little or no fat.

● *Energy and weight control:* Achieve and maintain a desirable body weight. To do so, choose a dietary pattern in which energy (caloric) intake is consistent with energy expenditure. To reduce energy intake, limit consumption of foods relatively high in calories, fats, and sugars, and minimize alcohol consumption. Increase energy expenditure through regular and sustained physical activity.

● *Complex carbohydrates and fiber:* Increase consumption of whole grain foods and cereal products, vegetables (including dried beans and peas), and fruits.

● *Sodium:* Reduce intake of sodium by choosing foods relatively low in sodium and limiting the amount of salt added in food preparation and at the table.

● *Alcohol:* To reduce the risk for chronic disease, take alcohol only in moderation (no more than two drinks a day), if at all. Avoid drinking any alcohol before or while driving, operating machinery, taking medications, or engaging in any other activity requiring judgment. Avoid drinking alcohol while pregnant.

Other Issues for Some People:

● *Fluoride:* Community water systems should contain fluoride at optimal levels for prevention of tooth decay. If such water is not available, use other appropriate sources of fluoride.

● *Sugars:* Those who are particularly vulnerable to dental caries (cavities), especially children, should limit their consumption and frequency of use of foods high in sugars.

● *Calcium:* Adolescent girls and adult women should increase consumption of foods high in calcium, including low-fat dairy products.

● *Iron:* Children, adolescents, and women of childbearing age should be sure to consume foods that are good sources of iron, such as lean meats, fish, certain beans, and iron-enriched cereals and whole grain products. This issue is of special concern for low-income families.

Source: *The Surgeon General's Report on Nutrition and Health,*
U.S. Department of Health and Human Services, Public Health Service, 1988

The Yo-Yo Syndrome. The cycle of gaining weight, then losing it on a diet, then gaining it again—often called the yo-yo syndrome—may be worse than not losing weight at all. For one thing, the cycle dieter loses muscle mass as well as fat while dieting, but gains back chiefly fat. For another, the body's metabolism—the rate at which it burns calories—appears to slow down with each bout of weight loss, making it easier to gain weight when individuals return to normal eating. As weight cycling continues, dieters must eat fewer and fewer calories to lose weight; meanwhile, they gain weight faster each time they start eating normally again.

Many weight control experts are now advocating that obese patients lose weight slowly (20 to 30 pounds over a yearlong period, for example) on a well-balanced diet of normal foods. It seems important for an obese individual to succeed the first time he or she tries to lose weight, and then to maintain the loss.

Obesity and High-Fat Diets. Two recent studies indicate that obesity in the United States may be linked to the high-fat U.S. diet. One of these studies compared the amount of fat on the bodies of a group of sedentary obese men with their usual food intake. Researchers found that it was not the number of calories that accounted for the amount of body fat but the proportion of fat in the diet—the more fat these men ate, the more body fat they had regardless of how many calories they took in. Similarly, another study reported that obese women ate more total fat than did nonobese women. There is evidence that dietary fats are converted to body fat more efficiently than are dietary carbohydrates, but more research is needed before this phenomenon is understood.

Apple Alert

Early in 1989 the U.S. Environmental Protection Agency said that daminozide, a chemical used on about 5 percent of red apples grown in the United States, poses a significant cancer risk to humans. Daminozide is used to make apples ripen uniformly on the tree and to extend their shelf life. It penetrates the flesh of the apple and cannot be washed or peeled off or eliminated by cooking. The EPA plans to remove the chemical, sold under the name Alar, from the market in 1990—not immediately, because interim test results do not show conclusively that it is an imminent danger to human health.

A report from the Natural Resources Defense Council (NRDC), an environmental group, claimed that the EPA had underestimated the cancer risk from Alar, particularly for children. As public alarm grew—to the extent that many school boards took apples out of school cafeterias—the EPA, the Food and Drug Administration, and the Agriculture Department declared that the NRDC's figures were flawed and that it was safe to eat apples. Consumers have limited options since it is impossible to tell if an apple has been treated with Alar. They can accept the word of government and other experts that Alar-treated apples are safe. They can buy green apples, which are not treated with Alar (some yellow apples are). Or they can shop at organic food stores or other stores that refuse to accept fruit that has been treated.

See also the feature articles A NEW LOOK AT MEAT *and* HOW TO PREVENT CHILDHOOD OBESITY *and the Spotlight on Health articles* FACTS ABOUT OAT BRAN *and* SAFETY AT THE SALAD BAR.

ELEANOR R. WILLIAMS, PH.D.

Obstetrics and Gynecology

The Pill and Breast Cancer: Is There a Link? • The Expanding Role of Ultrasound • Looking Through the Laparoscope

Breast Cancer and the Pill

Recent studies have reported an association between oral contraceptives and breast cancer, renewing earlier concerns over the safety of birth control pills. Breast cancer kills more than 43,000 U.S. women a year, and studies suggest that nearly 1 in 10 women will develop the disease at some point in their lives.

Today birth control pills contain less than half the amounts of the female sex hormones estrogen and progestin (which can contribute to the development of breast cancer) than they did when they were first marketed almost 30 years ago. The lower-dose pills have been shown to be safer and to cause fewer side effects, and in fact high-dose pills have recently been removed from the U.S. market.

Early studies that attempted to investigate the relationship between breast cancer and oral contraceptives were inconclusive. Some showed a higher incidence of cancer in women who took the pill, others a lower incidence, and still others showed no effect at all. But by the mid-1980s, several large epidemiological studies had been published that found no link at all between breast cancer and the pill. One important study conducted in 1985 and again in 1986 provided data on women in different risk groups who were taking oral contraceptives. It found no signifi-

cant increase or decrease in risk associated with the age at which women began using the pill, or with long-term use (more than 15 years). Nor did the risk increase for women under the age of 25 who used a pill with high progestin content, for those with a family history of breast cancer, or for those who took oral contraceptives before their first pregnancy. This study is significant because of the methodology used and the size of the sample. (In 1985 the study included 2,000 women with breast cancer and a similar number of controls—those free of breast cancer; in 1986 there were more than 4,500 women in each group.) The results convinced most physicians that the controversy had finally been settled and that they could once more dispense oral contraceptives without worrying about breast cancer.

Recently, however, new studies have again reported an association between use of oral contraceptives and breast cancer. One study linked long-term pill use with an increased risk of breast cancer in all women under the age of 45, another found an increased risk only in those women under 45 who took birth control pills prior to their first pregnancy, while a third found only those women with one child to be at greater risk.

Clearly, there is no agreement on who, if anyone, is at risk. Moreover, at least four more studies scheduled to be published in mid-1989 are expected to add to the confusion. Two reportedly show no increased risk of breast cancer, one shows some women are at risk, and another points to an overall increase in risk for all women who use the pill.

In an attempt to evaluate the risks and clear up the confusion, an advisory panel of the U.S. Food and Drug Administration analyzed the most recent reports. It concluded that there was insufficient evidence on which to assume that a definitive relationship existed between breast cancer and the pill. The panel therefore decided that there was no need at this time to change the warnings inserted in oral contraceptive packages. It did recommend, however, that more data be collected, and it endorsed a planned study by the National Cancer Institute, which would include 2,000 women and be completed sometime after 1992. The American College of Obstetricians and Gynecologists, concurring with the FDA panel, was also unwilling to change its opinion on the safety of the pill. The group found the new findings inconclusive and for the present will continue to rely on evidence from the older, larger studies.

New Uses for Ultrasound

Abdominal ultrasound has made an important contribution to the improvement of women's health, revolutionizing obstetric and gynecologic care. In the

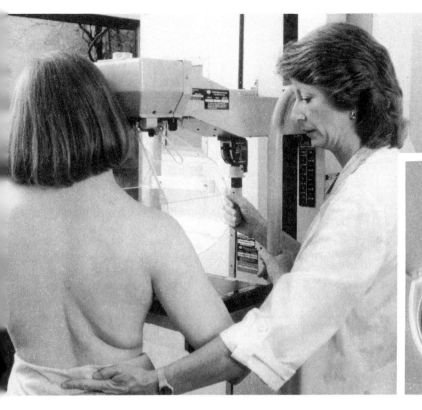

Evidence from recent studies linking oral contraceptives to breast cancer has been found inconclusive by a U.S. government panel (left, a mammogram checkup; below, the pill).

procedure, a transducer—an instrument like a microphone—is passed over the abdomen and produces sound waves, which are then translated into a two-dimensional image called a sonogram, which can be viewed on a screen. The procedure is painless and, unlike X rays, involves no risk of radiation damage.

A fetus can now be visualized with ultrasound and evaluated while it is in the womb. By the end of the second month of pregnancy, a sonogram can provide sufficient information for a physician to determine whether the pregnancy is normal. Ultrasound has become sophisticated enough to allow doctors to monitor the breathing, muscle tone, and movements of the fetus. They can also determine the degree of maturity of the placenta, the sex of the infant, and whether there is sufficient amniotic fluid surrounding the fetus. However, in the first eight weeks of pregnancy the image produced by abdominal ultrasound is not clear enough to evaluate whether a pregnancy is intrauterine or extrauterine.

Ultrasound has also made two prenatal tests, chorionic villus sampling and amniocentesis, safer and more effective. In both tests, ultrasound is used by the physician to guide the needle into the amniotic sac so that the fetus and other important structures can be avoided.

Abdominal ultrasound is also a valuable tool in gynecology, where it is used to evaluate pelvic structures. However, because pelvic structures in nonpregnant women generally lie deep in the pelvis, they are difficult to visualize and define in detail with an abdominal transducer. The thickness of the abdominal wall (how much fat there is) and the amount of feces and gas in the bowel can also alter and distort the image. Now, however, a transducer has been adapted for use in the vagina, greatly improving diagnostic capabilities—in both nonpregnant and pregnant women. When it is inside the vagina, this probe is close to uterine and ovarian structures and can provide an accurate image of the pelvis. A well-defined image of the gestational sac can be seen at 4½ weeks and a fetal heartbeat can be detected at 6 to 6½ weeks.

The new vaginal ultrasound technique also allows ectopic pregnancies—in which the embryo implants and grows outside the uterus (usually in one of the fallopian tubes)—to be identified at a very early stage. This allows doctors to perform surgery earlier, removing the embryo and preserving the fallopian tube. Vaginal ultrasound is also helpful in procedures used for obtaining eggs for in vitro fertilization.

Used as an adjunct to abdominal ultrasound, vaginal ultrasound, with continued improvement, may eventually allow physicians to determine whether an internal lesion or mass is benign or malignant without performing an invasive procedure.

Laparoscopic Surgery

Laparoscopy is a procedure in which a telescopic instrument (a laparoscope) is inserted into the abdomen through a small incision in the abdominal wall. Sometimes referred to as belly button surgery, this technique is frequently used for performing tubal ligations (a method of sterilization that involves tying the fallopian tubes so that sperm cannot reach an egg to fertilize it).

Surgical instruments have been modified so that they can be passed either through the laparoscope or through a separate puncture site. Because these instruments are long, using them is like operating through remote control; doctors must work with the instruments while peering through the laparoscope. A television monitor is sometimes attached to the laparoscope, allowing all technicians involved in the procedure to watch it on the screen. More important, surgical skills have been developed that make it possible to perform more delicate and intricate laparoscopic surgery. For example, in a woman with an ectopic pregnancy in which the fallopian tube has not ruptured, the tube can be opened, the embryo can be removed, and bleeding can be controlled—all through the laparoscope. At one time only unruptured ectopic pregnancies were operated on with the laparoscope. Today, though, many physicians are able to use laparoscopic surgery to treat even ruptured ectopic pregnancies if the woman has not suffered extensive internal bleeding.

Other technological advances have also helped expand the use of laparoscopy. For example, as noted above, vaginal ultrasound allows ectopic pregnancies to be diagnosed at a very early stage, making laparoscopic removal more feasible. Gynecologists who have become skilled in laparoscopy are using it to perform other surgical procedures, such as opening blocked fallopian tubes, removing fallopian tubes, ovarian cysts, and adhesions (scar tissue binding one organ to another), and treating endometriosis (a condition in which tissue from the endometrium—the membrane that lines the uterus—grows on the outside of the uterus or elsewhere in the pelvic cavity). Interestingly, when extensive surgical procedures are performed using the laparoscope, tissues heal beautifully, leaving little or no scar tissue.

Not all physicians are trained to use the laparoscope, which requires special skills as well as the proper instruments. Moreover, operating time is frequently longer than that required for a traditional abdominal operation. And at times technical difficulties make it impossible to complete a procedure through the laparoscope, and an abdominal procedure is needed anyway.

On the positive side, laparoscopy offers many advantages. The patient generally fares better, the costs—emotional and physical as well as financial—are markedly reduced, and the hospital stay is usually shorter. Some women are able to go home the day the procedure is performed, others within one to two days. Patients suffer less discomfort, feel better, and are not as sick or as weak as those who have standard abdominal surgery. Finally, the recovery period is markedly reduced; patients can generally go back to work within a week or two.

Laparoscopy is a technique still in its infancy. As more experience with it is acquired, its use will no doubt be extended to other surgical procedures.

See also the feature article HAVING A FIRST CHILD AFTER 35 *and the Spotlight on Health articles* OBSTETRICS AND MALPRACTICE *and* YEAST INFECTIONS.

JOHANNA F. PERLMUTTER, M.D.

Pediatrics

Reducing Deafness From Meningitis • Cause of Roseola Identified? • Preventing Asthma Attacks • Breast-Feeding and Childhood Cancer

Hearing Loss and Meningitis

Researchers from Dallas reported in October 1988 that early treatment with the drug dexamethasone can prevent deafness in children with bacterial meningitis, a life-threatening infection of the lining of the brain and spinal cord. Although effective antibiotics and other advances have reduced the mortality rate from bacterial meningitis to 5 percent, one-quarter of the victims of this disease still suffer severe long-term effects, such as hearing loss, seizures, and mental retardation. Scientists suspect that many of these complications are caused by a combination of brain swelling and intense inflammation in the nervous system. Dexamethasone (a type of steroid) was chosen for the study because it is known to reduce swelling of the brain and also to fight inflammation.

Two hundred children were divided into two groups: half received dexamethasone plus an antibiotic, while the other half were treated with the antibiotic alone. The investigators found that in patients who were given dexamethasone, fever disappeared more rapidly and inflammation was less severe than in those receiving just the antibiotic. More importantly, moderate or severe hearing loss developed in only 3.3 percent of dexamethasone-treated children, compared with 15.5 percent of patients not given the steroid medication. These results suggest that the early treatment of bacterial meningitis with dexamethasone as well as antibiotics may prevent significant hearing loss.

A Roseola Virus?

According to a 1988 report, Japanese scientists have discovered the cause of roseola, a common disease of young infants. Roseola is a distinctive illness, characterized by high fever lasting for three or four days and by a rash that appears as the fever goes away. Although doctors have long assumed that roseola is caused by a virus, until recently no one had been able to prove it. In 1986 scientists discovered a new virus, which was eventually named human herpesvirus-6. Since its discovery, this virus has been an infectious agent in search of a disease. But thanks to the Japanese investigators, the search may finally have ended.

The investigators took blood samples from infants with fever who were suspected of having roseola and subjected these samples to a variety of laboratory tests. As their fevers broke, four of the babies developed the typical rash of roseola. And in these same four babies' blood samples, the lab tests isolated a virus that seemed to be identical to human herpesvirus-6. Furthermore, all of the babies with roseola developed antibodies against human herpesvirus-6, another indication that they had been infected with the virus. Although the number of patients in the study was small, the results certainly suggest that human herpesvirus-6 is the cause of roseola.

Steroids to Prevent Asthma Attacks

A recent Canadian study concluded that giving the drug prednisone to young children with asthma at the first sign of a cold can prevent or reduce the severity of asthma attacks. In asthma, the most common chronic disease of childhood, the airways in the lungs become narrowed and get clogged with mucus, which results in the typical high-pitched sound we recognize as wheezing. Episodes of asthma can be triggered by an allergy, an infection, or other stimuli. Although most patients improve with medications (called bronchodilators) designed to open up the airways, some have frequent, serious attacks that require hospitalization. Steroids such as prednisone have been used for many years as a treatment for severe asthma. Though they are very effective, their long-term use is associated with a number of unpleasant side effects, including growth delay and a typical cherubic appearance. Short-term use does not provoke the side effects. Because many asthma attacks are triggered by upper respiratory infections (colds), the Canadian researchers examined whether a short course of prednisone, begun at the first hint of a cold, could prevent full-blown attacks of asthma.

Thirty-two children six years of age or younger who had had frequent, severe asthma attacks were divided into two groups. In the first year of the study, both groups received the same treatment: bronchodilators alone, supplemented with steroids if needed to treat a severe attack. In the second year of the study, however, one group was begun on a short course of prednisone (in addition to bronchodilators) as soon as any cold symptoms appeared, while the other group continued to receive bronchodilator therapy alone. The investigators found that the steroid-treated children spent far less time wheezing and had fewer asthma attacks, emergency room visits, and hospitalizations than did the group receiving only bronchodilators.

In view of major measles outbreaks, U.S. health officials have recommended stepped-up vaccinations for children. Here a two-year-old expresses her feelings.

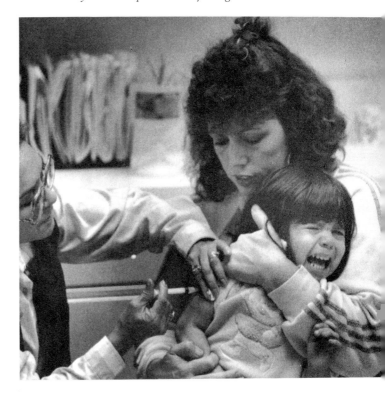

USE THE SAFETY SEAT SAFELY

You're a conscientious, safety-conscious parent. You wouldn't dream of letting your child ride in an automobile without buckling him/her into a safety seat—which you've bought as the best and safest of safety seats after consulting with other parents and the trusty salesperson at the mall. Therefore, you think, you've done the best you could to ensure that your child is effectively restrained and protected in the event of an accident. Right? Wrong! According to a recent on-the-scene study in Indiana (which has a mandatory child safety seat law) over 70 percent of the car seats the observers checked were being used incorrectly. Among the most common mistakes that parents were making were:

- Harnesses holding the children in place were too loose or not fastened at all.
- Seat belts holding the car seat frames in place were incorrectly threaded through the frames, so that the seat could lurch forward on impact. Occasionally, seat belts were not even used.
- Seats designed for infants (under 20 pounds) incorrectly had the babies facing forward instead of facing the rear.
- Seats with attachable parts—restraining bars, shields, or straps—didn't have them attached.

The moral is that it's not enough to stuff the child into the car seat; it has to be done right. It pays to read the instructions.

Eczema From Food Allergies

Food allergies may be more common in patients with eczema than was previously thought, according to a study published in 1988. Eczema, or atopic dermatitis, is a common skin rash best known for its itchiness and tendency to flare up at the slightest provocation. Despite the well-recognized association between eczema and certain kinds of allergies, the role played by food allergies has long been a controversial one.

To explore the issue further, researchers at the University of Arkansas tested 46 children with eczema for the presence of food allergy, using both skin tests and food challenges. In the food challenges, patients were fed various food substances (in a disguised form) and observed carefully for any serious reactions. Approximately 60 percent (28) of the patients had a positive skin reaction to one of the foods tested. Of the 28, over half had positive food challenges. Eggs, peanuts, and milk accounted for most of the positive reactions to food challenges. These reactions consisted of skin rashes, gastrointestinal symptoms, respiratory symptoms, or a combination of all three. The results of this study indicate that a significant proportion of children with eczema may have an underlying food allergy.

See also the feature article ALL ABOUT ALLERGIES.

Sickle-Cell Anemia

Researchers from Belgium recently reported on five cases in which children with severe sickle-cell anemia were cured by bone marrow transplants. Sickle-cell anemia is a hereditary blood disease that primarily affects blacks. In this condition, the red blood cells contain an abnormal type of hemoglobin (the pigment that carries oxygen), which causes them to become distorted, or sickle shaped, and stiff. These distorted cells create logjams in small blood vessels within the bones and certain organs, resulting in episodes of severe pain. People with sickle-cell anemia also are at risk for developing serious bacterial infections.

Bone marrow transplants, which involve replacing a person's diseased bone marrow with healthy marrow (often from another individual), are currently used to treat certain blood diseases, such as leukemia and aplastic anemia. The five children in the Belgian study (all from the central African nation of Zaire) were the first patients to undergo such transplants for the treatment of sickle-cell anemia.

In four of the five patients, the transplant was successful on the first attempt; the fifth child required a second transplant after the first one failed. Even though some of the patients experienced complications, most of these were not serious and improved with treatment. Despite the encouraging results, bone marrow transplants remain risky procedures, with a mortality rate as high as 25 percent. Since nowadays most children with sickle-cell anemia do well with conventional treatment, it is doubtful whether a bone marrow transplant is really worth the risk.

See also the Spotlight on Health article ANEMIA.

Breast-Feeding and Cancer

A provocative study conducted by the U.S. National Institute of Child Health and Human Development reported that infants who are breast-fed may have a lower risk of developing cancer later in childhood. Approximately 200 children from Denver, who had been diagnosed as having cancer when they were between 18 months and 15 years of age, were compared with a similar group of children who did not have cancer. All the children were classified according to the amount of time they had nursed during infancy: breast-fed for six months or more, breast-fed for less than six months, or never breast-fed. The investigators found that children who had nursed for more than six months had a lower risk of cancer than the other two groups. Although this information is preliminary, it supports the notion that breast-feeding in infancy offers a variety of benefits, some of which are yet to be discovered.

Measles Vaccine Guidelines

Federal health officials in the United States have proposed an extra measles shot for some infants. Measles was thought to be on the verge of eradication in the United States a decade ago, but in recent years there have been major outbreaks among infants under the usual vaccination age of 15 months and among schoolchildren whose vaccinations have not protected them. As many as 10 percent of vaccinated children are still susceptible to measles, according to the federal officials. In areas where there are repeated outbreaks of measles, the Centers for Disease Control now recommends that infants get a first measles vaccination at 9 months, to be followed by the usual measles-mumps-rubella shot at 15 months.

Benefits of Circumcision

Reversing a position it first took in 1971, the American Academy of Pediatrics issued a statement in March 1989 saying that there are medical advantages to circumcision of newborn boys, or removal of the foreskin from the penis. According to the academy's task force on circumcision, studies of babies born in U.S. Army hospitals between 1975 and 1984 showed that uncircumcised boys were almost 11 times as likely as circumcised boys to suffer urinary tract infections during their first 12 months. Furthermore, as the rate of circumcision dropped over the years, the incidence of infections increased. Such infections are a concern because the bacteria that cause them can spread through the blood, leading to meningitis and other serious conditions.

Because of possible flaws in the studies (which did not, for example, consider boys circumcised after leaving the hospital or in religious rites), the academy did not recommend routine circumcision. Instead, the academy said the decision should be made by parents in consultation with their doctors, taking into account religion, cultural attitudes, and tradition. The academy also stressed the importance of teaching uncircumcised boys to keep the foreskin area clean.

See also the feature articles How to Prevent Childhood Obesity *and* Sibling Rivalry *and the Spotlight on Health articles* Chicken Pox, Child Abuse, Children With AIDS, Dealing With a Colicky Baby, Dyslexia: A Reading Disorder, *and* Toilet Training.

RAYMOND B. KARASIC, M.D.

Public Health

New Evidence Linking Ultraviolet Light and Cataracts • Move to Regulate Computer VDTs • U.S. Radon Advisory

Ultraviolet Hazards

A December 1988 study of men who work on Chesapeake Bay found that those with more exposure to ultraviolet radiation—a component of sunlight—ran an increased risk of developing cataracts. A cataract is a clouding of the lens of an eye; it can seriously impair vision. Doubling the amount of exposure to short-wavelength ultraviolet light (ultraviolet beta, or UVB), which can cause sunburn and skin cancer, appeared to raise the risk of cortical cataracts—those occurring in the cortex surrounding the nucleus of the lens—by about 60 percent. The study provided new evidence that people with heavy exposure to sunlight need to protect their eyes. The researchers recommended wearing a hat with a brim, as well as close-fitting sunglasses capable of absorbing UVB rays. It remained unclear whether the average individual who engages in recreational swimming or skiing faces an increased chance of developing cataracts.

Scientists are becoming more and more concerned about the health effects of tanning machines. These machines generally use ultraviolet rays with longer wavelengths. Such radiation, known as ultraviolet alpha, or UVA, does not redden the skin as rapidly as UVB, but it does more harm to the skin's deeper layers. Moreover, tanning with the machines increases the effect of sunlight taken soon thereafter, and severe burns have resulted from sun bathing too quickly after using a tanning machine. (*See also the feature article* Safety in the Sun.)

Computer VDTs

Unions and certain elected officials have continued to call for regulation of VDTs—computer video display

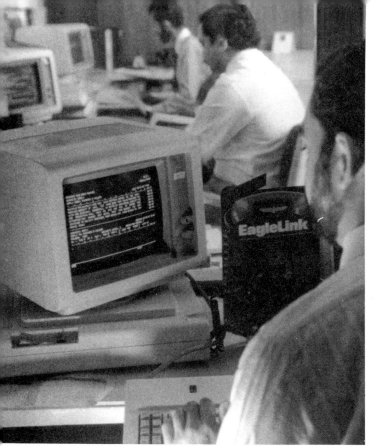

Complaints ranging from eyestrain to miscarriage from people who spend long hours in front of video display terminals have led to studies to determine whether computer screens are hazardous to health.

terminals—in the workplace. In June 1988 a New York county adopted a law mandating 15-minute rest breaks every three hours, special training, and specially designed office furniture for many workers using VDTs. The Suffolk County law, which applied to VDT operators who spend more than 26 hours a week in front of a screen in a company with at least 20 terminals, was reportedly the first in the United States to regulate VDT safety in industry. The measure encountered resistance from businesses, and court challenges were filed against it.

For years there have been complaints of vision problems (including eyestrain and cataracts), headaches, stiff necks, and back strain among VDT users. Some pregnant female users are said to have had miscarriages or to have given birth to infants with birth defects. It is extraordinarily difficult, however, to prove that these problems were caused by VDTs. A California study that was published in mid-1988 found that women in the first three months of pregnancy who used VDTs for more than 20 hours a week had almost twice the rate of miscarriages as women who used the terminals for less than 20 hours a week. But were VDTs or some other factor responsible? The

researchers said that clerical workers in the study had more miscarriages than did professional women. Many studies have shown that VDTs do *not* give off significant amounts of ionizing radiation—radiation that has enough energy to knock electrons out of atoms and thus is particularly hazardous to body tissues.

Radon Scare

In September 1988 the U.S. Environmental Protection Agency (EPA) and the surgeon general's office issued a public health advisory recommending that most people have their homes checked for radon gas. Testing was urged for all detached and row houses and for all apartments below the third floor. A federal law was enacted in October to help states establish programs to test homes and schools for the presence of the gas.

A colorless, odorless, radioactive gas produced in the earth's crust, radon seeps into basements through cracks, sumps, and open places in foundations. It is an especially serious potential problem during the winter, when houses are tightly sealed, since the concentration of radon may build up considerably. The gas may account for as many as 5,000 to 20,000 deaths from lung cancer in the United States each year. (About 142,000 people in the United States are estimated to die of lung cancer each year.)

Radon concentrations are usually given in terms of picocuries, which is a measure of radioactivity. If the peak concentration in a home is less than 4 picocuries in a liter of air (the minimum level for which the EPA recommends that corrective action be taken), the chances of producing lung cancer over a lifetime are extremely small, and probably nothing needs to be done. Many homes, however, have been found to have more than 20 picocuries, and levels over 100 picocuries have been detected in homes in certain areas of the country.

Lead Dangers

Lead pollution of the air has declined considerably in recent years because of the drop in use of leaded gasoline, but scientists seem to keep finding new sources of exposure to lead. Persistent ingestion of the substance can lead to such disorders as kidney damage and hearing loss. Lead is especially dangerous to children, in whom it can cause learning disabilities and even severe brain damage.

In late 1987 it was reported in testimony before a congressional subcommittee that water fountains may be a hazard, since many electric water coolers, including some used in schools, produce high levels of lead in the water. The offending coolers have lead-lined tanks or lead-containing solder in their lines. Coolers manufactured recently should be free of lead; however, older ones that remain in use could be hazardous.

Pottery bowls and pots made in developing nations are another potential lead source that many people are not aware of. In guidelines set in 1971, the U.S. Food and Drug Administration required American ceramic companies to use sufficiently high temperatures in glazing so that lead in ceramic dishware could not leach into food. Improperly glazed imported pottery, including coffee mugs, can still produce high lead concentrations in food. It is best not to store foods in imported pottery containers, nor in ceramic containers made in the United States before 1971. (*See also the Health and Medical News article* ENVIRONMENT AND HEALTH.)

Malignant Mesothelioma

In mid-1988 researchers reported on an unexpected cluster of cases of malignant mesothelioma in a New Mexico community of about 2,000 Pueblo Indians. Mesothelioma is a cancer of the membranes lining the lungs or intestine and usually comes from exposure to asbestos. The Pueblo Indians' risk of contracting this type of cancer was about 1,000 times as high as normal.

The researchers found that the Pueblo used asbestos extensively in the manufacture of silver jewelry. For example, asbestos mats, called pounding boards, insulated the worktable from the intense heat of the brazing torches and hot metal. The mats were cleaned by hitting and rubbing them together, thereby driving asbestos fibers into the air. Also, asbestos was used to whiten leather leggings and moccasins before ceremonial dances. Clumps of asbestos fibers that developed during the whitening were eliminated by slapping the legging against the table, again driving asbestos into the air. All five of the individuals with mesothelioma were ceremonial dancers, and four of them worked with silver.

Fifth Disease

An outbreak of what is called fifth disease occurred in Connecticut in 1988. The outbreak was concentrated in the city of Torrington in the northwest part of the state but was not limited to that area. Fifth disease is a common virus-caused illness that affects mostly children, in which case it is usually mild. Symptoms include a rash and slight fever. When a woman is infected during pregnancy, the chances of a miscarriage or stillbirth increase. Few outbreaks have been studied, so researchers were closely ex-

amining the Connecticut episode in hope of increasing their understanding of the disease's effects.

The illness's name came from the fact that it was the fifth rash-producing disease described. (The first four were measles, rubella, scarlet fever, and Duke's disease, which is a mild form of scarlet fever.) Although fifth disease was first reported in 1889, the causative agent, the B19 parvovirus, was not identified until the 1980s.

Vaccines

Despite the many successes medical science has achieved, developing a safe and effective vaccine is still a difficult task. Pertussis, or whooping cough, vaccines have come under fire in recent years for producing too many side effects, some of them severe. Scientists accordingly developed two new versions of pertussis vaccine. It was reported in 1988 that large-scale trials of the two vaccines in Sweden showed that both are safe but less effective than had been hoped.

A vaccine against infection with the bacterium *Haemophilus influenzae* type b has shown more regional variation in effectiveness than any other known

After finding dangerously high levels of radon in a significant number of residences, the U.S. Environmental Protection Agency urged Americans to have their homes tested for this colorless, odorless, and potentially harmful gas. Here, a home inspection service offers radon testing.

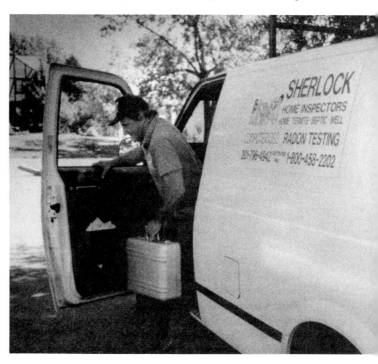

SAFE AT FIRST

Sliding into a base and getting called out is bad enough, but getting injured in the process makes it even worse. Base sliding is responsible for over 70 percent of all injuries sustained by recreational softball players (there are 40 million in the United States). But an orthopedic surgeon and his colleagues at the University of Michigan have come up with a way to reduce dramatically the number of injuries—by using breakaway bases that pop loose when hit hard by runner's foot or hand, reducing the force of the impact.

The researchers looked at accident reports from over a thousand games played by amateur softball enthusiasts, half of the games using standard stationary bases and half using breakaway bases. There were 45 sliding injuries in the games played with regular bases, mostly sprained or broken ankles. But only 2 sliding injuries occurred in all of the games played with breakaway bases.

Breakaway bases cost about $295 for a set of three—about double the price of standard bases. But they may be worth the extra cost if using them means that players won't be reduced to armchair athletes or have to hobble to postgame celebrations on crutches.

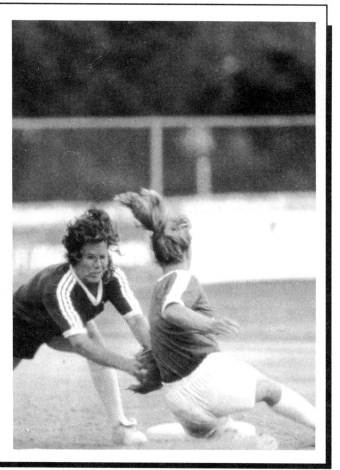

vaccine. The bacterium can be devastating in young children, causing meningitis and other problems. Studies that were reported in September 1988 found that the vaccine, which was licensed in the United States in 1985, was about 90 percent effective in Finland and in certain areas of the United States, but in other U.S. areas the vaccine's effectiveness was lower. In Minnesota, giving children the vaccine seemed to actually make them more likely to become infected with the germ. Minnesota consequently no longer uses the vaccine. Scientists have not yet found a satisfactory explanation for the regional variation. Meanwhile, an improved version of the vaccine, usable for younger children, was licensed in the United States in 1987.

Extensive trials in humans of a new vaccine against typhoid fever, a serious problem in many developing countries, showed very promising results. The new vaccine appears to be safer and easier to handle than previous typhoid vaccines and to be as effective as they are. Meanwhile, research continued on other new vaccines against typhoid.

Nutrition and Health

Mid-1988 saw the publication of the first report ever released by a U.S. surgeon general on nutrition and health. Identifying overconsumption of fat, especially saturated fat, as the most important dietary problem in the United States, the report recommended that food manufacturers increase the availability of products low in fat and cholesterol and advised Americans to eat foods low in these substances, such as leaner meats or fish and poultry, low-fat dairy products, and complex carbohydrates and fiber: whole grains, cereal products, vegetables (notably dried beans and peas), and fruits. A National Research Council report issued in early 1989 also recommended eating more complex carbohydrates and advised Americans to limit total fat intake to no more than 30 percent of total calories (less than 10 percent of which should be saturated fat), cholesterol to 300 milligrams daily, and salt to 6 grams daily. (*See also the Health and Medical News article* NUTRITION AND DIET.)

JAMES F. JEKEL, M.D., M.P.H.

Sexually Transmitted Diseases

Rebirth of the Condom • Chancroid Comeback • Treatment for Recurrent Herpes • Rising Incidence of Syphilis

Rebirth of the Condom

The rise in incurable sexually transmitted diseases (STDs) caused by the viruses that result in genital herpes and AIDS has invigorated sales of condoms, one of the oldest barrier forms of protection. Condoms offer some protection to people engaging in intercourse with infected or multiple partners. However, not all condoms are an effective barrier to the viruses. Natural membrane condoms, made from the intestines of sheep, have tiny pores through which the hepatitis B virus and the AIDS-causing human immunodeficiency virus (HIV) can pass. However, the natural membrane condoms probably prevent passage of the herpesvirus. Only latex condoms are an effective barrier to all of these agents, but the protection even they provide is not absolute. To be effective, the condom must be put on before any genital contact takes place. In addition, genital skin that is not covered by the condom may be infected, or the condom can break during intercourse or spill its contents if not removed properly after ejaculation. Oil-based lubricants such as petroleum jelly or vegetable oil weaken latex condoms and should not be used.

The effectiveness of condoms may be further improved by the addition of spermicides, such as nonoxynol-9. Spermicides—chemicals that kill sperm—also kill many sexually transmitted microorganisms, including HIV. The use of a spermicide-coated condom may thus offer more protection. Vaginal spermicides containing nonoxynol-9 also reduce the likelihood of infection by the bacteria that cause chlamydia and gonorrhea.

Chancroid Resurgence

Chancroid, an STD that for 30 years was rarely reported in the United States although it is common worldwide, has been making a comeback in the 1980s.

Between 1971 and 1980, an average of 878 cases of chancroid a year were reported by the U.S. Centers for Disease Control (CDC), but 4,998 cases were reported in 1987—the largest number since 1952. Outbreaks have occurred in California, Florida, and Pennsylvania and in New York City, Boston, and Dallas. Since many of the patients are prostitutes or migrant workers, traditional public health control methods, like tracing sexual contacts, are difficult to apply.

Chancroid is caused by the bacterium *Haemophilus ducreyi*. Infections result in genital ulcers or sores and enlargement of lymph glands in the groin area. Physicians believe that contracting chancroid, syphilis, or herpes may make a person more susceptible to contracting AIDS, because all three diseases can cause shallow ulcers that may facilitate the entry of HIV through the skin. Chancroid can be successfully treated with antibiotics, either injected or in pill form. In addition, the drug ciprofloxacin (brand name, Cipro) appears to be effective in treating chancroid when given in a single oral dose.

Acyclovir and Recurrent Herpes

Although there is no cure for genital infections caused by the *Herpes simplex* virus, the antiviral drug acyclovir (Zovirax), taken daily over a one-year period, has been shown to substantially reduce the number of recurrent episodes. This finding, reported in 1988, means that there may be a way to prevent recurrences of the painful blisters that form clusters of shallow ulcers.

A study conducted at 24 medical centers in the United States and Canada found that patients who took 400 milligrams of acyclovir orally twice a day for one year had an average of 1.8 recurrences of genital blisters during the year, in contrast to 11.4 recurrences for the untreated group. Patients taking acyclovir had few side effects. Acyclovir had already been shown to substantially shorten the duration of the initial herpes infection and to suppress recurrent infections when taken for a period of a few months. However, its safety and effectiveness if taken continuously for more than six months had not previously been known.

Antibiotic-Resistant Gonorrhea

Although the number of U.S. cases of gonorrhea is declining and most strains of the bacterium that causes the disease (*Neisseria gonorrhoeae*) are still susceptible to several common, low-cost antibiotics, an increasing number of strains have been appearing that are resistant to penicillin and other antibiotics. Since 1976, resistance to certain antibiotics has appeared in the

United States, principally the penicillins and the tetracyclines.

The most common type of resistance is caused by infection of the gonorrhea bacterium by a plasmid, a small bit of genetic material that instructs the bacterium to make an enzyme that breaks apart and destroys penicillin. Bacterial strains harboring the plasmid are called penicillinase-producing *Neisseria gonorrhoeae*, or PPNG. By 1987, PPNG had been reported in every state, with the total number of U.S. cases reaching 25,320.

The spread of antibiotic-resistant gonorrhea has created a definite economic problem. Aside from the medical complications that can arise from treatment failure, more money must be spent to monitor the spread of the resistant bacteria, and more expensive antibiotics are required to treat infected patients.

Syphilis on the Rise

Since 1986 the number of cases of syphilis reported in the United States has increased dramatically, after declining in the early 1980s. In 1987 a total of 35,147 cases of primary and secondary syphilis—the two

Condoms, once sold furtively by the druggist to male customers, are now openly displayed in convenience stores as a protection against AIDS and are purchased by women as well as men.

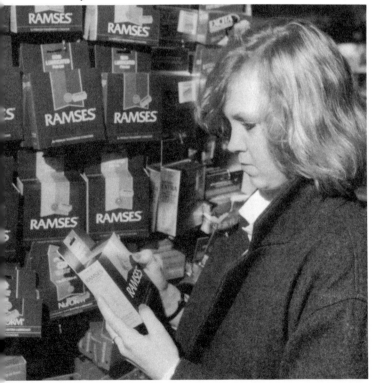

earliest stages of infection—were reported, which translates into 14.6 cases per 100,000 people, a 25 percent increase over the 1986 rate and the biggest one-year jump since 1960. Especially large increases were reported by California, Florida, and New York City.

Heterosexuals appear to account for most of the increase. (In the 1970s, 70 percent of male syphilis cases occurred among homosexual and bisexual men, but the incidence of STDs in homosexual men has dropped since the AIDS epidemic began.) Women showed the highest rate of increase, and this had repercussions on the number of babies born with syphilis. The 681 cases of congenital syphilis reported to the CDC in 1987 was the highest number in 15 years. Congenital syphilis is a serious disease that results in the death of 40 percent of afflicted children.

No one is certain why syphilis is increasing among heterosexuals. Interviews conducted in Philadelphia by public health workers suggested that prostitution in exchange for crack, the smokable form of cocaine, may be one reason. Another may be that new drug therapies for antibiotic-resistant gonorrhea are not as effective as penicillin against the bacterium causing syphilis. Yet another possible reason is that public health personnel are being diverted from treating syphilis and other STDs to contending with AIDS. Public health authorities warn that the genital ulcers caused by syphilis may facilitate the transmission of the AIDS virus.

See also the Health and Medical News article AIDS.
ROBERT C. NOBLE, M.D.

Skin

Vitamin D for Psoriasis • New Weapons in the Battle Against Wrinkles • Alpha-Interferon Approved to Treat Warts

Vitamin D and Psoriasis

New hope has arisen that vitamin D may be helpful in treating psoriasis. A chemically activated form of the vitamin has shown success as a therapy for this common skin disease.

For many years, scientists have speculated on a possible relationship between vitamin D and psoriasis. However, early attempts to treat the condition with vitamin D proved totally ineffective. The form of vitamin D used in the initial tests was the same form that is naturally absorbed from dietary sources or created in skin from the action of sunlight. Researchers now know that this form of vitamin D is inactive. To become active, it must be chemically altered in a series of reactions that take place in the liver and kidneys. The final result of these reactions is the active form of vitamin D, chemically known as 1,25 dihydroxy vitamin D3. When this active form of vitamin D is applied topically to the skin lesions of psoriasis patients, or when it is given orally, psoriasis improves. It has been shown that skin cells exposed to the active form of vitamin D slow their rate of replication. Because psoriasis is characterized by a greatly accelerated rate of replication of cells in the outermost layer of the skin, this inhibiting effect on cell replication may explain the drug's benefits.

Although it is not a cure, 1,25 dihydroxy vitamin D3 is an effective treatment for psoriasis, which is exciting news for the 1 to 2 percent of the population afflicted by the disease. Further investigation and understanding of how the drug works promises to give new insights into the causes of psoriasis.

Smoothing Wrinkles

People searching for products to reverse the physical, cosmetic effects of aging have had some new hope in recent months. The prescription drug tretinoin (sold under the U.S. brand name Retin-A, and as StieVAA and Vitamin A Acid in Canada) has been found to reduce fine wrinkles when applied topically to the skin. And in February 1988 the U.S. Food and Drug Administration (FDA) approved the use of a new substance to erase scars, such as those sometimes left from acne and chicken pox; the FDA was expected in 1989 to approve the substance to treat wrinkles as well. The substance was approved for both uses in Canada late in 1988.

The substance is a gelatin matrix implant, sold as Fibrel. It is made by mixing a portion of a patient's plasma with a gelatinous material. This mixture is then injected into the dermal layer beneath the wrinkle or scar. Fibrel is claimed to raise and repair damaged areas as well as to stimulate the growth of new tissue. At the time Fibrel was approved, there was only one other FDA-approved injectable wrinkle and scar modifier on the U.S. market, bovine collagen (sold as Zyderm or Zyplast). Fibrel's manufacturers claim it produces a longer-lasting improvement in appearance than bovine collagen. In one study, 79 percent of patients' scars showed continual improvement after two years. In contrast, bovine collagen is broken down by the body within two years, and patients need

new injections then to return the skin to its improved appearance. Fibrel also caused improvement in deeper wrinkles, on which tretinoin is not particularly successful. Furthermore, Fibrel is convenient because it is stable at room temperature and can be stored for more than two years before being mixed with plasma.

In the battle against wrinkles, only experience over time will establish the relative merits of cosmetic surgery, topical drugs like tretinoin, and injectable substances like bovine collagen and Fibrel.

See also the Spotlight on Health article THE RETINOIDS: WONDER DRUGS?

New Treatment for Warts

In June 1988 the FDA approved the use of alpha-interferon as a treatment for genital warts, which are a common and easily transmitted infection, affecting both men and women, that is caused by the human papilloma virus.

Interferon is a protein that is naturally produced by cells in the body in response to viral infection. In addition to having an antiviral effect, interferon has been shown to stimulate the immune system and to slow cell replication. Interferon exerts its antiviral effect by stimulating cells to produce other proteins that prevent viruses from reproducing. A logical therapeutic approach to genital warts was to amplify this natural defense system by producing large quantities of interferon in the laboratory through recombinant DNA technology and then directing it to the treatment of viral infections. Work in this area over the past decade has finally come to fruition in the form of a specific type of interferon, alpha-interferon. It is now sold in the United States under the brand name Intron A. (As of early 1989, it was not yet approved in Canada for treating genital warts.)

This form of alpha-interferon is in a solution, which is injected into the warts three times a week for three weeks. Treatment is currently limited by the fact that it is painful and expensive, although it is effective in curing or shrinking warts in more than 80 percent of patients. No uniformly effective therapy currently exists for genital warts—standard treatments include freezing the warts with liquid nitrogen, burning them with electric currents, or removing them through laser surgery—all of which can be painful and can leave scars. Furthermore, because studies have suggested a relationship between the human papilloma virus and cervical cancer, the demand for effective therapy has increased. Thus, even a partially effective new therapy has been welcomed by patients and physicians. The future may well bring more effective therapies using interferon technology in the treatment of viral infections. EDWARD E. BONDI, M.D.

Smoking

Warning About Nicotine Addiction •
New Smoking Regulations •
Tobacco Company Found Liable

Surgeon General's Report

Instead of presenting additional evidence of the effects of smoking on health, the annual Surgeon General's Report on the Health Consequences of Smoking that was issued in May 1988 addressed the issue of nicotine addiction. In his 618-page report, Dr. C. Everett Koop described smoking as being as addictive as using heroin or cocaine, explaining that this is why many people continue to smoke despite the known hazards of the habit. He characterized nicotine, the ingredient in tobacco that causes addiction, as a psychoactive (mood-altering) drug that can provide pleasurable effects while causing physical dependence. Koop called for labels warning of the addictive nature of tobacco to be added to the health warnings already required on tobacco packaging and advertisements. He also called for more research on ways to treat tobacco dependence, suggesting that such treatment should be covered by health insurance.

In January 1989 the surgeon general published a report entitled *Reducing the Health Consequences of Smoking: 25 Years of Progress,* in which he reviewed the advances made in curtailing smoking since the first annual report appeared in 1964. He warned that smoking remains the "single most important preventable cause of death" in the United States.

Research Update

Researchers continued to seek an understanding of the ways in which smoking is harmful to health and to look for ways to help the 70 to 90 percent of smokers who say they would like to quit. Japanese scientists reported a theory that may explain why smokers have an increased risk of heart disease. If the findings of animal research prove to hold true for humans, they said, tobacco smoke enhances the activity of low-density lipoproteins (or LDLs)—cholesterol-carrying particles in the blood—and thus increases one's risk for atherosclerosis, or hardening of the arteries.

Among findings that could lead to more successful stop-smoking strategies, researchers reported that heavy smokers (25 or more cigarettes per day) are more dependent on cigarettes than light smokers (15 or fewer cigarettes per day) and might benefit from specialized programs. It was also reported that when used properly, nicotine gum, which is available only by prescription in the United States, is effective in helping smokers kick the habit, especially when combined with physician counseling and follow-up.

New Smoking Restrictions

By the end of 1988, 43 states and 375 cities and counties in the United States had passed laws restricting smoking in some fashion. Among the most notable of these laws is one passed in New York City in January 1988, which limits smoking in a variety of public places. Businesses in the city that employ more than 15 people must have a written smoking policy and provide a smoke-free work area for all employees who request it. Restaurants seating over 50 people must now assign at least half their seats to a nonsmoking area, and indoor sports arenas must restrict smoking to no more than 50 percent of the lobby areas. Smoking is now forbidden in taxicabs.

Congress put a halt to smoking on all airline flights originating in the United States that are scheduled to last for two hours or less. The ban, which began on April 22, 1988, is in effect for a two-year trial period. The same legislation mandated that the Long Island Railroad and the Metro-North Commuter Railroad become smoke-free beginning February 15, 1988. Previously, trains on these metropolitan New York City commuter lines generally had one or more cars where smoking was allowed.

Northwest Airlines voluntarily carried the congressional smoking ban further, declaring all its domestic flights except those to Hawaii to be smoke-free. And Air Canada, which had begun to prohibit smoking on its short commuter flights in 1986, expanded its smoke-free policy to all flights in North America. Both airlines said their policies were arrived at after surveys showed that even passengers who smoke prefer no-smoking flights.

While passengers seemed to approve of Northwest's new policy, the tobacco industry was less enthusiastic. In April 1988 the food and tobacco conglomerate RJR Nabisco fired the New York advertising agency Saatchi & Saatchi DFS Compton, which had prepared the commercials announcing the airline's new policy. Saatchi & Saatchi had handled ads for nontobacco products for RJR.

Advertising

U.S. tobacco companies continued to spend heavily during 1988 to promote cigarettes; in 1986, the latest

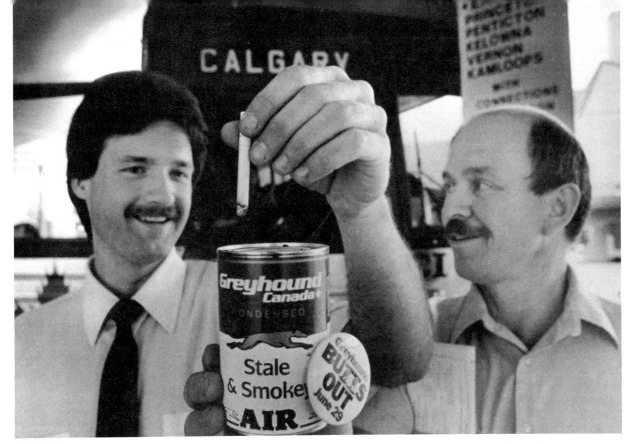

Before boarding the bus, a passenger complies with the new "butts out" policy on Greyhound Canada. Smoking restrictions are being applied by increasing numbers of public transportation companies in North America.

year for which figures are available, $2.4 billion was spent on advertising and promotion. In an effort to convince the public that smoking is still a popular habit, Philip Morris began a $5 million advertising campaign in June 1988, emphasizing the economic power of smokers. Using headlines designed to give the impression that smokers are an affluent and influential group, the campaign was based on information gathered from responses to a questionnaire distributed through the company's free-circulation quarterly magazine.

Professional pollsters and health experts criticized the use of information obtained in this way to authenticate such messages as "Today 21 million American smokers will go out to eat" and "$1 trillion is too much financial power to ignore." Some observers noted that despite this attempt to display the clout of smokers, U.S. tobacco consumption is declining at a rate of about 2 percent each year.

A ban on tobacco advertising in Canadian newspapers and magazines became effective January 1, 1989, with a similar ban for signs and billboards scheduled for 1991. The measure was supported in Parliament by all three of Canada's national political parties. Tobacco manufacturers are challenging the ban in court, claiming the law violates constitutional guarantees of free speech.

Tobacco Lobby

Tobacco companies and their lobbying organizations continued to spend large amounts of money in an effort to prevent the passage of antismoking legislation, opposing more than 200 proposed restrictive measures in 1988. Their efforts ranged from sending a lobbyist to testify at a city council meeting in St. Charles, Mo. (population 43,000), to mounting multi-million-dollar statewide media campaigns in Oregon and California.

Voters in Oregon defeated a November ballot proposal to ban smoking in virtually all enclosed public areas. The tobacco industry funded a campaign by Oregonians for Fair Choice that spent $2.7 million to oppose the measure, which would have been the strictest statewide law of its kind. About 60 percent of voters opposed the measure.

Tobacco interests had less success in a $22 million attempt to defeat a California ballot initiative known as Proposition 99. The measure, which passed by a 58 percent to 42 percent margin, increases the state's tax on cigarettes from 10 cents a pack to 35 cents a pack. The additional revenue is earmarked for education about the dangers of tobacco, medical care of the uninsured, and research on tobacco-related diseases.

BREAKING THE HABIT

There may be as many ways to stop smoking as there are ex-smokers. These tips are adapted from the booklet *Clearing the Air: How to Quit Smoking...and Quit for Keeps*, prepared by the U.S. National Cancer Institute.*

Ways of Quitting

Set a target date for stopping completely—perhaps a special day such as your birthday or anniversary.

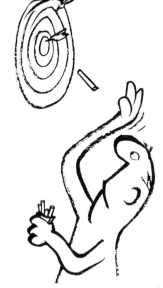

Postpone lighting your first cigarette one additional hour each day.

Don't empty your ashtrays. The sight and smell of stale butts will be very unpleasant.

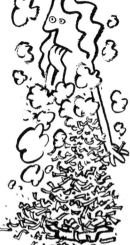

After You've Quit

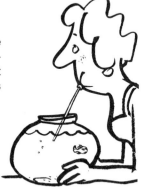

For the first two to three weeks, drink large quantities of water and fruit juice (but avoid sodas that contain caffeine).

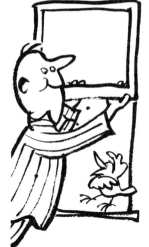

Develop a clean, fresh nonsmoking environment around yourself—at work and at home.

Find new habits that require you to use your hands.

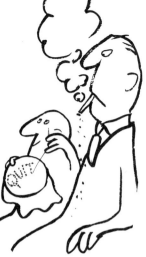

*Copies of the booklet are available, free of charge, from:
National Cancer Institute, Building 31, Room 10A24, 9000 Rockville Pike, Bethesda, MD 20892 (1-800-4-CANCER).

Liability Ruling

The first loss of a product liability suit by a tobacco company came in June 1988, when a federal jury in Newark, N.J., awarded $400,000 to the husband of a woman who had died of lung cancer. She had smoked a pack and a half of cigarettes daily for 40 years. The award was based on the jury's finding that before warning labels were placed on tobacco products there had been an express warranty that cigarettes were safe, and that the Liggett Group, the cigarette manufacturer found liable, was aware of the danger of smoking and should have advised its customers accordingly. (The Federal Cigarette Labeling and Advertising Act went into effect in 1966; it requires that cigarette packages carry labels warning of potential health hazards.)

The much-publicized trial lasted for four months and forced cigarette manufacturers to make public thousands of pages of previously confidential documents. Some of this material demonstrated that tobacco companies had privately acknowledged the link between smoking and cancer and other diseases as early as the 1940s, although they had publicly disclaimed such knowledge. (Throughout the trial the defendants maintained that there is no proven link between smoking and cancer.) The availability of this evidence was expected to generate more product liability suits against tobacco companies in the future. It also inspired a congressional subcommittee chaired by Representative Thomas Luken (D, Ohio) to hold hearings on allegedly deceptive advertising practices by tobacco marketers. This subcommittee has jurisdiction over the Federal Trade Commission, which is responsible for regulating print and broadcast advertising.

Death Certificates

In January 1989, Oregon and Utah revised their death certificates to ask doctors to specify if tobacco use contributed to death. State health officials hoped that the new forms would produce statistics to clarify who in the population is smoking and what the focus of public health programs should be to dissuade more people from smoking. Opponents of smoking welcomed the revisions for their symbolic value, saying they might encourage doctors to urge patients to stop smoking and might aid in liability suits against tobacco companies; the tobacco industry called the added questions meaningless because the certificates represent only a doctor's opinion or estimate. The American Medical Association urged other states to update their death certificates similarly.

BARBARA SCHERR TRENK

Teeth and Gums

Oral Health in Children • Periodontal Disease Treatments • AIDS Inhibitor in Saliva • Composite Fillings for Back Teeth

Fewer Cavities in Kids

In a follow-up to a similar survey conducted by the U.S. National Institute of Dental Research in 1979-1980, dentists who examined nearly 40,000 children across the country in 1986-1987 found that the marked downward trend in dental decay in children in the United States is continuing. Half of the youngsters 5 to 17 years old are now completely free of dental decay. In contrast, in 1979-1980, 36.6 percent of the children were decay-free; in the early 1970s the figure was only 28 percent. Not only is there a dramatic increase in the number who have no cavities or fillings, but those who still suffer tooth decay have fewer tooth surfaces affected—down from an average of five per child in 1980 to three in 1987. The reduction in new decay occurred mostly in cavities that form between the teeth—a 54 percent decrease between 1980 and 1987. Decay on the biting surfaces of the back teeth dropped 32 percent during this period.

The success in reducing tooth decay in children so effectively, especially the decay between the teeth, is due largely to the widespread use of different forms of fluoride—in drinking water and in dietary supplements during tooth formation, as well as in toothpastes, rinses, and topical applications. The increasing use of plastic sealants on the biting surfaces of the permanent back teeth of young children is having a major effect on protecting those highly susceptible tooth surfaces.

Most of the dental decay in the 5 to 17 age group now appears to occur in only about 20 percent of the children, who make up a highly susceptible, decay-prone group. Once the factors that contribute to these children being at high risk are determined, public health programs can be developed that will address their dental needs. Much research is being directed to developing simple tests for decay susceptibility that will identify the high-risk individuals. In addition, with the marked improvement in dental health in the younger segment of the U.S. population, attention is shifting to additional means of reducing decay in the older population, which did not have the benefits that the fluoride generation does. In the offing are new fluoride formulations, new antibacterial agents, and decay-reducing sugar substitutes such as xylitol. Xylitol-sweetened chewing gums are already widely used in many parts of the world.

Periodontal Disease Treatments

Significant advances have recently been made in treating periodontitis, the advanced form of gum, or periodontal, disease. As a result of improvements in oral hygiene devices and techniques, greater personal attention to plaque control, and wider use of antibacterial rinses, there has been a significant decrease in gingivitis (inflammation of the gums), the early form of periodontal disease. However, with people living longer and keeping their teeth longer, they are at increasing risk for the more serious periodontitis, which is characterized by loss of the connective tissue fibers and bone that anchor the teeth to the jaws. As the disease progresses, deep pockets form between the supporting tissues and the tooth roots, the teeth loosen, and eventually they are lost. During 1988 significant advances were made in techniques to slow down the rate of bone loss and to replace the lost connective tissue that attaches to the root, as well as to increase the level of bony support for the teeth.

Drug for Bone Loss. Nonsteroidal anti-inflammatory drugs may be one way to help reduce bone loss. These aspirin-like drugs have been widely used as pain relievers and for treating symptoms of arthritis. Because of reports that people using such agents over a long period of time have less periodontal disease, researchers investigated one of the new drugs in this group, called flurbiprofen. They found it to be particularly effective in reducing the rate of alveolar (jaw) bone loss in experimental periodontal disease (induced using a special diet) in dogs and monkeys. A three-year study of flurbiprofen's effect on humans was also encouraging, showing that flurbiprofen significantly slowed the rate of alveolar bone loss; a larger, multicenter study is currently under way. The drug, under the name Ansaid, has already been approved for treating arthritis patients, but its approval for periodontal disease will have to await the outcome of the current trials and the authorization of the U.S. Food and Drug Administration.

Experimental Treatments. In advanced forms of periodontal disease, only rarely do new connective tissue fibers grow and attach to the root surface to replace the tissue destroyed by the disease process. A new experimental technique shows promise of markedly increasing the likelihood of reattachment of connective tissue. This new technique, called guided

tissue regeneration, involves a special membrane, which has pores of a specific size, that is placed between the root and the gum tissues. The membrane (which later has to be removed) prevents unwanted gum tissue from growing around the root, while allowing the migration and growth of new tissue cells and fibers that attach to the root. Several studies have indicated that the technique can work. Researchers hope that by refining the procedure and using different types of membrane materials that do not have to be removed, they will be able to increase the success rate. Researchers are also investigating the use of a natural protein, fibronectin, that enhances the adhesion of cells to the root. A preliminary study of periodontal patients showed promising results one year after treatment.

Some dentists have begun using a variety of artificial materials to fill defects in the supporting bone caused by periodontal disease, in addition to the natural bone grafts they have traditionally relied on. Materials such as synthetic hydroxyapatite and beta-tricalcium phosphate are already used to build up the bony ridges that remain after a tooth has been pulled to help anchor artificial dentures. The use of such synthetics to repair periodontal defects is increasing, but it is still an experimental procedure, and none of the materials available has been sufficiently tested to judge how well they will work over the long term. Newer materials go beyond just repairing bone defects: they may actually stimulate or induce new bone formation. Their use in periodontal patients is still preliminary but promising, since they offer hope of reversing the bone destruction caused by periodontal disease.

Saliva and AIDS

Saliva may play an active role in hindering the virus that causes AIDS, according to recent research. This may help explain why, despite evidence that saliva is one of the body fluids that can carry the virus, there is no evidence that AIDS has actually been transmitted by saliva. Intensive study of household members who freely shared dishes, glasses, towels, and other items with AIDS patients has not revealed any transmission of the disease. (Dentists and hygienists, appropriately, use gloves, masks, and protective glasses when treating patients to avoid contact not so much with saliva but with the blood that can result from various dental procedures, such as periodontal treatment or tooth extraction.)

The failure of saliva to transmit AIDS has been attributed to the low level of the virus in the fluid. However, a recent study by researchers at the National Institute of Dental Research indicates that saliva may actually play an active role in protecting against the virus. The researchers found that components of saliva can actually bind to the virus and inhibit it from infecting lymphocytes—white blood cells that are part of the immune system and are usually attacked by the virus. A study of secretions collected from the different salivary glands indicates that the submandibular-sublingual glands located beneath the tongue are largely responsible for saliva's inhibitory effect. The researchers now want to identify the specific component of saliva responsible for inhibiting the AIDS virus and learn how it works to bind the virus.

Aesthetic Fillings for Back Teeth

Cavities in the back teeth may now be filled using materials similar to those used in the front teeth, instead of the familiar—and unattractive—metal fillings. Over the last decade the development of new plastic (composite) materials for filling cavities and techniques for bonding them to the teeth allowed dentists to restore front teeth in very aesthetic ways. But the use of these materials for filling back teeth had been limited because of concern over their ability to withstand the stress of heavy biting pressure and to retain their form. Their susceptibility to decay at their margins of contact with the tooth was also not known. As a result, silver and gold fillings remained the preferred materials for back teeth.

In 1988, after five years of stringent testing, two materials won acceptance by the Council on Dental Materials of the American Dental Association for safety and effectiveness in filling back, or posterior, teeth. The council warns that the posterior composites should not be used for large fillings where they are subject to heavy stress, and dentists who use the new materials must be meticulous in following the correct procedures for inserting the composites. With further improvements in composition and techniques for bonding the composites to the inner portion of the teeth, these aesthetic fillings could replace metal fillings in many situations.

Dental Fear

Despite the tremendous improvements in dental procedures and anesthetics in recent years, fear of the dentist is still common. Just how widespread dental fear is, however, was not known. In 1988 the findings were reported of the first U.S. study in more than 30 years to examine the epidemiology of dental fear. Over 1,000 residents of Seattle, Wash., were asked how they rated their feelings toward dental treatment. Some 20 percent of the respondents indicated high

dental fear, with 13.2 percent somewhat afraid, 4.2 percent very afraid, and 3.0 percent terrified. Females were 1.8 times more likely than males to report high fear. There were no significant differences in fear levels between white and nonwhite respondents or between affluent and nonaffluent respondents. Two-thirds of those surveyed reported that they had acquired their fear in childhood. Injections and drilling were the most feared dental procedures.

Because dental fear results in long intervals between visits to the dentist, delays in making appointments, and chronic cancellations—all of which exacerbate dental problems—more attention is being given to treating dental phobias and to teaching dentists how to reduce their patients' anxiety. Dental schools are placing an increasing emphasis on teaching students to display empathy and friendliness and to communicate better.

See also the Spotlight on Health articles FLUORIDATION: A SUCCESS STORY *and* WHAT ARE DENTAL IMPLANTS?

IRWIN D. MANDEL, D.D.S.

World Health News

AIDS Around the World • Diseases of Affluence • Cholera Outbreak in India • Animals Spreading Rare Illnesses

AIDS

Without doubt, AIDS—acquired immune deficiency syndrome—was the disease that captured the most attention worldwide in 1988 as the number of cases continued to mount.

Cases in Europe. Statistics presented at the June 1988 international AIDS conference in Sweden showed that the number of AIDS cases reported in Europe had surpassed 12,000 and was doubling every 11 months. The estimates of the number of persons in 30 European countries who were infected with the human immunodeficiency virus (HIV) that causes AIDS varied from 300,000 to 800,000. The World Health Organization estimated in January 1989 that there had been more than 350,000 cases of clinical AIDS worldwide since the epidemic began, including reported and unreported cases.

In Europe, as in the United States, it appears that intravenous drug abuse is becoming more important as a route of transmission of HIV. The proportion of AIDS cases among European drug abusers—who contract the virus by sharing unsanitary needles—rose from 7 percent in 1985 to about 30 percent in 1988, with France, Spain, and Italy reporting even higher percentages.

However, a new government report from Britain suggested that more British men and women had been infected with HIV through heterosexual intercourse than had previously been assumed. It had been thought that the number of cases of heterosexually acquired HIV infection in all of Britain was about 400, but the new report placed it nearer to 3,000 in England alone. That number would account for a very high proportion of the estimated 12,000 people in Britain who are HIV carriers or have full-blown cases of AIDS. However, studies suggest that with proper warning and precautions, heterosexual transmission may be kept to a low level. A Dutch study that followed the wives of 13 male hemophiliacs who had acquired HIV through infected blood products found no evidence of HIV transmission to the wives.

Africa and Asia. African nations have begun to participate more fully in AIDS information and control efforts after years of hesitancy brought about in part by the frequent accusation that AIDS began in Africa. The origins of AIDS now appear to be more complex than originally thought, and certainly many other

An Indian mother spoon-feeds her son, one of thousands of victims of a cholera epidemic that claimed more than 200 lives in the New Delhi area in 1988.

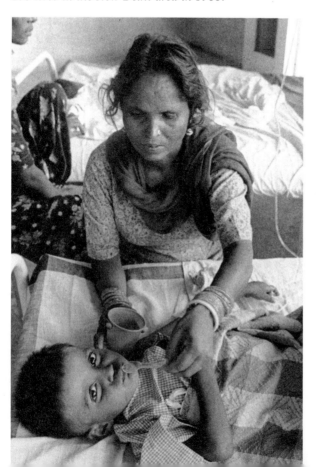

nations, including the United States, have contributed to its spread. Moreover, the potential disruption by AIDS of the central African nations appears to be so great—there are even fears for the ultimate survival of certain countries—that many Africans are now convinced they must join the worldwide effort to control the disease.

A report from Australia on the transmission of HIV through breast milk raised troubling problems for Africa as well as other regions of the world. The report documented six cases of AIDS infection in children of women who themselves became infected with HIV only after giving birth and who apparently then transmitted the virus to their infants through breast-feeding. This information is worrisome because in many parts of the world, including Africa, breast-feeding is a necessary method of infant feeding, since it has proven nutritional advantages and confers protection against infectious diseases. In addition, in many poor countries the water that is mixed with powdered formula or local foods is apt to be contaminated, which poses a health risk to children. Yet in areas with a high incidence of HIV infection, breast-feeding may cause many infants to acquire HIV infection and, eventually, AIDS. This could become an almost insoluble problem for the promotion of health among children. For now, evidence shows that most cases of AIDS in African children come not from breast-feeding but from unscreened blood transfusions administered to those seriously ill from anemia due to malaria.

The prevalence of HIV has been increasing in many Asian countries, but it remains low in comparison with Africa or the Americas. High HIV infection rates in Asia are found mostly in big cities where the majority of carriers are prostitutes and intravenous drug users.

See also the Health and Medical News article AIDS.

Diseases of Affluence

If there were any remaining doubts that diet, personal habits, and life-style are related to the incidence of heart disease, those doubts should be eliminated by the evidence from nations that have undergone recent improvement in the standard of living. In the decade from the period 1972-1974 to the period 1982-1984, the death rate from heart disease rose by more than 50 percent in Romania (the country has since undergone an economic downturn and has stopped reporting its mortality data). Spain, Yugoslavia, Hungary, Poland, Bulgaria, Greece, and Czechoslovakia also showed significant increases in deaths from heart disease, and it is believed that the Soviet Union experienced a similar trend.

Other "diseases of affluence" have also appeared in many countries. High rates of hypertension are reported in such areas as central Africa, Brazil, and Hungary. Cirrhosis of the liver from high alcohol intake is common and increasing in the Soviet Union and Eastern bloc nations. Lung cancer rates are increasing in both Western and developing nations.

Almost certainly these increases in disease rates are largely caused by the increasing use of the accoutrements of affluence: diets high in saturated animal fats and salt, cigarette smoking, excessive alcohol intake, and decreasing manual labor. Obesity is becoming more common in countries where the rate of heart disease is increasing. Some health experts believe that overeating in some countries may be in reaction to chronic wartime and postwar food shortages.

According to the World Health Organization, cigarette smoking in Africa has almost doubled and beer drinking has increased to six times what it was a decade ago. More than 95 percent of the people in Papua New Guinea smoke, as do more than 70 percent of the men in many other nations, such as Indonesia, Bangladesh, South Korea, and the Philippines. Smoking rates are very high in the world's most populous country, China. By contrast, smoking rates in the United States have been gradually dropping, by about 2 percent per year.

The amount of tar—a carcinogen found in tobacco—is much higher in many non-U.S. cigarettes than in those sold in the United States. However, the United States has been contributing to the worldwide increase in smoking with rapidly growing foreign cigarette sales, fueled by aggressive advertising. Some countries are upset with these developments; Nigeria, for one, is planning to ban all cigarette advertising.

Cholera Epidemic

Annual summer monsoon rains in India caused drains and sewers to overflow and pollute drinking water in New Delhi, the capital of India. The befouled water set off a major outbreak of cholera in July 1988, mostly among poor people living in unauthorized shantytowns near the Yamuna River that goes through New Delhi. Government officials reported in early August 1988 that more than 200 people, many of them children, had died, and at least 11,000 more had required treatment. Hospitals in the area were extremely overcrowded, with two or three persons to a bed.

To replace the heavy losses of fluid and salt caused by the severe form of diarrhea that characterizes cholera, patients are given water, sugar, and salts intravenously or orally. There is no antibiotic treatment, but previously healthy patients usually recover if rehydration therapy is prompt and sufficient.

Soviet Mystery Disease

Eighty-two children were hospitalized in the Ukrainian city of Chernovtsy with a mysterious disease that made their hair fall out. The children ranged in age from infants to 15-year-olds. Soviet health officials denied any problems in the air, water, or food, and they also denied the disease could be related to the 1986 Chernobyl nuclear power plant disaster, although Chernovtsy is only about 280 miles away. By early 1989 officials did not know either the cause of or the cure for this problem.

Rift Valley Fever

A relatively uncommon but serious viral disease called Rift Valley fever—so named because it was first discovered in Kenya's Rift Valley—recently appeared in western Africa in Senegal and Mauritania. The infection, which can cause encephalitis, hemorrhagic fever, or blindness in human beings and hepatitis in animals, is usually spread by mosquitoes. In the Senegal-Mauritania outbreak, 245 cases and 28 deaths were reported, making it one of the most serious outbreaks of the disease ever recorded for people. The epidemic apparently was caused, in part, by increased mosquito activity along the Sénégal River following the construction of the Diama Dam. It did not come as a complete surprise, as there had been cases of the disease earlier in southern Mauritania. In fact, the outbreak seemed to confirm predictions that the construction of the dam would have serious public health consequences.

Poker Players' Pneumonia

In the Nova Scotia city of Halifax, an outbreak of an unusual pneumonia occurred among 12 poker players following a game during which a cat, infected with Q fever, gave birth to three kittens in the same room as the poker game. (One of the poker players subsequently died.) Q fever is an uncommon illness caused by the microorganism *Coxiella burnetii*. It usually affects domesticated animals, such as cattle, sheep, and goats, and sometimes wild animals, such as rabbits. *C. burnetti* is found in large concentrations in the placenta and amniotic fluid of infected animals; during and after birth, the organism is dispersed into the air and may be inhaled by humans or animals, possibly leading to contamination. Ordinarily Q fever is a rural disease, but the fact that an urban cat was the reservoir for this outbreak raises questions as to whether the disease may become more prevalent in urban areas.

JAMES F. JEKEL, M.D., M.P.H.

Contributors

Abelson, David C., D.D.S. Senior Research Associate, Center for Clinical Research in Dentistry, Columbia University School of Dental and Oral Surgery, New York City. WHAT ARE DENTAL IMPLANTS?

Beutler, Ernest, M.D. Chairman, Department of Basic and Clinical Research, Scripps Clinic and Research Foundation; Clinical Professor of Medicine, University of California, San Diego. ANEMIA.

Biller, Henry B., Ph.D. Professor of Psychology, University of Rhode Island. CHILD ABUSE.

Boettcher, Iris F., M.D. Clinical Instructor, Division of Geriatrics, State University of New York, Buffalo. AGING AND THE AGED (coauthor).

Bondi, Edward E., M.D. Associate Professor, Department of Dermatology, University of Pennsylvania. SKIN; THE RETINOIDS: WONDER DRUGS?

Callender, David L., M.D. Resident in Otolaryngology, Baylor College of Medicine, Houston. EARS, NOSE, AND THROAT.

Cendron, Marc, M.D. Instructor of Urology, University of Pennsylvania. IMPOTENCE: A TREATABLE PROBLEM (coauthor).

Charash, Bruce D., M.D. Assistant Professor of Medicine, Division of Cardiology, New York Hospital-Cornell Medical Center, New York City. HEART AND CIRCULATORY SYSTEM (coauthor).

Cohen, Lynne. Ottawa-based writer. GOVERNMENT POLICIES AND PROGRAMS (CANADA).

Cowart, Virginia. Principal, Medical Information Service; Contributing Editor, *Physician and Sports Medicine*. FAMILY PLANNING; HOW DRUGS ARE APPROVED; MEDICAL TECHNOLOGY.

Davis, Sharon Watkins, M.P.A. Director, Cancer Information Service, Project Coordinator, Community Clinical Oncology Program, Fox Chase Cancer Center, Philadelphia. CANCER (coauthor).

Deitch, Mark. Medical writer and editor. OBSTETRICS AND MALPRACTICE.

Engstrom, Paul F., M.D. Vice President for Cancer Control, Fox Chase Cancer Center, Philadelphia; Professor of Medicine, Temple University Medical School. CANCER (coauthor).

Fink, Max, M.D. Professor of Psychiatry, State University of New York; Attending Psychiatrist, University Hospital, Stony Brook, N.Y. UPDATE ON "SHOCK" THERAPY.

Fisher, Jeffrey, M.D. Assistant Professor of Medicine, Division of Cardiology, New York Hospital-Cornell Medical Center, New York City. HEART AND CIRCULATORY SYSTEM (coauthor).

Hammill, Hunter, M.D. Assistant Professor, Department of Obstetrics and Gynecology, Baylor College of Medicine, Houston. YEAST INFECTIONS.

Hanno, Philip M., M.D. Associate Professor of Urology, University of Pennsylvania; Chief, Division of Urology, Philadelphia Veterans Administration Medical Center. IMPOTENCE: A TREATABLE PROBLEM (coauthor).

Hume, Eric L., M.D. Assistant Professor, Department of Orthopaedic Surgery, Rothman Institute, Thomas Jefferson University, Philadelphia. BONES, MUSCLES, AND JOINTS.

Jekel, James F., M.D., M.P.H. Professor of Epidemiology and Public Health, Yale University School of Medicine. AIDS; PUBLIC HEALTH; WORLD HEALTH NEWS.

Karasic, Raymond B., M.D. Assistant Professor of Pediatrics, University of Pittsburgh. CHICKEN POX; DEALING WITH A COLICKY BABY; PEDIATRICS.

Katz, Paul R., M.D. Fellowship Coordinator, Division of Geriatrics, State University of New York, Buffalo; Medical Director, Nursing Home Care Unit, Buffalo Veterans Administration Medical Center. AGING AND THE AGED (coauthor).

Lichtendorf, Susan S. Medical science journalist. DETECTING CANCER EARLY.

Mandel, Irwin D., D.D.S. Professor of Dentistry, Director, Center for Clinical Research in Dentistry, Columbia University School of Dental and Oral Surgery, New York City. FLUORIDATION: A SUCCESS STORY; TEETH AND GUMS.

Markowitz, Milton, M.D. Professor of Pediatrics, Associate Dean of Student Affairs, University of Connecticut School of Medicine. RHEUMATIC FEVER.

Maugh, Thomas H., II, Ph.D. Science Writer, Los Angeles *Times*. GENETICS AND GENETIC ENGINEERING.

McLellan, A. Thomas, Ph.D. Director of Clinical Research, Psychiatry Service, Philadelphia Veterans Administration Medical Center; Associate Professor, Department of Psychiatry, University of Pennsylvania. DRUG ABUSE (coauthor).

Meyerhoff, Michael K., Ed.D. Executive Director, The Epicenter Inc. (The Education for Parenthood Information Center), Wellesley Hills, Mass. TOILET TRAINING.

Moreno, Jonathan D., Ph.D. Professor of Pediatrics and of Medicine, Director, Division of Humanities in Medicine, State University of New York Health Science Center, Brooklyn. BIOETHICS; THE RIGHT TO DIE.

Moses, Hamilton, III, M.D. Associate Professor, Department of Neurology, The Johns Hopkins Medical Institutions; Vice President for Medical Affairs, The Johns Hopkins Hospital. BRAIN AND NERVOUS SYSTEM.

Noble, Robert C., M.D. Professor of Medicine, Division of Infectious Diseases, University of Kentucky College of Medicine. SEXUALLY TRANSMITTED DISEASES.

O'Brien, Charles P., M.D., Ph.D. Chief, Psychiatry Service, Philadelphia Veterans Administration Medical Center; Professor and Vice Chairman, Department of Psychiatry, University of Pennsylvania. DRUG ABUSE (coauthor).

Pelot, Daniel, M.D. Associate Clinical Professor, Division of Gastroenterology, Department of Medicine, University of California, Irvine. DIGESTIVE SYSTEM; HEMORRHOIDS.

Perlmutter, Johanna F., M.D. Assistant Professor, Department of Obstetrics and Gynecology, Harvard Medical School. OBSTETRICS AND GYNECOLOGY.

Repka, Michael X., M.D. Assistant Professor, The Johns Hopkins University; Consultant, Howard University, Washington, D.C.; Consultant, Sinai Hospital, Veterans Administration Medical Center, Baltimore. EYES.

Rodman, Morton J., Ph.D. Professor of Pharmacology, Rutgers University, New Brunswick, N.J. MEDICATIONS AND DRUGS.

Rotherham, James A. Staff Director, U.S. House of Representatives Subcommittee on Domestic Marketing, Consumer Relations, and Nutrition. GOVERNMENT POLICIES AND PROGRAMS (UNITED STATES).

Rubinstein, Arye, M.D., Ph.D. Professor of Pediatrics, Microbiology, and Immunology, Director, Division of Allergy and Immunology, Albert Einstein College of Medicine, Bronx, N.Y. CHILDREN WITH AIDS.

Sims, Dorothea F. Former Co-chairperson, Committee on Health Delivery, National Diabetes Advisory Board; former member, American Diabetes Association Board. DIABETES (coauthor).

Sims, Ethan A. H., M.D. Professor Emeritus of Medicine, University of Vermont;

Attending Physician, Medical Center Hospital of Vermont. DIABETES (coauthor).

Smith, Pat Costello. Free-lance writer and editor. SJOGREN'S SYNDROME.

Sollee, Natalie D., Ph.D. Instructor, Harvard Medical School. DYSLEXIA: A READING DISORDER.

Spiegel, David, M.D. Associate Professor of Psychiatry and Behavioral Sciences, Director, Psychiatry Clinic, Stanford University School of Medicine. MENTAL HEALTH.

Thro, Ellen. Science writer specializing in environmental and medical topics. ENVIRONMENT AND HEALTH.

Trenk, Barbara Scherr. Writer specializing in health issues. SMOKING.

Williams, Eleanor R., Ph.D. Associate Professor, Department of Human Nutrition and Food Systems, University of Maryland. FACTS ABOUT OAT BRAN; NUTRITION AND DIET.

Woody, George E., M.D. Chief, Substance Abuse Treatment Unit, Philadelphia Veterans Administration Medical Center; Clinical Professor, Department of Psychiatry, University of Pennsylvania. DRUG ABUSE (coauthor).

Zetterman, Rowen K., M.D. Chief, Section of Digestive Disease and Nutrition, University of Nebraska Medical Center; Associate Chief of Staff for Research, Veterans Administration Medical Center, Omaha. LIVER.

Index

Page number in *italics* indicates the reference is to an illustration.

A

AARP, *see* American Association of Retired Persons
Abortion
adolescents, 249
Canada, 286–287
fetal tissue research and transplants, 246
health effects, 286
prematurity due to multiple, 168
RU 486, *278*, 279
see also Miscarriage (spontaneous abortion)
Absenteeism
employee fitness-wellness programs, effect of, 111
Absinthe
hallucinations, 164
Abuse, *see* Child abuse and neglect
Accidents
eye injuries, 276
softball base sliding injuries, 318
Accutane, *see* Isotretinoin
ACE inhibitors, *see* Angiotensin-converting enzyme inhibitors
Acesulfame potassium
artificial sweetener, 307
Acetaldehyde
alcohol-cancer link, 282
Acetaminophen
aspirin substitute, 50, 57
medicine cabinet supplies, 218
Acetylsalicylic acid
aspirin, 47–48
Aci-jel
yeast infections, 190
Acitretin
psoriasis, 238
Acne
isotretinoin, 180, 236–238
sunlight, 9–10
Acquired immune deficiency syndrome, *see* AIDS
ACS, *see* American Cancer Society
Actigall, *see* Ursodiol
Acute nonlymphocytic leukemia
mitoxantrone, 299
Acyclovir
chicken pox, 231
herpes, 319
ADA, *see* American Dental Association
Addiction
cocaine treatment, 266–267, 305
famous persons, 163–165
nervous system, 253–255
nicotine, 256, 322
see also Alcoholism; Drug abuse
Adenomatous polyps
colorectal cancer, 263
Adipocytes
fat cells, 120
Adolescents
abortion consent, 249
AIDS, 201
aspirin risks, 57
asthma, 97
hospitalized, 188
obesity, 128
older parents, 149
Adoption
manic-depression, 139
obesity, 121
schizophrenia, 303
Adrenal glands
Parkinson's disease, 255
Adrenaline, *see* Epinephrine

Adult respiratory distress syndrome (ARDS)
skeletal trauma, 249
Advertising
aspirin as heart attack preventive, 54–56
childhood obesity, 125
meat, 38–39
tobacco, Canada, 287–288, 323
tobacco, Nigeria, 329
tobacco, U.S., 322–323
Advil, *see* Ibuprofen
Aerobic exercise
dance, 80–82, 88–90, 91–93
walking, 290
Aerosol pentamidine, *see* Pentamidine
Affluence, *see* Socioeconomic conditions
Africa
AIDS, 328
hypertension, 329
Rift Valley fever, 329
smoking, 329
Age
adult chicken pox, 230–231
AIDS and HIV infection, 243
allergies, 96, 97, 102, 103
asthma, 97
cancer death rates, 256
cancer screening, 227–229, 264
child abuse victims, 193
delayed childbearing, 144–155
fluoridation for adults, 195, 326
impotence, 234
long-term-care insurance, 69
mammography, 227, 260
maternal, and prematurity, 168
pernicious anemia, 183
shoulder problems in middle age, 250–251
smoking habits, 256
toilet training, 224
under 30, trauma as cause of death, 249
see also Aging and the aged; specific age groups
Aging and the aged, 240–242
air pollution, 269
cancer death rates, 255
dental implants, 213
depression and suicide, 135
heatstroke, 269
long-term care, 58–69
Medicare Catastrophic Coverage Act, 283–285
periodontitis, 326
right-to-die cases, 209, 247
sibling relationship, 23
skin, 6, 14, 236, 237–238, 321
sunstroke, 13
see also Age; Medicare
Agriculture, U.S. Department of
beef grading and labeling, 39, 41
AIDS, 242–246
allergies, 103
Canadian experimental drug policy, 288
children, 199–201
drug abuse, 265–266, 267, 327–328
experimental drugs, 180, 201, 288, 297–298
premature infants, 170
saliva, 326–327
sexually transmitted diseases, relationship to, 319, 320
tissue research, 247
U.S. government policies, 267, 285–286
worldwide epidemic, 327–328

Air Canada
smoking regulations, 322
Airlines
smoking restrictions, 322
Air pollution
drought and heat wave, 269–273
lead, 316
sources, 272–273
Alar, *see* Daminozide
Alberta
abortion, 287
nurses' strike, *287*, 288
Albuterol
allergies and asthma, 101
Alcohol consumption
absinthe hallucinations, 163
cancer, 282
coronary heart disease, 292
impotence, 234
manic-depression symptoms, 141
maternal, prematurity due to, 168
recommended limitation, 306, 309
stroke, 252
worldwide affluence, 329
see also Alcoholism
Alcoholic hepatitis
medications and drugs, 294
Alcoholics Anonymous, 267
Alcoholism
famous persons, 160, 165
folic-acid deficiency, 183
ALD, *see* Assistive listening device
Allergies, 94–103
aspirin, 56–57
eczema, 314
infant colic, 184–185
photosensitive reactions, 7, 14
toilet training, 225
vaginal itching, 189
Alpha-interferon
genital warts, 298, 321
Kaposi's sarcoma, 245, 299
leukemia, 298, 299
lymphoma, 281
Alprazolam
anxiety, 138
Alveolar bone loss
flurbiprofen, 326
Alzheimer's disease
dementia, 240
family stress, 61
genetic engineering, 281
genetics, 240–241
long-term-care insurance, 69
transmission, 241
AMA, *see* American Medical Association
Amblyopia
retinopathy of prematurity, 276
American Academy of Pediatrics
circumcision, 315
dance as therapy, 92
American Association of Retired Persons
long-term-care planning, 59, 60
American Cancer Society
cancer, early detection, 226, 227
colorectal cancer screening, 263–264
mammography, 260
Pap tests, 227
American College of Obstetricians and Gynecologists
malpractice insurance, 204–205
oral contraceptives and breast cancer, 310
Pap tests, 227

American Dental Association
back teeth fillings, 327
fluoride, 196
aerobic exercise, 82, 93
American Heart Association
cardiovascular deaths, 50
dietary fat and cholesterol, 36, 177
American Home Products Corporation
Dalkon Shield, 277
American Medical Association
AIDS treatment, 244
allergy testing, 99
obstetrical malpractice, 206
smoking, 325
American Psychiatric Association
electroconvulsive therapy, 198
Amish
manic-depression, 139–140
Amitriptyline
depression, 138
Amniocentesis
delayed first pregnancy, 152
Down's syndrome, 282
sonography, 311
Amphetamines
impotence, 234
Amputation
leg, blood vessel blockage in, 297
Anabolic steroids, *see* Steroids
Anafranil, *see* Clomipramine
Analgesics
medicine cabinet supplies, 218
see also specific analgesics
Anaphylactic reaction
allergies, 97, 101
Anatomy of Melancholy, The, 131
Anemia, 181–183
HIV-infected blood transfusions, 328
premature infants, 172
see also Sickle-cell anemia
Anencephaly
babies' organ transplants, 247
Anesthesia
dental implants, 214
electroconvulsive therapy, 198
Angina pectoris
aspirin, 53
silent ischemia, 292
Angioplasty, balloon, *see* Balloon angioplasty
Angiotensin-converting enzyme inhibitors (ACE)
hypertension, 300
kidney disease, 261
Animals
allergies, 96, 100
Lyme disease, 78–79
Q fever, 329
Anisakis simplix
intestinal infections, 264–265
Ankylosing spondylitis
aspirin, 50
diclofenac, 302
Anorexia nervosa
infertility, 150
St. Catherine of Siena, 165
Ansaid, *see* Flurbiprofen
Antacids
medicine cabinet supplies, 219
Antibiotics
cattle-growth stimulation, 44
cefuroxime axetil, 298
Lyme disease, 73, 78
meningitis, 312
mupirocin, 298
photosensitive reaction, 7
sexually transmitted diseases, 319

strep infection, 212
topical, 218
yeast infections, 189
Antibodies
AIDS, 243, 244, 245
allergies, 96, 98, 99
anemia, 182
chicken pox, 230
hepatitis, 294
herpesvirus, 313
HIV, 201
Sjogren's syndrome, 223
Anticancer drugs, *see*
Chemotherapy
Anticoagulants
aspirin, interaction with, 56
Antidepressant drugs
cocaine addiction, 266
fluoxetine, 301
impotence, 234
manic-depression, 140, 141–
142, 198
Anti-Drug Abuse Act of 1988,
267–268
Antifungal agents
ringworm, 299
yeast infections, 189–190, 299
Antigens
allergies, 96
rheumatic fever, 211
Antihistamines
allergies, 100
colds, 219
Anti-inflammatory drugs
nonsteroidal, 302, 326
Anti-oncogenes, *see* Genetics
Anxiety
dance, reducing with, 92
dental visits, 327
depression, 134, 138
exercise, reducing with, 242
impotence, 234
locus coeruleus, 304
side effect, drug, 138
toilet training, 224, 225
tranquilizing drugs, 138
see also Stress, emotional
Apnea
premature infants, 169
Apo-Ranitidine, *see* Ranitidine
Apples
daminozide, 309–310
Apraclonidine
glaucoma laser surgery, 303
Archer, Bill
Medicare Catastrophic Coverage
Act, 284
ARDS, *see* Adult respiratory
distress syndrome
Arms
trauma treatment, 250
Arotinoid ethyl ester
antitumor, 238
Arsenic poisoning
Napoleon Bonaparte, 163
Arteries, *see* Atherosclerosis;
Coronary arteries
Arteriography
penile, 235
Arthritis
allergies, 103
aspirin, 48, 50, 56, 218
dance therapy, 93
Lyme disease, 72, 77
medications and drugs, 302–
303, 326
rotator cuff tear, 250–251
Sjogren's syndrome, 221, 222
sunlight, 9
Arthrography
knee diagnosis, 250
shoulder diagnosis, 250–251
Arthroplasty
shoulder reconstruction, 251
Arthroscopy
knee diagnosis, 250
Artificial feeding
bioethics, 208–209, 247

Artificial heart
U.S. government programs,
293–294
Artificial insemination
older women, 150, 152
Artificial sweeteners, *see*
Sweeteners, artificial
Asbestos
lung cancer, 229
malignant mesothelioma, 317
Asia
AIDS, 328
Aspirin, 46–57
coronary artery restenosis, 289
heart attack victims, 291
medicine cabinet supplies, 218
Reye's syndrome link, 218, 231
rheumatic fever, 211
stroke prevention, 252
sunburn, 13
tainted, 220
Assistive listening device (ALD)
hearing loss, 265
Astemizole
allergies, 100
Asthma
air pollution, 273
allergies, 97
aspirin, 57
dance therapy, 93
steroids, 313
sunlight, 9
tests, 99
AT&T Communications
employee fitness-wellness
programs, 111–112, 116
Atherosclerosis
impotence, 234, 235
nutrition and diet, 306
smoking, 322
Athletics, *see* Sports
Ativan, *see* Lorazepam
Atopic dermatitis, *see* Eczema
Australia
lead, levels in children, 274
Autoimmune diseases
diabetes, 260–262
hemolytic anemia, 181–182
HIV-related, 199–201
Prosorba Column, 295–296
Sjogren's syndrome, 221–223
Automobiles, *see* Gasoline; Seat
belts
Autopsy
in history, 158, 160, 162
Awards
cancer research, 257, 258–260
Axid, *see* Nizatidine
Azidothymidine
AIDS, 201, 244
FDA regulations, 180
AZT, *see* Azidothymidine

B

Babies, *see* Infants
Bach, Johann Sebastian
cause of death, 162
Back
employee fitness-wellness
programs, 106, 111
Bacon
dietary fat, 45
Bacteria
chicken pox skin infection, 231
children with AIDS,
susceptibility to, 199, 200
Lyme disease, 73–75
salad bar contamination, 232–
233
sexually transmitted diseases,
319–320
streptococcus, 210–211, 212
tooth decay, 194
vaccines, 298, 317–318
vaginal balance, 190
see also specific bacteria and
bacterial diseases

Bactroban, *see* Mupirocin
Baked goods
food allergies, 103
oat bran, 177
recommended intake, 306
Baldness
minoxidil, 302
Soviet mystery disease, 329
Ballet dancers
aerobic exercise, 85, 89, 90
ovulation problems, 150
Balloon angioplasty
blocked blood vessels, 240, 297
coronary arteries, 289
heart attack, 291
Balloon valvuloplasty
heart valves, 240, 289–290
Ballroom dancing, 83, 90
Band-Aids
medicine cabinet supplies, 220
Barbiturates
impotence, 234
Basal cell carcinoma, 8–9
Baseball, *see* Softball
Base sliding
injuries, 318
Basophils
allergies, 97
Bathrooms
medicine cabinet, 220
safety devices for the
handicapped, 29
toilet training, 224–225
Battered child syndrome, *see*
Child abuse and neglect
Baulieu, Etienne-Emile
RU 486, 278
Bayer AG
aspirin, 48
B cells (B lymphocytes)
AIDS, 199, 200
Beaches
sunscreens, 10
Beclomethasone
allergies and asthma, 101
Beef, 35–45
saturated fat, 306
Beefalo, 40
Beef Industry Council
advertising campaign, 39
Beethoven, Ludwig van
ailments and autopsy, *161,*
162–163
Behavior
abused child, 193
allergies changing, 103
cancer prevention, 256
delayed childbearing, life-style
changes and, 147–149
diabetes and life-style, 261, 262
drug abuse, 305
hospitalized children, 188
hospital visitor, 186–188
infant colic, 184–185
life-style modification, wellness
programs, 104–117
manic-depression, 130–143
maternal life-style and
prematurity, 168
neuropsychology, 216
obesity and life-style, 125, 126
obsessive-compulsive, 301
sibling competition, 16–23
stroke and life-style, 251
toilet training regression, 225
Type A, 134, 289
Behavioral therapies
cocaine addiction, 266–267,
305
impotence, 235
liquid protein diet, 307–308
Bellini, Vincenzo
liver abscess, 162
Bennett, William
antidrug program, 268
Bentsen, Lloyd
Medicare Catastrophic Coverage
Act, 284–285
Benzophenes
sunscreens, 10

Bereavement
immune system, 304
Bergasol
tan accelerator, 15
Berol USA
employee fitness-wellness
program, 177
Beta-amyloid
Alzheimer's disease, 241
Beta blockers
hypertension, 293
Beta-carotene
lung cancer prevention, 256
Beta-interferon
leukemia, 281
lymphoma, 281
Bilirubin
jaundice, 170
Bioethics, 246–249
premature infants, 174
right-to-die cases, 207–209
Biogen Inc.
pig growth hormone, 39
Biological response modifiers
cancer treatment, 257–258
Biopsy
cancer, 228
Sjogren's syndrome, 223
Biotechnology, *see* Genetic
engineering
Bipolar disorder, *see* Manic-
depression
Birth control, *see* Family planning
Birth control pills, *see* Oral
contraceptives
Birth defects
AIDS, 199–201, 266
chicken pox, 231
congenital syphilis, 320
delayed childbearing, 152
drug side effects, 180, 237–238
phenylketonuria, 283
premature infants, 170–172
prenatal tests, 152, 282
retinoids, 180, 237, 238
Birth order
sibling rivalry, 18
see also Only children
Birth rate
older women, 149–150
Black, G. V.
fluoridation, 194
Black, Sir James W.
Nobel Prize, 259
Blacks
hypertension drugs, 300
prostate cancer risk, 229
sickle-cell anemia, 182, 314
skin and ultraviolet light, 9
Bladder, urinary
cancer risk factors, 229
toilet training, 224–225
Bleeding
anemia, 181, 183
aspirin hazards, 56, 57
dressings, 220
genital, and IUDs, 278
newborn infant's brain, 170
nose, 222
rectal, 202
skeletal trauma, 249, 250
see also Hemophilia
Blepharospasm
botulinum toxin, 276
Blindness, *see* Visual impairment
Blisters
herpes, 319
Blood
aspirin and platelet buildup, 54
stool, 170, 227, 228, 256, 264
see also Anemia; Bleeding;
specific blood component
Blood clots
artificial heart valves, 300
aspirin, 51
fat embolism syndrome, 249
medications and drugs, 291
oral contraceptives, 251
stroke, 251–252

Blood pressure
dance, lowering with, 82
debrisoquine, 281–282
employee fitness-wellness
  programs, lowering with, 111
exercise, lowering with, 242
impotence, 234, 235
Blood pressure, elevated, *see*
  Hypertension
Blood sugar
diabetes, 262
exercise, lowering with, 242
Blood transfusions
AIDS, 243, 328
children with AIDS, 200
non-A, non-B hepatitis, 294
premature infants, 170, 172
Blood vessels
allergies, 97
aspirin, 52–54
hemorrhoids, 202–203
lasers for blocked, 297
penile erection, 234, 235
retinopathy of prematurity, 171,
  275
ultraviolet light, 6, 14
**Blue Cross and Blue Shield
  Association**
employee fitness-wellness
  programs, 111, 116
B lymphocytes, *see* B cells
B19 parvovirus
fifth disease, 317
Body temperature, *see*
  Temperature, body
Boerhaave, Hermann
autopsy, 158
Bone cancer
genetics, 281
Bone marrow
anemia, 181, 182, 183
sickle-cell anemia, 314
transplants, 183, 314
Bones, 249–251
dental implants, 213–214
periodontal loss, 326
retinoids, 237
see also Osteoporosis
Book **(Kempe),** 165
Borellia burgdorferi
Lyme disease, 74
Boric acid
yeast infections, 190
Borowski, Joe
Canadian abortion policy, 287
Borysenko, Joan
psychoneuroimmunology, *304*
Boswell, James
gonorrhea, 158
Bottle-feeding, *see* Infant formula
Botulinum toxin
eye squint and eyelid spasm,
  276
Bovine collagen
wrinkles and scars, 321
Bowel
hemorrhoids, 202–203
laxatives, 219
Sjogren's syndrome, 222
toilet training, 224–225
ulcerative colitis, 302
see also Stools
Bradykinin
pain, 49
Brahms, Johannes
liver cancer, 162
Braille, 30, 33
Brain, 251–255
Alzheimer's disease, 240
death, 207, 247
dyslexia, 215–216
electroconvulsive therapy, 198
encephalitis, 231
exercise, effect of, 242
fetal tissue transplants, 246, 255
HIV transmission to, 244
mental illness, sites linked to,
  304
see also Anencephaly; Brain
  damage; Strokes

Brain damage
cerebral palsy, 253
children with AIDS, 200
lead, 316
mental illness, 304
obstetrical malpractice, 205–
  206
premature infants, 170
stroke, 252
Bran, *see* Oat bran
Brazil
AIDS, 244
Bread, *see* Baked goods
Breakfast cereals
oat bran, 176–177
Breast cancer
chemotherapy, 256, 257
fenretinide, 238
genetics, 281
mammography, 227, 260, 284
mitoxantrone, 299
oral contraceptives, 310, *311*
pregnancy, 151
risk factors, 229
RU 486, 279
screening, 226, 227, 229, 260
Breast-feeding
allergy protection, 103
cancer prevention, 314–315
childhood obesity prevention,
  126–127
HIV transmission, 201, 328
infant colic, 184
older child's jealousy, 21
premature infants, 169
Breathing abnormalities
premature infants, 169, 171–
  172
wheezing, 97, 102, 313
Britain, *see* Great Britain
British Columbia
abortion, 286
doctors' fees, 289
Bronchodilators
allergies and asthma, 101, 313
Bronchopulmonary dysplasia
premature infants, 174
Bronx (N.Y.)
children with AIDS, 201
Burgdorfer, Willy
Lyme disease, 73–74
Burkitt's lymphoma
Jason Gaes, 258
Burton, Robert, 131
Bypass surgery
coronary artery, 240, 300
penile, 235

C

Calamine lotion, 218–219
chicken pox, 231
Calcium
dietary recommendations, 309
Calcium antagonists, *see* Calcium
  blockers
**Calcium blockers (calcium
  antagonists)**
stroke, 253
California
cigarette tax, 323
colorectal cancer and genetics
  study, 263–264
human tissue ownership, 247
Salmonella-infected eggs, 264
syphilis, 320
California State University
aerobic benefits of dance, 88
Calories
dance, burned by, 90
dietary recommendation, 309
fat, 177, 306, 309, 318
meat and poultry, 36, 37
obesity, 121–129
Canada
abortion, 286–287
AIDS, 244, 288

alcoholic hepatitis study, 294
aspirin trademark, 48
astemizole, 100
asthma research, 313
carotid surgery study, 252
children with AIDS, 199
dyslexia testing and programs,
  216, 217
employee fitness-wellness
  programs, 106, 111
experimental drugs, 245, 288
fluoridation, 195
gelatin matrix implant (Fibrel),
  321
government drug approval
  procedure, 178, 288
government policies and
  programs, 283–286
greenhouse effect, 270–272
Huntington's disease screening,
  282
Lyme disease, 75
medications and drugs, 288,
  298, 299
Q fever, 329
smoking regulations, 287, 322,
  323
tobacco advertising ban, 287–
  288
tretinoin, 236
Canada Life Assurance Company
employee fitness-wellness
  program, 111
**Canadian Cooperative Study
  Group**
aspirin and stroke study, 50, 53
Cancer, 255–260
alcohol, 282
allergies, 103
anti-oncogenes, 259, 280
asbestos, 317
breast-feeding, lowering risk
  with, 314–315
daminozide, 309–310
dietary fat and cholesterol, 36
early detection, 226–229
employee fitness-wellness
  programs, preventing with, 111
head and neck tumors, 266
infertility, 150–151
medications and drugs, 299
nuclear wastes, 273
nutrition and diet, 256, 306
retinoids, 236, 237, 238
see also Carcinogens;
  Chemotherapy; specific types
  of cancer; specific organs and
  tissues
Candida albicans
yeast infections, 189–190, 299
Canesten, *see* Clotrimazole
Cannell, John J., *259*
Canthaxanthin
tanning pills, 15
Caplan, Elinor
Ontario healthcare costs, 288
Capua, Raymond de, 165
Carbamazepine
mania, 138, 142
Carbohydrates
government recommendations,
  309, 318
Carbon dioxide
greenhouse effect, 270–272
Carcinogens
asbestos, 317
daminozide, 309–310
nuclear waste, 273
ultraviolet light, 6–9
Carcinoma, *see* Cancer
Cardiac arrhythmia, *see* Heartbeat,
  abnormal
**Cardiopulmonary resuscitation
  (CPR)**
heart attacks, 291
Cardiovascular disorders, *see*
  Coronary heart disease; Heart
  attack; Heartbeat, abnormal;
  Strokes
Caries, dental, *see* Tooth decay

Carotid endarterectomy
stroke, 252
Cataracts
cornea transplant, 277
famous persons, 162
ultraviolet light, 7, 15, 315
Catastrophic health insurance act,
  see Medicare Catastrophic
  Coverage Act
Catatonia
electroconvulsive therapy, 197
Cats
allergies, 96, 100, 101
Q fever, 329
CAT scan, *see* CT scan
Cattle, *see* Meat; Milk and milk
  products
Cavernosography
impotence, 235
Cavities, tooth, *see* Tooth decay
CDC, *see* Centers for Disease
  Control
Ceftin, *see* Cefuroxime axetil
Cefuroxime axetil
respiratory infections, 298
Centers for Disease Control, U.S.
AIDS, 243, 285
chancroid, 319
children with AIDS, 199, 200,
  201
fitness-wellness programs, 107
fluoridation, 196
Lyme disease, 75
measles vaccine, 315
nuclear waste, 273
Salmonella-infected eggs, 264
Central nervous system, *see* Brain;
  Nervous system
Ceramics
lead, 317
Cereals
oat bran, 176–177
Cerebellum
encephalitis, 231
Cerebral palsy
Christopher Nolan, 253
obstetrical malpractice, 205–
  206
Cervical cap, 278–279
Cervix, uterine
barrier contraceptives, 278–279
cancer, early detection, 226–
  227, 229
cancer, risk factors, 229
cancer and infertility, 150
prematurity due to
  abnormalities, 168
Cesarean deliveries
malpractice, 204
older mothers, 154–155
CFCs, *see* Chlorofluorocarbons
Chagas' disease
garbled DNA, 282
Challenge tests, *see* Inhaled
  challenge; Oral challenge
Chancroid, 319
Chemoprevention
cancer, 256
Chemotherapy
anemia, 183
breast cancer, early, 257
head and neck cancer, 266
leukemia, 299
multidrug resistance, 256–257
Chenix, *see* Chenodiol
Chenodiol
gallstones, 302
Chernobyl nuclear accident
mysterious children's disease,
  329
Chewing gum
nicotine, 322
xylitol, 326
Chiaie, Stephano
fluoridation, 194
Chianina, 40
Chicken, *see* Poultry
Chicken pox, 230–231
children with AIDS, 200
Reye's syndrome, 57, 218

Child abuse and neglect, 191–193
  premature babies, 174
  toilet training, 224
Childbirth
  aspirin, 49, 56
  delayed first pregnancy, 151–155
  HIV transmission, 200–201
  malpractice, 204–206
  postpartum depression, 165
  RU 486 and labor induction, 279
Children, 312–315
  AIDS, 199–201, 243, 328
  allergies and asthma, 94, 96, 97, 103, 313–314
  aspirin risks, 57, 218
  cancer, 227, 258, 259, 266, 280
  chicken pox, 230–231
  cholesterol, 293
  cochlear implants, 266
  congenital syphilis, 320
  diabetes, 260
  dyslexia, 215–217
  eye injuries, 276
  fifth disease, 317
  fluoridation, 194–196, 325
  Hib bacteria vaccine, 298, 317–318
  hospitalized, 188
  hospital visits by, 186
  idiopathic thrombocytopenic purpura, 295
  immune system, 305
  lead poisoning, 274, 316–317
  Lyme disease, 71–79
  medications and drugs, 298
  medicine cabinet safety, 218, 220
  nutrition and diet, 309
  obesity, 118–129
  older parents, 149
  rheumatic fever, 210–212
  sibling rivalry, 16–23
  Soviet mystery disease, 329
  sun exposure, 12–13
  toilet training, 224–225
  tooth decay, 325
  visual impairment, 259, 275–277, 280
  see also Adolescents; Child abuse and neglect; Infants; Newborn infants
China
  RU 486, 279
  smoking, 329
Chlamydia
  spermicides, 319
Chlordiazepoxide
  anxiety, 138
Chlorofluorocarbons
  greenhouse effect, 270
Cholera
  epidemic, *328,* 329
Cholesterol
  alcohol, 292
  atherosclerosis and impotence, 234
  children, 293
  dance, lowering level with, 82
  employee fitness-wellness programs, lowering level with, 111
  gallstones, 295, 302
  meat, 35–41, 45
  oat bran, lowering level with, 176–177
  oil labeling, 307
  retinoids, 237
  saturated fats, 306–307, 318
Chopin, Frederic
  tuberculosis, 160
Chorea
  rheumatic fever, 211
  see also Huntington's disease
Chorionic villus sampling
  delayed first pregnancy, 152
  Down's syndrome, 282
  sonography, 311

Chromosomes
  chromosome 5 and colorectal cancer, 281
  chromosome 5 and schizophrenia, 303
  chromosome 21 and Alzheimer's disease, 241
  manic-depression, 130–143
  miscarriage, 152
Chronic lymphocytic leukemia, 182
Churchill, Winston
  manic-depression, 132
CIC, *see* Circulating immune complexes
Cigarette smoking, *see* Smoking
Cimetidine
  allergies, 100
  peptic ulcers, 302
Cipro, *see* Ciprofloxacin
Ciprofloxacin
  chancroid, 319
Circle K Corporation
  employee medical coverage, 112
Circulating immune complexes (CIC)
  Prosorba Column, 295–296
Circulatory system, 289–294
Circumcision
  benefits, 315
  HIV transmission preventive, 244
Cirrhosis, liver
  hepatitis, 294–295
  worldwide increase, 329
Cis-platinum
  head and neck cancer, 266
Civil liberties
  AIDS, 201, 245–246, 285
  random drug testing, 267
Clean Water Act
  lead, 274
Climate, *see* Weather
Clomipramine
  obsessive-compulsive disorder, 301
Clostridium perfringens
  food poisoning, 233
Clothing
  yeast infections, 190
Clotrimazole
  yeast infections, 189
CMVIG, *see* Cytomegalovirus immune globulin
Cocaine
  AIDS, 265
  nervous system effects, 253–254, 305
  treatment, 266–267, 305
Cocaine Anonymous, 267
Cochlear implants
  hearing loss, 265–266
Coconut oil
  saturated fat, 307
Colchicine
  cirrhosis, 294
Colds
  asthma, 313
  home remedies, 219
Coleridge, Samuel Taylor
  opium use, 165
Colic, 184–185
Colitis
  mesalamine, 302
Colon
  ulcerative colitis, 302
  see also Stools
Colon cancer
  genetics, 260, 262–263, 281
  insoluble fiber, 176
  risk factors, 229
  screening, 226, 227, 228, 229, 256, 264
Colostomy
  premature infant, 171
Common cold, *see* Colds

Communication
  computer aid, 30
  dance therapy, 92
Commuter railroads
  smoking regulations, 322
Complexion
  ultraviolet light, 9, 229
Computerized tomography, *see* CT scan
Computers
  cancer research database, 257
  learning disabilities, 30
  video display terminals, 315–316
Conditioned responses, *see* Behavioral therapies
Condoms
  AIDS, 244, 286, 319, *320*
  effective use, 319
Congress, U.S.
  AIDS legislation, 246, 285
  Medicare Catastrophic Coverage Act, 283, 284–285
  smoking regulations, 322
  tobacco lobby, 323
Conjunctivitis
  allergies, 97
  premature infants, 170
Connecticut
  fifth disease, 317
  Lyme disease, 72, 73, 75
Connective tissue
  Sjogren's syndrome, 221–222
Conroy, Claire
  right-to-die case, 208–209
Consent documents
  electroconvulsive therapy, 198
  living will, *208,* 209
Constipation
  fiber, dietary, 176
  hemorrhoids, 202–203
  laxatives, 219
  Sjogren's syndrome, 222
  toilet training, 225
Consumer Products Safety Commission
  tanning machines, 14
Consumers and consumer protection
  meat grading and labeling, 41–45
  nursing homes, 63–64
  tanning machines, 14
Consumers Union
  long-term-care insurance, 68–69
Contact dermatitis
  patch test, 99
Contact lenses
  corneal replacement, 277
Continuing care community
  elderly, 69
Contraceptives, *see* Family planning; Oral contraceptives
Control Data Corporation
  employee fitness-wellness program, 107, 111, 112, 114–115
Cooking, *see* Food preparation
Cornea
  transplant, 277
  ultraviolet light, 7, 12, 15
Coronary arteries
  clot dissolvants, 291
  fish oil pills, 289
  restenosis, 289
  silent ischemia, 292
Coronary artery bypass surgery
  artificial heart valves, blood clot prevention in, 300
  elderly, 240
Coronary heart disease
  affluence and rising European incidence of, 328
  alcohol, 292
  aspirin, 47, 50–56
  children, prevention in, 293
  dietary fat and cholesterol, 36, 306
  employee fitness-wellness programs, 106, 111

  exercise, prevention with, 242
  Henry VIII, 161
  smoking, 293
  stroke, 252
  Type A, B personality, 289
CorTemp, 301
Cortex
  schizophrenia, 304
Corticosteroids
  allergies and asthma, 101
  see also Steroids
Cosmetics
  allergies, 96, 99
  photosensitive reaction, 7
  sunscreens, 10
  see also Toiletries
Costs of healthcare, *see* Healthcare costs
Council on Dental Materials
  back teeth fillings, 327
Couney, Martin
  neonatal intensive care, 167
Counseling, *see* Psychotherapy
Coxiella burnettii
  Q fever, 329
CPR, *see* Cardiopulmonary resuscitation
Crabbe, George
  opium use, 165
Crack
  AIDS, 265
  nervous system effects, 254
  prostitution, 320
Craven, Lawrence L.
  aspirin and heart attack, 51
Crib death, *see* Sudden infant death syndrome
Cromolyn sodium
  allergies, 100–101
Crossbreeding
  livestock, 40
Crossed eyes
  botulinum toxin, 276
  retinopathy of prematurity, 276
Crying, *see* Tears
Cryotherapy
  hemorrhoids, 203
  retinopathy of prematurity, 171, 275–276
CT scan
  joint fracture repair, 251
  premature infants, 170
Customs Service, U.S.
  drug testing, 267
CVS, *see* Chorionic villus sampling
Cyclo-oxygenase
  aspirin inhibition, 49
Cyclophosphamide
  anemia, 182
Cyclosporine
  diabetes, 260, 261
Cyclothymia, 133
Cytomegalovirus immune globulin (CMVIG)
  immune system, 298
Cytomegalovirus infections
  ganciclovir, 245, 298
Cytotoxic testing
  food allergies, 99
Cytovene, *see* Ganciclovir

D

Dairy products, *see* Milk and milk products
Dalkon Shield, 277
Dallas, Andrea Maddox
  aerobic dance benefit, 91
Dallas Independent School District
  employee fitness-wellness program, 111
Dam-Burst of Dreams, 253
Daminozide
  apples, 309–310

Damminix
 Lyme disease, 79
Dance, 80–93
Dance/movement therapy, 92–93
Dapsone
 anemia, 182
Darwin, Erasmus, 137
Database, *see* Computers
Datril, *see* Acetaminophen
Day care
 child abuse and neglect, 191
 elderly, 59
Daylight, *see* Sunlight
Daytop Village (Rockaway, N.Y.),
 266
ddC, *see* Dideoxycytidine
Deafness, *see* Hearing loss
Dean, H. Trendley
 fluoridation, 195
Death and dying
 anencephalic infants and organ
  transplants, 247
 bereavement, 304
 famous people's causes, 156–
  165
 heart attack, 291
 organ life extension, 248–249
 right-to-die cases, 207–209,
  247
Death certificates
 tobacco use, 325
Death rates
 AIDS, 243
 alcoholic hepatitis, 294
 aspirin overdose, 57
 breast cancer, 310
 cancer, 226, 255, 262–263
 cardiovascular disorders, 36,
  50–51, 53–54
 depressives' suicides, 134–135
 dietary factors, 286, 306
 electroconvulsive therapy, 198
 heart disease, 252, 328
 heat wave, 269
 hypertension, men using
  medication, 293
 lung cancer, 316
 maternal and older pregnancy,
  155
 meningitis, 312
 sickle-cell anemia and bone
  marrow transplants, 314
 skin cancer, 9
 stroke, 251, 252
 trauma, 249
Debrisoquine
 toxic reactions, 281–282
Decay, tooth, *see* Tooth decay
Decongestants
 allergies, 100
 colds, 219
Deer
 Lyme disease, 73, 75, 79
Defense Nuclear Facilities Safety
 Board
 toxic wastes, 273
Defibrillator
 heart attacks, 291
Dementia
 Alzheimer's disease, 240
Dementia praecox, *see*
 Schizophrenia
Dental implants, 213–214
Dental surgery
 AIDS, 326
 implants, 213–214
Dental survey
 fear of dentist, 327
Dentistry, *see* Teeth and gums
Deodorants, *see* Toiletries
Deoxyribonucleic acid, *see* DNA
Depo-Provera
 injectable contraceptive, 279
Depression, 130–143
 allergies, 103
 brain lesions, 304
 electroconvulsive therapy, 197–
  198
 exercise, reducing with, 242
 immune system, 304

impotence, 234
medications and drugs, 138,
 140, 141–142, 301
Parkinson's disease, 255
postpartum, 165
sunlight, 9
De Quincey, Thomas
 opium use, 165
Dermatology, *see* Skin
DES, *see* Diethylstilbestrol
Desipramine
 cocaine addiction, 266
Developing countries, *see* World
 health news
Dexamethasone
 meningitis, 312
Diabetes, 260–262
 exercise, 242
 fetal tissue transplants, 246, 261
 impotence, 234
 maternal, prematurity due to,
  168
 nutrition and diet, 306
 oral medications and aspirin
  interaction, 56
 pregnancy, 153–154
 stroke, 251
 yeast infections, 189
Diagnosis
 AIDS, 245
 allergies, 98–99
 autoimmune hemolytic anemia,
  182
 cancer, 226–229, 260, 264
 chicken pox, 230
 children with AIDS, 199–200,
  201
 food allergies, 103
 historical figures' illnesses, 156–
  165
 HIV, 200, 245
 impotence, 234–235
 joint problems, 250–251
 Lyme disease, 71–72, 77–78
 manic-depression, 141
 rheumatic fever, 211
 Sjogren's syndrome, 221, 222–
  223
 sonography, 310–311
Diama Dam (Africa)
 Rift Valley fever, 329
Diaper rash
 petroleum jelly, 218
Diaphragm
 cervical cap comparison, 278–
  279
Diarrhea
 cholera, 329
 fish parasites, 265
 medicine cabinet supplies, 219
 Salmonella-infected eggs, 264
 toilet training, 225
Diclofenac
 arthritis, 302–303
Dideoxycytidine (ddC)
 AIDS, 244
Diet, *see* Nutrition and diet
Diet and Health
 National Research Council
  report, 306, 318
Diethylstilbestrol (DES)
 side effects, 180
Diet pills
 abuse, 254
Digestive system, 262–265
 cancer drugs, 299
 food intolerance and allergies,
  102–103
 infant colic, 184–185
 medications and drugs, 302
 medicine cabinet supplies, 219
 premature infant, 170–171
 Sjogren's syndrome, 221, 222
Dihydroxyacetone
 tan accelerator, 15
Dipyridamole
 blood clots and artificial heart
  valves, 300
Dirty Dancing **(movie),** 84

Disabled persons, *see*
 Handicapped persons
Discharge, vaginal
 yeast infection, 189
Disco dancing, 90
Discrimination
 AIDS, 201, 245–246, 267, 285
Dissociation
 trauma, 305–306
Diuretics
 hypertension, 293, 300
DNA
 alcohol-cancer link, 282
 kinetoplastids, 282
Doctors, *see* Physicians
DOE, *see* Energy, U.S.
 Department of
Dopamine
 depression, 304
 manic-depression, 140
 Parkinson's disease, 255, 301
Down's syndrome
 Alzheimer's disease, 241
 delayed childbearing, 152
 prenatal testing, 152, 282
Doxepin
 depression, 138
Dresser, Heinrich
 aspirin, 48, 49
Dressings
 medicine cabinet supplies, 220
Drinking, *see* Alcohol
 consumption; Alcoholism
Drought
 greenhouse effect, 270–272
Drug abuse, 265–268
 AIDS, 245, 327–328
 female AIDS victims, 201, 244
 impotence, 234
 literary figures, 165
 manic-depression symptoms,
  141
 maternal, prematurity due to,
  168
 nervous system effects, 253–
  255, 305
 treatment, 305
Drugs and medications, *see*
 Medications and drugs;
 specific medications
Dry mouth
 drugs and side effects, 138, 142
 radiation therapy, effect of, 266
 Sjogren's syndrome, 221–223
Duncan, Isadora
 modern dance, 85
Durable power of attorney, 209
Dust
 allergies, 96, 97, 100, 101
Dyes
 skin, 15
Dying, *see* Death and dying
Dyslexia, 215–217
Dysphagia
 head and neck cancer surgery,
  266
Dysthymia, 133

E

Eager, J. M.
 fluoridation, 194
Earle, James, 158
Ears, 265–266
 Sjogren's syndrome, 222
 see also Hearing loss
Eating habits, *see* Nutrition and
 diet
Eating problems, *see* Anorexia
 nervosa
ECG, *see* Electrocardiogram
Eclampsia
 delayed childbearing, 153
ECM, *see* Erythema chronicum
 migrans
Economics, *see* Healthcare costs;
 Socioeconomic conditions

ECT, *see* Electroconvulsive therapy
Ectopic pregnancy
 IUDs, 278
 laparoscopy, 312
 sonography, 311
Eczema
 food allergies, 94–96, 314
Edelman, Toby
 nursing homes, 64
Edison, Thomas
 dyslexia, 217
Education
 children with AIDS, 201
 developmental disabilities and
  prematurity, 174
 dyslexia, 216 -217
 parenthood, 193
 toilet training, 224–225
Eggs
 allergies, 103, 314
 Salmonella, 264
Einstein, Albert
 dyslexia, 217
Ejaculation, 234
Elavil, *see* Amitriptyline
Elbow
 trauma treatment, 250
Eldepryl, *see* Selegiline
Elderly population, *see* Aging and
 the aged
Electrocardiogram
 portable machine, 291, 292
 silent ischemia, 292
Electroconvulsive therapy, 197–
 198
 manic-depression, 140, 143
Electronic fetal monitoring
 malpractice fears, 204, 205
Electroshock therapy, *see*
 Electroconvulsive therapy
Elion, Gertrude B.
 Nobel Prize, 257, 258–259
El Niño
 heat wave, 270, 272
Embolism, *see* Fat embolism
 syndrome
Emergency medical treatment
 heart attacks, 291
 hospital, 13
 medicine cabinet supplies, 218–
  220
Emery, Lynne
 dance benefits, 88, 89, 91
Emotional abuse
 children, 191, 193
Emotions
 dance and well-being, 92–93
 dissociation, 305–306
 parents of premature infants,
  172–173
 sibling rivalry, 16–23
 silent ischemia, 292
 sunlight, 9
 see also Stress, emotional
Employment
 drug testing, 267
 fitness-wellness programs, 104–
  117
 smoking policy, 287, 322
 see also Occupational safety
  and health
Employment Assistance Programs,
 115
Encephalitis
 chicken pox, 231
Endometriosis
 infertility, 150
 laparoscopy, 312
 RU 486, 279
Endometrial cancer
 early detection, 227–228
 risk factors, 229
Endorphins
 exercise, 91
Energy, U.S. Department of
 nuclear plants hazards, 273
Environmental Protection Agency
 (EPA)
 daminozide, 309–310
 global warming, 271

lead, 274
Lyme disease, 79
radon, 256, 316
Environment and health, 269–274
lead, 316–317
obesity, 125
radon, 316, *317*
Sjogren's syndrome, 223
Enzymes
anemia, 182
EPA, *see* Environmental Protection
Agency
Epidemics
AIDS, 242–246, 285–286, 327–
328
cholera, *328*, 329
Epiglottitis
meningitis, 298
Epikeratophakia
cornea transplant, 277
Epinephrine
anaphylactic reactions, 98
EPO, *see* Erythropoietin
Erection
impotence, 234–235
Erythema chronicum migrans
(ECM)
Lyme disease, 72–78
Erythema nodosum
Mozart, 162
Erythrocytes, *see* Red blood cells
Erythropoietin
anemia, 181, 182–183
Esophagus
cancer, 256
Estrogen
breast cancer, 256
impotence, 234
oral contraceptives and strokes,
251–252, 310
women's skills, 281
Ethics, *see* Bioethics
Etretinate
birth defects, 237
skin disorders, 237, 238
Europe
AIDS, 327–328
diseases of affluence, 328–329
Euthanasia
right-to-die cases, 209
Exercise
childhood obesity, 128, 129
dance, 80–93
diabetes, 242, 261, 262
elderly, 242
employee fitness-wellness
programs, 104–117
handicapped persons, 32–33
heat-sensitive pacemaker, 296–
297
infertility, 150
silent ischemia, 291–292
walking, 290
Experimental drugs
AIDS-related, 180, 201, 244–
245, 288, 297–298
FDA approval, 180
External fixators
leg fractures, 249–250
Eye cancer
genetics, 259, 280
ultraviolet light, 7
Eyes, 275–277
AIDS-related infections, 245,
298
allergies, 97
glaucoma surgery, 303
medications and drugs, 245,
298, 303
premature infants, 170, 171
protection, 12, 14–15, 315
retinoblastoma, 259, 280
Sjogren's syndrome, 221–223
video display terminals, 315–
316
see also Cataracts; Visual
impairment

F

Fallopian tubes
ectopic pregnancy, 278, 311,
312
infertility, 150
laparoscopy, 312
False teeth, *see* Dental implants
Familial colonic polyposis
genetics, 263
Family
care for aging, 58–69
child abuse and neglect, 191–
193
children with AIDS, 201
consent documents, 198, 209
delayed childbearing, *144*, 146–
147
manic-depression, 137–140
medicine cabinet, 218–220
obesity, 125–127
right-to-die cases, 208–209
sibling rivalry, 16–23
see also Genetics; Parents
Family planning, 277–279
delayed first pregnancy, 144–
155
sterilization, 312
see also Oral contraceptives
Farsightedness
epikeratophakia, 277
Fast food
nutritious alternatives, 128
Fat, body
cells, 120–121
dance, 82
see also Obesity
Fat, dietary
cancer, 256, 262
childhood obesity, 127, 128,
129
meat and poultry, 35–45
obesity, 309
recommended allowance, 177,
306, 309, 318
stearic acid, 306–307
stroke, 251
Fat embolism syndrome
fracture complication, 249
Fathers
child abuse and neglect, 192–
193
older fathers, 147–149
Fatty acids
saturated fats, 306
Faulkner, William
alcohol abuse, 165
FDA, *see* Food and Drug
Administration
Fear, *see* Anxiety
Federal Cigarette Labeling and
Advertising Act, 325
Federal Trade Commission
aspirin advertising, 56
Feed Materials Production Center
(Fernald, Ohio)
toxic wastes, 273
Female health, *see* Obstetrics and
gynecology; Pregnancy;
Women
Feminine hygiene sprays
yeast infections, 189
Fertility, *see* Infertility; Pregnancy
Fertility drugs
multiple births, 155
Fetus
chicken pox, 231
deaths and stillbirth, 153
electronic monitoring, 204, 205
HIV transmission, 200–201
Lyme disease, 78
prenatal tests, 152, 282, 310–
311
tissue transplants, 246, 255, 261
Fever
aspirin, 49

Fiber, dietary
cancer prevention, 256, 262
hemorrhoids, 202
oat bran, 176–177
supplements, 306
U.S. surgeon general's
recommendations, 306, 309,
318
Fibrel, *see* Gelatin matrix implant
Fibroids
delayed childbearing, 154
Fibronectin
periodontal disease, 326
Fifth disease, 317
First aid
heart attacks, 291
medicine cabinet supplies, 218–
220
Firstborn, *see* Birth order; Only
children
Fish
allergies, 103
raw, intestinal infections from,
264–265
Fish oils
coronary artery reblockage, 289
Fitness, *see* Physical fitness
Fitzgerald, F. Scott
cause of death, 160
5-fluorouracil
head and neck cancer, 266
Florida
no-fault obstetrical insurance,
206
right-to-die cases, 207–208
syphilis, 320
Flu, *see* Influenza
Flunisolide
allergies and asthma, 101
Fluoride, 194–196
Sjogren's syndrome, 223
tooth decay prevention, 325–
326
U.S. surgeon general's
recommendations, 309
Fluoxetine
depression, 138, 142, 301
Flurbiprofen
periodontal bone loss, 326
Folic acid
pernicious anemia, 183
Folk dancing, 88, 92
Folk medicine
salicin, 48
Fonda, Jane
aerobic dance videos, 82
Food allergies, 94, 96, 99, 102–
103
eczema, 314
Food and Drug Administration
acesulfame potassium (Sunette),
307
AIDS-related drugs, 179, 180,
245
alpha-interferon, 321
aspirin-cardiovascular link, 53,
56
botulinum toxin, 276
cervical cap, 278
cytotoxic self-test kits, 99
drug approval procedure, 178–
180
erythropoietin, 182–183
flurbiprofen, 326
gelatin matrix implant (Fibrel),
321
lead in ceramics, 317
medical technology, 295–297
medications and drugs, 297–
301
methamphetamine, 254
oil labeling, 307
oral contraceptives, 310
ParaGard IUD, 277
Prosorba Column, 295
raw fish parasite, 264
retinoids, 237–238
sunscreens, 10
tanning products, 14, 15

Food contamination
apples, 309–310
eggs, 264
fish, 264–265
lead in ceramic dishware, 317
salad bar, 232–233
Food intolerance, 102
Food poisoning
food allergy confused with, 102
Reiter's syndrome, 103
salad bar, 232–233
symptoms, 233
Food preparation
egg safety, 264
fish safety, 264
meat, 45
oat bran, 177
salad bar safety, 232–233
Foods, *see* Nutrition and diet;
specific foodstuffs
Forest fires
heat wave and drought, 270
Forests
greenhouse effect, 270, 272
Formula, infant, *see* Infant formula
Fractures
treatment, 249–250
France
RU 486, 279
tan accelerator, 15
Fraternal twins
delayed pregnancy incidence,
155
Freezing, *see* Cryotherapy
Friedreich's ataxia
genetics, 281
Fruits
daminozide in apples, 309–310
recommended intake, 306, 318
salad bar, 233
FTC, *see* Federal Trade
Commission
Fungus
yeast infections, 189–190, 299
Furadantin, *see* Nitrofurantoin

G

Gaes, Jason, 258
Galaburda, Albert M.
dyslexia study, 216
Gallstones
medications and drugs, 295,
302
Games
handicapped persons, 33
Gamma globulin
children with AIDS, 201
Ganciclovir
AIDS-related eye infection, 245,
298
Gardner's syndrome
genetics, 263
Garner, James
beef advertising, 39
Gas, intestinal
infant colic, 184–185
see also Heartburn
Gasoline
emissions pollution, 272, 316
Gastroesophageal reflux
premature babies, 174
Gastrointestinal tract, 262–265
aspirin intolerance, 56–57
fiber, dietary, 176
folic acid deficiency, 183
food allergies and intolerance,
102, 314
infant colic, 184–185
medicine cabinet supplies, 219
premature infants, 170–171
see also Digestive system
Gauguin, Paul
absinthe hallucinations, 163

Gelatin matrix implant
  wrinkles and scars, 321
Gender
  aspirin and stroke prevention,
    252
  dental visit anxiety, 327
  depression incidence, 133, 139
  hormones and skill differences,
    281
  rheumatic fever incidence, 211
  sibling rivalry, 20, 21
  Sjogren's syndrome, 222
  toilet training, 224
**General Motors Cancer Research
  Foundation**
  awards, 259–260
Genetic engineering, 280–283
  alpha-interferon, 298
  cancer, 256, 257–258
  diabetes, 261
  erythropoietin, 182–183
  interferon, 321
  meat products, 37–38, 39–41
Genetics, 280–283
  allergies, 94
  Alzheimer's disease, 240–241
  anemias, 181–183
  colorectal cancer, 259–260,
    262–263
  diabetes, 261
  dyslexia, 216
  manic-depression, 137–140
  Marfan's syndrome, 163
  obesity, 121, 124–125
  personality, 303
  rheumatic fever, 210
  schizophrenia, 303
  sickle-cell anemia, 182, 314
  skin cancer, 257
  stroke, 251
  thalassemia, 183
Genital ulcers
  HIV transmission, 244
  sexually transmitted diseases,
    319
Genital warts
  alpha-interferon, 298, 321
Gentian violet
  yeast infections, 190
George III
  insanity, 158–159
George Washington University
  aspirin research, 50
Gerhardt, Charles Frédéric
  acetylsalicylic acid, 47
Geriatrics, *see* Aging and aged
German measles, *see* Rubella
Geschwind, Norman
  dyslexia study, 216
Gestational diabetes
  delayed pregnancy, 154
Gingivitis
  decrease, 326
GI tract, *see* Gastrointestinal tract
Glands
  Sjogren's syndrome, 221–223
  see also specific glands
Glaucoma
  laser surgery medication, 303
  retinopathy of prematurity, 276
Gleason, Jimmie
  obstetrics and malpractice, 204–
    205, 206
Global warming, *see* Greenhouse
  effect
Glucose
  diabetes, 261–262
  stroke, 253
Glucose-6-phosphate kinase
  anemia, 182
Glutathione
  chemotherapy resistance, 257
Goggles
  Sjogren's syndrome, 223
  tanning machines, 14–15
Golde, David W.
  human tissue ownership issue,
    247, *248*

Gonorrhea
  antibiotic-resistant, 319–320
  historical figures, 158
  spermicides, 319
Gout
  aspirin, 56
**Government policies and
  programs, Canadian,** 286–289
  drug approval procedure, 178
  dyslexia testing and programs,
    216–217
  tobacco advertising ban, 323
**Government policies and
  programs, U.S.,** 283–286
  AIDS, 245–246
  artificial heart, 293–294
  drug abuse, 267
  dyslexia testing and programs,
    216–217
  egg inspection and grading, 264
  environmental, 273–274
  FDA approval procedure, 178–
    180
  fetal tissue transplants, 246
  meat grading and labeling, 41–
    45
  nutrition reports, 306, 309, 318
  smoking restrictions, 322
  see also Law; specific
    governmental bodies
Goya, Francisco
  lead poisoning, 163
Grading, meat, *see* Labeling
Graft procedures, *see*
  Transplantation of organs and
  tissues
Graham, Martha
  modern dance, 85
Grasses, *see* Trees and grasses
Great Britain
  AIDS, 328
Greenhouse effect, 270–272
Greyhound Canada
  smoking restrictions, *323*
Groupe Roussel Uclaf
  RU 486, 279
Growth hormones
  lean meat, 39–40
Guided immunology, *see*
  Psychoneuroimmunology
Guided tissue regeneration
  periodontal disease, 326
Gum, *see* Chewing gum
Gums, *see* Periodontal disease;
  Teeth and gums
Gynecology, *see* Obstetrics and
  gynecology
Gyne-Lotrimin, *see* Clotrimazole
GynoPharma
  ParaGard IUD, 277–278

H

Habits, *see* Behavior
Haemophilus b conjugate vaccine
  Haemophilus influenzae type b
    infection, 298
Haemophilus ducreyi
  chancroid, 319
**Haemophilus influenzae type b
  (Hib) bacteria**
  vaccine, 298, 317–318
Hahn, Lorrain
  ballroom dancing, 88–89
Hair, *see* Baldness
Haldol, *see* Haloperidol
Hallucinations
  absinthe, 163–164
  electroconvulsive therapy, 197
  medieval mystics, 165
**HALO (Health Awareness/Lifestyle
  Orientation),** 112–114, 116
Haloperidol
  psychosis, 138

Hamburgers
  dietary fat and cholesterol, 38,
    39, 45
Hand
  trauma treatment, 250
Handel, George Frederick
  cataracts and stroke, 162
Handicapped persons
  Christopher Nolan, 253
  dance, 92
  technological aids, 24–33
  see also specific handicapping
    condition
**Hanford nuclear power plant
  (Wash.)**
  toxic wastes, 273
Harris, Elaine
  Sjogren's syndrome, 221, 223
Harvard University
  beta-carotene studies, 256
  Physicians' Health Study
    Research Group, 52–53, 54
Hay fever, 96, 97
HDLs, *see* High-density
  lipoproteins
Head
  tumors, 266
Headaches
  allergies and migraines, 103
**Health and Human Services, U.S.
  Department of**
  Ethics Advisory Board, 246
  fetal cell transplants, 246
Healthcare costs
  antibiotic-resistant gonorrhea,
    320
  Canadian government policies,
    288, 289
  children with AIDS, 201
  dental implants, 213
  nursing home, 60–61, 67–69
  obstetrical malpractice, 204
  premature infants, 174
  unhealthy life-styles, 106–107,
    109, 111, 112, 117
  U.S. government policies, 283–
    285
**Health Care Financing
  Administration, U.S.**
  nursing homes, 164
Health facilities
  elderly people, 59–69
  workplace, 104–117
  see also Hospitals
Health insurance
  employee fitness-wellness
    programs, 106–116
  HIV screening, 246
  long-term care, 67–69
  see also Medicare
**Health Insurance Plan of Greater
  New York (HIP)**
  mammography study, 260
Health maintenance organizations
  employee fitness-wellness
    programs, 107, 114–116
Health personnel
  HIV infection, 244
  home aides for the elderly, 59–
    60
Health promotion programs, *see*
  Physical fitness
Hearing aids
  types and innovations, 265–266
Hearing loss
  famous persons, 162
  lead, 316
  meningitis, 312–313
  technological aids, 265–266
Heart, 289–294
  Lyme disease, 72, 76
  rheumatic fever, 210, 211–212
  transplants, 247, 301
  see also Coronary heart disease;
    Heart attack; Heartbeat,
    abnormal; Heart defects;
    Heart rate; Heart valves
Heart attack
  aspirin and streptokinase, 291
  aspirin prevention, 51–52, 53

  balloon angioplasty, 291
  blood clot dissolvants, 291
  cocaine, 254
  employee fitness–wellness
    programs, prevention with,
    111–112, 113
  oral contraceptives, 293
  risk, alcohol as lowering, 292
  sudden death, emergency
    prevention of, 291
  Type A survival rate, 289
  women, 292, 293
Heartbeat, abnormal
  cocaine, 254
  pacemaker, 296–297
Heartburn
  aspirin, 56
  medicine cabinet supplies, 219
Heart defects
  premature infants, 171–172
Heart disease, *see* Coronary heart
  disease
Heart rate
  exercise target, 82, 93
Heart valves
  balloon valvuloplasty, 289–290
  surgical replacement, 240, 300
Heatstroke
  heat wave deaths, 269
Heat wave
  greenhouse effect, 269–271
Hemingway, Ernest
  alcohol abuse, 165
Hemoglobin
  anemia, 181, 182, 183
Hemolytic anemia, 181–182
Hemophilia
  AIDS transmission, 328
  aspirin hazard, 56
  children with AIDS, 201
Hemorrhages, *see* Bleeding
Hemorrhagic stroke
  aspirin treatment, 52–53
Hemorrhoids, 202–203
  anemia, 183
  fiber, dietary, 176
  Napoleon Bonaparte, 163
Hennekens, Charles H., *52*
Henry VIII
  cause of death, 161
Hepatitis
  virus, 294, 319
Herbicides, *see* Pesticides and
  herbicides
Hereditary spherocytosis
  anemia, 182
Heredity, *see* Genetics
Hernia, *see* Inguinal hernia
Heroin
  AIDS, 263, 265, 266, 267
Herpes simplex viruses
  acyclovir, 319
Herpesvirus
  chicken pox, 230
  roseola, 313
Herpes zoster, *see* Shingles
Heterosexuality
  AIDS, 243–244, 265, 328
  syphilis rate, 320
  see also Prostitution
Hib bacteria
  Haemophilus influenzae
    conjugate vaccine, 298
Hib TITER, *see* Haemophilus b
  conjugate vaccine
High blood pressure, *see*
  Hypertension
High-density lipoproteins (HDLs)
  alcohol, 292
  oat bran, 177
HIP, *see* Health Insurance Plan of
  Greater New York
Hip
  fracture treatment, 250
Hippocrates
  aspirin, 48
  depression, 131
Hismanal, *see* Astemizole

Histamine
allergies, 97, 103
see also Antihistamines
Historical persons
causes of death, 156–165
Hitchings, George H.
Nobel Prize, *257,* 258–259
HIV (human immunodeficiency virus)
AIDS, 242–246
breast-feeding, transmission of, 201, 328
British heterosexuals, 328
children with AIDS, 199–201
condoms, 319
see also AIDS
HIV-II (human immunodeficiency virus type two)
characteristics, 242–243
Hives
allergies, 97, 102
aspirin-related, 57
HMOs, *see* Health maintenance organizations
Hoffmann, Felix
aspirin, 48, *49*
Home care
AIDS, 285
elderly, 59–60, 69
Medicare coverage, 283–284
Home medical tests
cancer detection, 226, 227, 228
cytotoxic kits, 99
diabetes blood glucose levels, 262
HIV antibody, 245
Home medicine cabinet, 218–220
Homosexuality
syphilis rate, 320
see also AIDS
Hormones
allergy, 96
animal, growth, 39–40
contraceptives, 277, 279
electroconvulsive therapy, 198
gender-linked skills, 281
see also specific hormones
Hospice care
Medicare coverage, 283
Hospitals
AIDS patients, 245
Canadian government policies, 288
emergency room treatment, 13
HIV transmission, 244
Medicare reimbursement, 283–284
neonatal intensive care, 167–168, 173
obstetrical malpractice, 206
visitors, 186–188
Hostility
sibling, 16–23
Hudson Institute
AIDS study, 243
Human immunodeficiency virus, *see* HIV, HIV-II
Humidity
sunstroke, 13
Huntington's disease
screening program, 282
Hyaline membrane disease, *see* Respiratory distress syndrome
Hydrocephalus
premature infants, 170
Hydrocortisone
hemorrhoids, 202–203
medicine cabinet supplies, 218
Hypertension
affluence and worldwide incidence, 329
medications and drugs, 293, 299–300
pregnancy, 54, 152–153, 168
stroke, 251
Hypnosis
posttraumatic stress disorder, 306
Hypomania, 133, 134

Hypothalamus
electroconvulsive therapy, 198
prostaglandin production, 49
Hypothermia
internal thermometer, 301
sunstroke, 13
Hysteria
medieval mystics, 165
Hytrin, *see* Terazosin

I

Ibuprofen
aspirin substitute, 50, 57
medicine cabinet supplies, 218
Ice
polar melting, 271
sprain swellings, 220
Idiopathic thrombocytopenic purpura (ITP)
Prosorba Column, 295–296
IgE, *see* Immunoglobulin E
IgG, *see* Immunoglobulin G
Imagery
mental illness, 304
musculoskeletal problems, 250–251
Imipramine
depression, 138
Immune system
allergies, 96, 103
anemias, 182, 183
aspirin, 47, 50
chicken pox, 231
children with AIDS, 199–201
mind, 304–305
premature infants, 170
Prosorba Column, 295–296
rheumatic fever, 211
sickle-cell anemia, 314
Sjogren's syndrome, 221–223
tissue research, 246
ultraviolet light effect, 6–7
see also AIDS
Immune therapy
allergies, 101
cancer, 256, 257–258
Immunization
chicken pox, 231
measles, *313,* 315
see also Vaccines
Immunoglobulin E (IgE)
allergies, 96, 99, 102
Immunoglobulin G (IgG)
Prosorba Column, 295–296
Immunoglobulins
children with AIDS, 200
Immunosuppression
cytomegalovirus immune globulin, 298
Medicare coverage, 284
Impetigo
mupirocin, 298
Implants
adrenal medullas for Parkinson's disease, 255
contraceptive, 279
dental, 213–214
ear, 265–266
insulin pumps, 262
penile, 235
skeletal trauma, 250
wrinkles and scars, 321
Impotence, 234–235
Incubator
premature babies, 169, 173
India
cholera epidemic, *328,* 329
Indians, American
Pima Indians, obesity in, 124
Pueblo, malignant mesothelioma in, 317
Indigestion, *see* Heartburn

Indocin IV, *see* Indomethacin
Indomethacin
premature infants, 172
INDs (investigational new drugs), *see* Experimental drugs
Infant formula
AIDS, 328
allergies, 103
colic, 185
premature infants, 169
Infants
AIDS, 199–201, 266, 328
anencephalic organ transplants, 247
breast-feeding and cancer prevention, 314–315
colic, 184–185
eye muscle surgery, 276
fluoride, 196
food allergies, 102, 103
haemophilus b conjugate vaccine, 298
measles vaccine, *313,* 315
medicine cabinet supplies, 218
obesity prevention, 126–127
premature, 166–174
roseola, 313
seat belts, 314
see also Newborn infants
Infection
chicken pox complication, 231
children with AIDS, 199–201
genital tract and sexual dysfunction, 234
medications and drugs, 297–299
penile prostheses, 235
premature infants, 168, 170
toilet training, 225
urinary tract and circumcision, 315
wound, 218
yeast, 189–190, 299
Infertility
delayed pregnancy, 149–151
internal thermometer, 301
sperm allergy, 96
vaginal ultrasound, 311
Inflammation
allergies, 94–96
aspirin, 49–50
rheumatic fever, 211–212
shinsplints, 82
Influenza
aspirin risk, 57
Informed consent, *see* Consent documents
Infrared coagulation
hemorrhoids, 203
Inguinal hernia
premature infants, 173
Inhaled challenge
allergy/asthma testing, 99
Inhalers
allergies and asthma, 100–101
Inheritance, *see* Genetics
Insanity, *see* Mental health
Insecticides, *see* Pesticides and herbicides
Insects
bite and sting allergies, 96, 101
food contamination, 233
global warming, 272
Insoluble fiber
gastrointestinal system, 176
Insulin
diabetes, 260–262
Medicare coverage, 284
Insulin-dependent diabetes mellitus (Type I diabetes), 260, 261
Insurance, *see* Health insurance; Liability
Intal, *see* Cromolyn sodium
Integrated Genetics, Inc.
Huntington's disease screening, 282

Intensive care
neonatal, 167–168, 173, 174
visitors, 188
Intercourse
AIDS transmission, 201, 244, 328
condoms, 319
impotence, 234–235
vaginal dryness, 221, 222, 223
yeast infection, 189, 190
Interferon
genital warts, 298, 321
Kaposi's syndrome, 245, 299
leukemia and lymphoma, 281, 298, 299
Interleukin-2
cancer, 257
Intermediate care facility, 61
Intestines, *see* Digestive system
Intrauterine device (IUD)
infertility, 150
ParaGard, 277–278
Intravenous drug users, *see* Drug abuse
Intron A, *see* Alpha-interferon
In vitro fertilization
multiple births, 155
vaginal ultrasound, 311
Iopidine, *see* Apraclonidine
Ireland
fluoridation, 195
Iron
anemia, 181, 183
dietary requirement, 36, 309
Ischemia, *see* Silent ischemia; Transient ischemic attacks
Islets of Langerhans
transplants, 261
Isocarboxazid
depression, 138
Isotretinoin
acne, 236, 238
birth defects, 180, 237–238
FDA labeling requirement, 180, 238
skin cancer, 238, 256
Isotrex, *see* Isotretinoin
Itching
allergies, 97
chicken pox, 230, 231
eczema, 314
hemorrhoids, 202
yeast infections, 189, 190
ITP, *see* Idiopathic thrombocytopenic purpura
IUD, *see* Intrauterine device
IVF, *see* In vitro fertilization
Ixodes ticks
Lyme disease, 74, 76

J

Jarvik-7 artificial heart
funding, 293–294
Jaundice
newborn infants, 169–170
Jaw
bone loss, 326
dental implants, 213
Jealousy
sibling, 16–23
toilet training regression, 225
Jobes, Nancy Ellen
right-to-die case, 209
Joffrey, Robert, 93
Johnson, Virginia E.
AIDS and heterosexuals, 243
impotency, 235
Johnson & Johnson
employee fitness-wellness program, 111, 116, 117
Joints, 249–251
rheumatic fever, 211
Sjogren's syndrome, 221
see also Arthritis

Juvenile rheumatoid arthritis
Lyme disease, 72

K

Kansas
malpractice and obstetrician
shortage, 204–205
Kaposi's sarcoma
experimental drugs, 245, 299
Keats, John
opium use, 165
tuberculosis, 159–160
Kelvin 500 pacemaker
heat–sensitive, 296–297
Kempe, C. Henry
child abuse and neglect, 191
Kempe, Margery
hysteria and postpartum
depression, 165
Ketoconazole
yeast infections, 190
Kidneys
anemia, 182–183
aspirin hazards, 56
diabetes, 261
lead, 316
Mozart's death, 162
transplants, 298
Kinetoplastids
garbled DNA, 282
King Broadcasting Co.
employee fitness–wellness
program, 117
Knees
arthography and arthroscopy,
250
Knudson, Alfred G., Jr.
cancer research award, 259
Koop, C. Everett, *285*
abortion, 286
nutrition report, 286, 306, 309,
318
smoking, 322
Kraepelin, Emil
manic–depression, 133

L

Labeling
aspirin, 53, 57
cigarettes, 287, 322, 325
isotretinoin, 180, 238
meat, fat content, 36, 41–45
oil, saturated fat content, 307
Labor (childbirth)
aspirin, 48, 56
delayed pregnancy, 154
RU 486, induction with, 279
Lacrisert
Sjogren's syndrome, 223
Lactose
intolerance, 102
Lamb, 37, 38, 42
Landmark College (Putney, Vt.)
dyslexia, 217
Language, *see* Communication
Laparoscopy
obstetrics and gynecology, 312
Large intestine, *see* Colon
Larynx
cancer, 256
Lasers
blocked blood vessels, 296, 297
glaucoma surgery, 303
hemorrhoid therapy, 203
Latex
condoms, 319
Law
abortion legislation, 249
AIDS, 246, 285
Anti-Drug Abuse Act, 267–268
cancer research, 256

child abuse and neglect, 191
cigarette warning labels, 325
consent documents, 198, 209
dyslexics' protection, 217
Federal Cigarette Labeling and
Advertising Act, 325
Medicare Catastrophic Coverage
Act, 283–285
nontreatment of the dying, 246–
247
obstetrical malpractice, 205
right-to-die cases, 207–209
Safe Drinking Water Act, 274
smoking regulations, Canada,
287
smoking regulations, U.S., 322
video display terminals, 316
see also Congress, U.S.;
Government policies
and programs, Canadian;
Government policies and
programs, U.S.
Laxatives
hemorrhoids, 203
medicine cabinet supplies, 219
LDLs, *see* Low-density lipoproteins
L-dopa
anemia, 182
Parkinson's disease, 301
Lead poisoning
ceramics, 317
children, 274, 316–317
Goya's death, 163
Learning disabilities
computer aids, 31
dyslexia, 215–217
Legs
blocked blood vessels, 297
bone fractures, 249–250
paralysis treatment, 250
softball base-sliding injuries, 318
Legumes
cholesterol lowering, 176, 177
Lens (glasses)
implant, 277
protective, 14–15, 277
sunglasses, 12, 317
Lesions, brain
depression, 304
Leukemia
anemia, 182
children, 227
genetics, 281
medications and drugs, 281,
298, 299
risk factors, 229
tissue research, 247
Levodopa, *see* L-dopa
Lewis, Sinclair
alcohol abuse, 165
Liability
obstetrics, 204–206
tobacco industry, 325
Librium, *see* Chlordiazepoxide
Life-style, *see* Behavior;
Socioeconomic conditions
Life-sustaining treatment
organs for transplants, 246,
247–249
premature infants, 167–174
right-to-die cases, 207–209,
247
Light, *see* Sunlight; Ultraviolet
light
Light treatment, *see* Phototherapy
Lincoln, Abraham
manic–depression, 132
Marfan's syndrome, 163
Lipoproteins, *see* High-density
lipoproteins; Low-density
lipoproteins
Liquid protein diet
weight loss, 307–308
Lisinopril
hypertension, 300
Lithium
manic–depression, 138, 140,
142
Liver, 294–295
aspirin hazards, 56

disorder, as cause of famous
people's death, 162
missing enzyme and drug
reactions, 282
newborn infants, 170
retinoids, toxicity of, 237
soluble fiber, 176
tanning pills, 15
yeast infection medication, 190
Livestock, *see* Meat; Milk and milk
products; Poultry
Living will, *208*, 209
Lobbying
tobacco industry, 323
Locus coeruleus
depression, 304
**Loma Linda University Medical
Center**
anencephalic infants, 247
Lorazepam
anxiety, 138
Lothery, Cliff
dance, 91
Lotion, *see* Calamine lotion
Low-density lipoproteins (LDLs)
oat bran, 177
smoking, 322
Low-fat diet
cancer, 256, 262
children, 125–129
oat bran, 176–177
recommendations, 306, 309,
318
workplace, 116
Low-impact aerobics, 82
Lubricants
condoms, 319
Ludiomil, *see* Maprotiline
Luken, Thomas
tobacco advertising, 325
Lung cancer
beta-carotene, 256
death rates, 255
genetics, 281
liability suit, 325
radon, 256, 316
risk factors, 229
worldwide increase, 328
Lungs
children with AIDS, 200
ozone pollution, 272–273
premature infants, 169, 174
skeletal trauma, 249
see also Pneumonia;
Tuberculosis
Lupus, *see* Subacute lupus
erythematosus; Systemic lupus
erythematosus
Lyme disease, 70–79
Lymphatic system
chancroid, 319
Lymphocytes
children with AIDS, 199–200
saliva and AIDS transmission,
326–327
Sjogren's syndrome, 221, 223
tumor-infiltrating, 257
Lymphoid interstitial pneumonia
children with AIDS, 200
Lymphoma
genetics, 281
medications and drugs, 299

M

Macrophages
AIDS drugs, 244
**Magnetic resonance imaging
(MRI)**
muscoskeletal problems, 250–
251
Malaysia
tropical oils, 307
Male health, *see* Men
Malignant melanoma
ultraviolet light, 9, 12–13
warning signs, 9, 228

Malignant mesothelioma
asbestos, 317
Malpractice
obstetrics, 204–206
Mammography
early cancer detection, 227,
229, 256, 260, *311*
Medicare coverage, 284
Manic-depression, 130–143
electroconvulsive therapy, 197–
198
Schumann, Robert, 162
MAO inhibitors, *see* Monoamine
oxidase inhibitors
Maprotiline
depression, 138
Marfan's syndrome
Lincoln, Abraham, 163
Marplan, *see* Isocarboxazid
Martyrdom
medieval mystics, 165
**Massachusetts Eye and Ear
Infirmary**
anti-oncogenes, 280
Mast cells
allergies, 96–97, 100
Masters, William H.
AIDS and heterosexuals, 243
impotency, 235
Mauritania
Rift Valley fever, 329
Mayonnaise
bacterial growth, 233
McCarthy, Joseph R.
alcohol abuse, 165
McKay, Frederick S.
fluoridation, 194
McKee Baking Company
employee fitness-wellness
program, 117
Measles
children with AIDS, 200
vaccine, *313*, 315
Meat, 34–45
saturated fat, 307
Medicaid
home healthcare, 60
nursing homes, 67
Medical costs, *see* Healthcare
costs
Medical ethics, *see* Bioethics
Medical insurance, *see* Health
insurance
Medical malpractice, *see*
Malpractice
Medical technology, 295–297
artificial heart, 293–294
dental implants, 213–214
handicapped, aids for the, 24–
33
hearing aids, 265–266
heart pumping device, 248
implantable insulin pumps, 261–
262
musculoskeletal diagnosis and
treatment, 250–251
portable electrocardiogram, 291
see also names of specific
medical and surgical
techniques
Medical tests at home, *see* Home
medical tests
**Medicare Catastrophic Coverage
Act,** 67, 283–285
Medicare, U.S.
Catastrophic Coverage Act,
283–285
home healthcare, 60
mammography, 284
nursing homes, 67
Medications and drugs, 297–303
AIDS, 201, 244–245, 288, 297–
298
alcoholic hepatitis, 294
allergies, 100–101
alveolar bone loss, 326
anemia, 182, 183
antidepressants for drug
addiction, 266

aspirin, 46–57, 252, 289, 291
blood clot dissolving, 291
Canada, 288
cancer, 259, 266
cancer and premature
  menopause, 151
chicken pox, 231
diabetes, 260, 261
diabetes-linked kidney failure,
  261
eye problems, 276
expiration date, 220
FDA approval procedure, 178–
  180
fertility and multiple births, 155
hemorrhoids, 203
hypertension, 293
impotence, 234
infant colic, 185
interferons, 281, 298, 299, 321
manic-depression, 138, 140–
  142
Medicare coverage, 283, 284
medicine cabinet supplies, 218-
  220
photosensitive reaction, 7
retinoids, 236–238, 256
rheumatic fever, 211–212
RU 486, *278*, 279
skin, 321
stroke, 253
yeast infections, 189–190, 299
see also Side effects of
  therapeutic agents;
  names of specific drugs and
  specific disorders
Medicine cabinet, 218–220
Medieval mystics, 165
Melancholia, 131, 133
Melanin, 6, 15
Melanoma, *see* Malignant
  melanoma
Mellaril, *see* Thioridazine
Membranes
  anemia, 181–183
Memory
  Alzheimer's disease, 240
  electroconvulsive therapy, 143,
    198
  Parkinson's disease, 255
  stroke, 251
Men
  alcohol and coronary heart
    disease, 292
  aspirin-cardiovascular link, 51,
    53
  cancer tests, 228
  depressed elderly suicides, 135
  eye injuries, 276
  HIV risk, 244
  impotence, 234–235
  infertility, 151
  recommended nutrients, 36–37
  stroke, 252
  yeast infections, 190
  see also Fathers; Gender
Meningitis
  children with AIDS, 200
  dexamethasone, 312–313
  Lyme disease, 72, 76
  urinary tract infections, 315
  vaccines, 298, 317–318
Menopause
  endometrial tissue testing, 227–
    228
  premature, and cancer drugs,
    151
Menstruation
  anemia, 183
  effects on women's skills, 281
  hormone contraceptives, 279
  infertility, 150
  premenstrual syndrome, 96
  yeast infections, 189, 190
Mental health, 303–306
  abused child, 191, 193
  dance, 81, 91–93
  exercise, improvement with,
    242

historical figures, 159, 162,
  163–164
manic-depression, 130–143
medications and drugs, 301–
  302
psychiatric ward visitors, 188
Mental retardation
  dance therapy, 92
  Down's syndrome, 152, 241,
    282
  meningitis, 312
  phenylketonuria, 283
Mesalamine
  ulcerative colitis, 302
Mescaline
  Huxley, Aldous, 165
Metabolism
  quick weight loss and gain, 309
  obesity, 121–125
Metaprotenorol
  allergies and asthma, 101
Methacholine
  allergy testing, 99
Methadone
  AIDS prevention, 267
  heroin, 266
Methamphetamine, *see* Speed
Methane
  greenhouse effect, 270
Methyl tert-butyl ether
  gallstones, 295
Metolazone
  hypertension, 300
Metoprolol
  hypertension, 293
Metro Gel, *see* Metronidazole
Metronidazole
  rosacea, 299
Mice
  Lyme disease, 79
Michaels, Margaret Kelly
  child abuse, 191
Michigan
  fluoridation study, 195
Miconazole
  yeast infections, 189
Migraines
  allergies, 103
Milk and milk products
  allergies, 103, 314
  children's diet, 127
  fluoride supplements, 196
  infant colic, 184–185
  lactose intolerance, 102
  yogurt for yeast infections, 190
  see also Breast-feeding; Infant
    formula
Mind, *see* Behavior; Brain;
  Emotions; Mental health
Minnesota
  abortion consent law, 249
Minors, *see* Adolescents
Minoxidil
  baldness, 302
**Miscarriage (spontaneous
  abortion)**
  diethylstibesterol, 180
  fifth disease, 317
  older women, 152
  video display terminals, 316
Mites
  allergies, 101
Mitoxantrone
  leukemia, 299
Modern dance, 85, 89
Moisture Seekers, The, 223
Moisturizers
  medicine cabinet supplies, 218
  Sjogren's syndrome, 223
  sunlight, 11, 13
Mold
  allergies, 96, 101
  food contamination, 232–233
Moles, *see* Warts
Monistat, *see* Miconazole
Monoamine oxidase inhibitors
  depression, 138, 301
Mood, *see* Depression; Emotions
Mood-swing disorder, *see* Manic-
  depression

Moore, John
  human tissue ownership, 247,
    248
Mortality rates, *see* Death rates
Mosquitoes
  Rift Valley fever, 329
Mothers
  AIDS-infected children, 199–
    201
  infant colic, 185
  older mothers, 147–149
  see also Adoption; Breast-
    feeding; Parents; Pregnancy;
    Single parenthood
Mouth, *see* Dry mouth; Oral
  cancer; Teeth and gums
Mouth washes
  fluoride, 195, 196
Mozart, Wolfgang Amadeus
  terminal illness, 162
MRI, *see* Magnetic resonance
  imaging
Mucus
  hemorrhoids, 202
Mulroney, Brian
  abortion, 287
Multiple births
  delayed pregnancy, 155
  see also Twins
Multiple sclerosis
  impotence, 234
  manic-depressive symptoms,
    141
Mupirocin
  impetigo, 298
Muscle relaxants
  electroconvulsive therapy, 198
Muscles, 249–251
  dance, 81, 82, 89
  eyelid closure, 276
  infant colic, 185
  quick weight loss and gain, 309
Musset, Alfred de
  syphilis, 162
My Book for Kids With Cansur,
  258
Mycelex, *see* Clotrimazole
Myclo, *see* Clotrimazole
Myelography
  spinal cord diagnosis, 250–251
Mykrox, *see* Metolazone
Myopia, *see* Nearsightedness
Mysticism
  medieval martyrs, 165

N

Naftifine
  ringworm, 299
Naftin, *see* Naftifine
nAnB hepatitis, *see* non–A, non–B
  hepatitis
Napoleon Bonaparte
  cause of death, 163
Naproxen
  aspirin substitute, 57
Narcotics, *see* Drug abuse;
  specific kinds of narcotics
Nardil, *see* Phenelzine
Nasal congestion, *see* Nose
Nasalcrom, *see* Cromolyn sodium
Nasal smears
  allergy testing, 99
Nasal sprays
  allergies, 100, 101
  infection transmission, 219
  insulin, 262
National Academy of Sciences
  AIDS report, 245–246, 285
  dietary fat report, 35–36, 39,
    44–45
  see also Nutrition Research
    Council
**National Association of Insurance
  Commissioners**
  HIV screening, 246
National Cancer Act of 1971, 256

National Cancer Institute
  cancer prevention and
    treatment, 255, 256, 257
  oral contraceptives and breast
    cancer study, 310
National Cash Register Company
  employee fitness-wellness
    program, 112
**National Center for Health
  Statistics**
  cancer survey, 256
National Dance Association, 82
National Eye Institute
  retinopathy of prematurity, 275
National Health Interview Survey
  cancer survey, 256
**National Heart, Lung, and Blood
  Institute**
  heart attacks, 291
National Heart Savers Association
  saturated fats, 307
**National Institute of Child Health
  and Human Development**
  breast-feeding and cancer
    prevention, 314–315
**National Institute of Dental
  Research**
  saliva inhibition of AIDS virus,
    326–327
  tooth decay survey, 194, 325
National Institute of Drug Abuse
  cocaine use, 254
**National Institute of Mental
  Health**
  exercise, 91, 92
National Institutes of Health
  artificial heart, 293–294
  cervical cap, 278
  cochlear implants, 266
  dietary fat and cholesterol, 36
  diabetes and blood glucose
    control, 261
  fetal tissue transplants, 246
National Pork Producers Council
  advertising campaign, 38
National Research Council
  nutrition and health report, 306,
    318
Native Americans, *see* Indians,
  American
**Natural Resources Defense
  Council**
  daminozide, 309–310
NDAs (new drug applications), *see*
  Experimental drugs
Nearsightedness
  epikeratophakia, 277
  retinopathy of prematurity, 276
NEC, *see* Necrotizing enterocolitis
Neck
  tumors, 266
Necrotizing enterocolitis
  premature infants, 170–171
Needles
  AIDS-prevention exchange
    program, 245, 267
  drug users' sharing, AIDS and,
    265, 267, 327–328
  implantable insulin pump, 262
NEF, *see* Nutritional Effects
  Foundation
Neisseria gonorrhoeae
  antibiotics, 319–320
Neonatal intensive care unit, 167–
  168, 173, 174
Neonates, *see* Newborn infants
Nervous system, 251–255
  chicken pox complication, 230,
    231
  children with AIDS, 200
  fetal tissue transplants, 246
  Lyme disease, 72, 76
  medications and drugs, 301–302
  neuropsychology, 216
  premature infants, 170
  rheumatic fever, 211
Neurology, *see* Brain; Nervous
  system
Neuropsychology
  dyslexia, 216

Neurotic depression, 133
Neurotransmitters
depression, 304
drug abuse, 305
electroconvulsive therapy, 198
Newborn infants
AIDS, 199–201, 244, 266, 328
anencephalic, and organ
transplants, 247
circumcision, 315
colic, 184–185
congenital syphilis, 320
deaths, and maternal
hypertension, 153
food allergies, 103
low birth weight, 151, 153
phenylketonuria, 283
prematurity, 167–174, 275–276
New Brunswick
abortion, 287
New Jersey
right-to-die cases, 207, 208–209
tobacco liability suit, 325
New York City
AIDS, 201, 265, 266
children's cholesterol-lowering
experiment, 293
smoking restrictions, 322
syphilis, 320
right-to-die cases, 209, 247
Nicotine, *see* Smoking
Nicotine gum
smoking addiction, 322
Nigeria
cigarette advertising, 329
Nightingale, Stuart L.
FDA approval procedure, 1/8
NIH, *see* National Institutes of
Health
Nishizuka, Yasutomi
cancer research award, 259,
260
Nitrofurantoin
anemia side effect, 182
Nitrogen oxides
emissions limitation, 272
Nizatidine
peptic ulcer, 302
Nizoral, *see* Ketoconazole
NMDA blockers
stroke, 253
Nobel Prize
cancer research, *257,* 258–259
No-fault insurance
obstetrical malpractice, 206
Nolan, Christopher, 253
non-A, non-B hepatitis
virus, 294
**Non-insulin-dependent diabetes
mellitus (type II diabetes),**
261, 262
Nonoxynol-9
spermicide, 319
**Nonsteroidal anti-inflammatory
drugs**
arthritis, 302–303
periodontal bone loss, 326
Norepinephrine
depression, 304
Noristerat
injectable contraceptive, 279
Norpramin, *see* Desipramine
Northwest Airlines
smoking regulations, 322
Nose, 265–266
allergies, 97, 99, 100, 101
congestion, aspirin-related, 57
Sjogren's syndrome, 221, 222
sunburn, 12
Novantrone, *see* Mitoxantrone
Nova Scotia
Q fever, 329
Novocimetine, *see* Cimetidine
NRDC, *see* Natural Resources
Defense Council
NSAIDs, *see* Nonsteroidal anti-
inflammatory drugs
Nuclear magnetic resonance, *see*
Magnetic resonance imaging

Nuclear power
Chernobyl accident, 329
employee drug testing, 267
toxic wastes, 273
Nuprin, *see* Ibuprofen
Nurses
Alberta strike, *287,* 288
homecare for elderly, 59–61
Medicare coverage of services,
283–284
Nursing (lactation), *see* Breast-
feeding
Nursing homes, *58,* 61–68
Medicare coverage, 283–284
Nussbaum, Hedda
child abuse, 191, 192
Nutrients
meat, 36–37
see also specific kinds of
nutrients
Nutritional Effects Foundation
meat labeling, 44
Nutrition and diet, 306–310
affluence-linked diseases, 328
American Heart Association
recommendation, 36, 177
artificial feeding, 208–209, 247
cancer prevention, 256, 262,
281
childhood obesity, 125–129
employee food pavilions, 116
fluoride supplements, 196, 325
food allergies, 94–96, 97–98,
102–103, 314
hemorrhoids, 202
meat, 34–45
National Research Council
report, 306, 318
oat bran, 176–177
phenylketonuria, 283
premature infants, 169
retinopathy of prematurity, 276
salad bar safety, 232–233
stroke, 251
U.S. surgeon general's report,
286, 306, 309, 318
yeast infections, 190

O

Oat bran, 176–177
Oatmeal
cholesterol lowering, 176–177
Obesity
children, 118–129
dance, 92
diabetes, 242, 261, 262
employee fitness-wellness
programs, 107, 111
hemorrhoids, 202
high-fat diet, 309
liquid protein diet, 307–308
older women's pregnancy
complications, 154
stroke, 251
weight loss, approach to, 309
worldwide increase, 329
yeast infections, 190
Obsessive-compulsive disorder
clomipramine, 301
Obstetrics and gynecology, 310–
312
delayed first pregnancy, 144–
155
malpractice, 204–206
Pap test, 226–228
see also Childbirth; Pregnancy;
Women
Occupational safety and health
eye injuries, 276
fitness-wellness programs, 104–
117
nuclear weapons plants, 273
video display terminals, 315–
316
worksite allergies, 96, 99

O'Connor, Mary
right-to-die case, 247
Octreotide
digestive system cancers, 299
Oculinum, *see* Botulinum toxin
Ode to a Nightingale, 165
Odors
yeast infection, 189
**Office of National Drug Control
Policy, U.S.,** 268
Ohio
toxic wastes, 273
Oils
labeling, 307
saturated fat, 306–307
Older population, *see* Aging and
the aged
Oleic acid
cholesterol, 306
Olive oil
cholesterol, 306, 307
Oncogenes, *see* Genetics
O'Neill, Eugene
alcohol abuse, *163,* 165
1,25 dihydroxy vitamin D3
psoriasis, 321
Only children
delayed childbearing, 146
Ontario
abortion, 286
healthcare costs, 288
Open-heart surgery, *see* Coronary
artery bypass surgery; Heart
valves
Opium
literary figures, 165
Opticrom, *see* Cromolyn sodium
Oral cancer
prevention and research, 256
risk factors, 229
Oral challenge
food allergy testing, 99, 103,
314
Oral contraceptives
breast cancer, 310, *311*
folic-acid deficiency, 183
heart attacks, 293
stroke, 251–252
Oral surgery, *see* Dental surgery
Oregon
smoking policies, 323
Organ transplants, *see*
Transplantation of organs and
tissues
Orthopedics, 249–251
Orton, Samuel
dyslexia, 215
Osteoarthritis
medications and drugs, 302
Osteomyelitis
Henry VIII, 161
Osteoporosis
dancing to prevent, 89–90
exercise to prevent, 242
Ovaries
cancer, 151, 229
infertility, 150–151
Overeaters Anonymous
aerobic dance, 92
Over-the-counter medications
allergies, 100
medicine cabinet supplies, 218–
220
Overweight, *see* Obesity; Weight
Oxygen
electroconvulsive therapy, 198
hemoglobin, 181, 182, 183
Ozone
layer, depletion effects, 8
pollution, 270, 272, 273

P

PABA (para-aminobenzoic acid)
sunscreens, 10
Pacemaker
heat-sensitive, 296–297

Pacific rockfish (red snapper)
intestinal infections, 264
Pacific salmon
intestinal infections, 264
Pacifier
infant colic, 185
Pain
aspirin, 47–49
electroconvulsive therapy, 198
hemorrhoids, 202, 203
infant colic, 184–185
medications, 218
sickle-cell anemia, 182
urination and yeast infection,
189
Paint
lead content, 274
Palermo, Claire
Lyme disease, 77
Palmer, Earl A.
retinopathy of prematurity, 275
Palmitic acid
cholesterol, 306, 307
Palm oil
saturated fat, 307
Pancreas
cancer drug, 299
cancer risk factors, 229
transplants, 261
Pancreatitis
cancer risk, 229
historical figures, 158
Pantex (Amarillo, Texas)
toxic wastes, 273
Pap test
cancer screening, 226–227,
229, 256
contraceptive use
contraindication, 278, 279
ParaGard Copper T 380A
IUD, 277–278
Paralysis
cocaine and spinal cord stroke,
254
stroke, 251
surgical treatment, 250
Paranoia
methamphetamine, 255
Paraplegia
surgical treatment, 250
Parasitic diseases
garbled DNA, 282
raw fish, 264–265
vulval itching, 189
Parents
adolescent abortion consent,
249
aging, care of, 58–69, 148, 149
child abuse and neglect, 191–
193
childhood obesity, 125–126
delayed childbearing, 144–149
dyslexic child, 216–217
infant colic, 185
premature infants, 172–173,
174
sibling rivalry, 16–23
see also Mothers
Parents Anonymous, 193
Parethesia
dental implants, 214
Parkinson's disease
adrenal medulla implants, 255
electroconvulsive therapy, 197
fetal tissue transplants, 255
medications and drugs, 301
substantia nigra, 304
Parnate, *see* Tranylcypromine
Passive smoking, *see* Secondhand
smoke
Patch test
allergies, 99
Patents
aspirin, 48
Patient consent, *see* Consent
documents
Patterson, John H.
employee fitness-wellness
program, 112

PCBs, *see* Polychlorinated biphenyls
PCP, *see* Pneumocystis carinii pneumonia
PDQ (Physician Data Query)
  cancer research database, 257
Peanuts
  allergies, 103, 314
Pediatrics, 312–315
  see also Adolescents; Children; Infants; Newborn infants
Pelvic inflammatory disease (PID)
  infertility, 150
  ParaGard IUD, 277
Pelvis
  fracture treatment, 250
  sonography, 311
Penicillin
  gonorrhea, 319–320
  Lyme disease, 73, 78
  rheumatic fever, 212
Penincillinase-producing *Neisseria gonorrhoeae*
  antibiotic-resistant gonorrhea, 319–320
Penis
  circumcision benefits, 244, 315
  condoms, 319
  erection physiology, 234
  see also Impotence
Pentamidine
  AIDS-related pneumonia, 244–245, 298
Pentam 300, *see* Pentamidine
Peptic ulcers
  nizatidine, 302
Peptides
  electroconvulsive therapy, 198
Peptol, *see* Cimetidine
Percutaneous transluminal coronary angioplasty, *see* Balloon angioplasty
Perfume
  photosensitive reaction, 7
Periodontal disease
  bone loss, 326
  guided tissue regeneration, 326
Perlmutter, Abe
  right-to-die case, 207–208
Permethrin
  Lyme disease, 79
Persantine, *see* Dipyridamole
Personality
  Alzheimer's disease and changes in, 240
  drug abuse and changes in, 254
  dyslexia, 216
  genetics, 303
  hypomania, 133, 134
  Type A/Type B, 134, 289
  see also Behavior; Emotions; Self-esteem
Personality disorders, *see* Mental health
Personnel, health, *see* Health personnel
Pertofrane, *see* Desipramine
Pertussis, *see* Whooping cough
Pesticides and herbicides
  Lyme disease, 79
PET, *see* Positron emission tomography
Peterson, David
  Ontario healthcare costs, 288
Petroleum jelly
  diaper rash, 218
Pets, *see* Animals
Peyronie's disease
  impotence, 234
P-glycoprotein
  chemotherapy resistance, 257
Pharmaceuticals, *see* Medications and drugs
Phenelzine
  depression, 138
Phenylketonuria (PKU)
  diet, 283
Philip Morris Co.
  cigarette advertising, 323

Philippines
  tropical oils, 307
Photoaging
  tretinoin, 237–238
  ultraviolet light, 6, 14
Photosensitive reactions
  medications and drugs, 7
Phototherapy
  newborn infant jaundice, 170
Physical examination
  allergy diagnosis, 98
  cancer, early detection, 227–229
  dyslexia, 216
  exercise program for elderly, 242
Physical fitness
  dance, 80–93
  delayed first pregnancy, 155
  elderly, 242
  employee fitness-wellness programs, 104–117
  see also Exercise; Nutrition and diet
Physically disabled persons, *see* Handicapped persons
Physician Data Query, *see* PDQ
Physicians
  antismoking, 259
  Canadian government policies, 288–289
  cancer research database, 257
  malpractice, 204–206
  obstetrician shortage, 204–205
  see also Physical examination; specialty of practice
Physicians' Health Study Research Group
  aspirin study, 52–53, 54
PID, *see* Pelvic inflammatory disease
Pima Indians
  metabolism/obesity study, 124
Pituitary gland
  electroconvulsive therapy, 198
  impotence, 234
  infertility, 150
PKC, *see* Protein kinase C
PKU, *see* Phenylketonuria
Placebo
  food allergy testing, 99
Placenta
  childbirth complications, 151, 153
Platelets, blood
  aspirin, 54
Plutonium
  nuclear plant leaks, 273
Pneumocystis carinii pneumonia
  children with AIDS, 200
  experimental drugs, 244–245, 298
Pneumonia
  AIDS-related, 200, 244–245, 298
  chicken pox complication, 231
  Q fever, 329
  skeletal trauma, 249
  trimetrexate, 180
  vaccine, 298
  see also Lymphoid interstitial pneumonia
Poisoning
  anemia, 182
  aspirin, 57
  famous persons, 163
  food, 102, 103, 232–233
  lead, 274, 316–317
  medicine cabinet antidotes, 219–220
Pollen
  allergies, 96, 97, 99
Polychlorinated biphenyls (PCBs)
  nuclear power wastes, 273
Polycystic ovarian disease
  infertility, 150
Polyps
  colorectal, 263–264

Population Council of New York
  ParaGard IUD, 277–278
Porcine somatotropin (PST)
  genetic engineering, 39–40
Pork, 37, 38, 39, 42
Porphyria
  George III, 158–159
Positron emission tomography
  schizophrenia, 304
Postal Service, U.S.
  home HIV antibody tests, 245
Postpartum depression
  Kempe, Margery, 165
Posttraumatic stress disorder
  dissociation, 305–306
Potassium
  hypertension drugs, 300
Pottery, *see* Ceramics
Poultry, 37, 38
Power of attorney
  living will, 208, 209
Power plants
  greenhouse effect, 271–272
  see also Nuclear power
Prednisone
  anemia, 182
  asthma, 313
Preeclampsia
  hypertension, 54, 152–153
Pregnancy
  alcoholic beverages, 309, 318
  aspirin, 48, 49, 56
  chicken pox, 230–231
  delayed first, 144–155
  ectopic, 278, 311, 312
  electroconvulsive therapy, 197
  fifth disease, 317
  hemorrhoids, 202
  HIV infection, 200, 201
  Lyme disease, 78
  malpractice fears, 204–206
  phenylketonuria, 283
  preeclampsia, 54
  prematurity, 168–169
  prenatal tests, 152, 282, 310–311
  prostaglandins, 48–49
  video display terminals, 316
  yeast infections, 189, 190
  see also Abortion; Birth defects; Childbirth; Fetus; In vitro fertilization; Miscarriage
Premature aging, *see* Photoaging
Prematurity, 166–174
  retinopathy of prematurity, 275–276
Prenatal tests
  delayed pregnancy, 152
  Down's syndrome, 282
  sonography, 310–311
Presidential Commission on the Human Immunodeficiency Virus Epidemic
  antidiscrimination law, 285
Prevention Leadership Forum
  worksite fitness-wellness activity, 105–106
Preventive medicine
  cancer early detection, 226–229
  dance, 80–93
  fluoridation, 194–196
  safety in sun, 4–15
  worksite fitness-wellness programs, 104–117
  see also Nutrition and diet
Priapism
  impotence, 234
Prick test
  allergies, 98–99, 103
Prinivil, *see* Lisinopril
Prizes, *see* Awards
Proctosigmoidoscopy
  cancer screening, 228, 229, 264
Progestasert
  hormone-releasing IUD, 277–278
Progesterone, *see* Progestin
Progestin
  oral contraceptives, 310

ProHIBiT, *see* Haemophilus b conjugate vaccine
Propylthiouracil
  alcoholic hepatitis, 294
Prosorba Immunoadsorption Treatment Column
  idiopathic thrombocytopenic purpura, 295–296
Prostacyclin
  aspirin, 54
Prostaglandins
  aspirin, 48–49, 54, 56
Prostate cancer
  early detection, 228
  risk factors, 229
Prostheses
  penile, 235
Prostitution
  drug abuse and sexually transmitted diseases, 320, 328
Protein
  dietary requirement, 36–37
  hemoglobin, 181, 183
  infant colic, 184, 185
  liquid diet, 307–308
  64K autoantibody, 261
Protein kinase C (PKC)
  cancer cell development, 260
Provocation and neutralization test
  allergies, 99
Prozac, *see* Fluoxetine
Pseudogenes
  garbled DNA, 282
Pseudoterranova decipiens
  intestinal infections, 264–265
Psoralen
  skin cancer, 15
Psoriasis
  retinoids, 237, 238
  sunlight, 9
  vitamin D, 320–321
Psychology and psychiatry, *see* Behavior; Mental health; Psychotherapy
Psychoneuroimmunology
  mind and immune system, 304–305
Psychosis
  drugs, 138, 255
  electroconvulsive therapy, 197–198
  mania, 134
  see also Schizophrenia
Psychotherapy
  abusive parents, 193
  cocaine addiction, 266
  dance, 92
  families of children with AIDS, 201
  impotence, 235
Psychotic mania, 134
Public health, 315–318
  AIDS, 242–246, 265–266, 285–286, 327–328
  children with AIDS, 199, 201
  dental hygiene, 325
  sexually transmitted diseases, 319–320
Public Health Service, U.S.
  AIDS, 285–286
  aspirin and Reye's syndrome, 57
  fluoridation, 195, 196
  lead effects on children, 274, 275
Pueblo Indians
  asbestos and malignant mesothelioma, 317
Pulmonary disease, *see* Lungs; Pneumonia; Tuberculosis
Pulmonary lymphoid hyperplasia, *see* Lymphoid interstitial pneumonia
Pyrogens
  body temperature, 49
Pyruvate kinase
  anemia, 182

343

Q

Quadriplegia
  surgical treatment, 250
Quilts and quiltmaking
  AIDS memorial, *243*
Quinlan, Karen Ann
  right-to-die case, 207

R

Race walking, 290
Radiation
  anemia, 183
  immune system, effect on, 6–7
  leukemia risk, 229
  nuclear wastes, 273
  radon, 256, 316
  video display terminals, 316
Radiation therapy
  head and neck cancer, 266
Radioallergosorbent test, *see* RAST
Radon
  house testing, 316, *317*
  lung cancer, 256, 316
Ragweed, 96, 99
Railroads
  drug testing, 267
  see also Commuter railroads
Ranitidine
  allergies, 100
Rape
  posttraumatic stress disorder, 305
Rash
  allergies, 97, 102
  chicken pox, 230–231
  eczema, 314
  fifth disease, 317
  Lyme disease, 72, 73, 76
  roseola, 313
  see also Hives
RAST (radioallergosorbent test)
  allergies, 99
Rb gene
  retinoblastoma, 280
RDA, *see* Recommended Daily
  Dietary Allowances
Reagan, Ronald
  abortion, 286
  AIDS, 246, 285
  bioethics, 246
  Medicare Catastrophic Coverage
  Act, 283
Recombinant DNA technology,
  see Genetic engineering
Recommended Daily Dietary
  Allowances
  cancer prevention, 256
  fat, 177
  meat, 36
Rectum
  cancer screening, 227, 228
  colorectal cancer, 259–260,
  263–264, 281–282
  hemorrhoids, 202–203
Red blood cells (erythrocytes)
  anemia, 181–183
Rehabilitation Act of 1973, 217
Relapse prevention, *see* Behavioral
  therapies
Respirator
  anencephalic infant's organ
  transplants, 248
  premature babies, 167–168, 169
  right-to-die cases, 207–208
Respiratory distress syndrome
  (RDS)
  premature infants, 169
Respiratory system
  allergies, 94, 96, 97, 99–100,
  314
  children with AIDS, 200

  medications and drugs, 298
  premature infants, 169, 174
  see also Lung cancer
Restaurants
  salad bars, 232–233
  smoking restrictions, 322
Retardation, mental, *see* Mental
  retardation
Retina
  AIDS-related infection, 245, 298
  premature babies, 171
Retin-A, *see* Tretinoin
Retinoblastoma
  genetics, 259, 280
Retinoids, 236–238
  skin cancer prevention, 256
  see also Tretinoin
Retinopathy of prematurity, 171
  freezing technique, 275–276
Retirement communities, *see*
  Continuing care community
Retrovir, *see* Azidothymidine
Reye's syndrome
  aspirin link, 57, 218, 231
  chicken pox complication, 231
Reynolds, Debbie
  aerobic dance videos, 82
Rheumatic fever, 210–212
Rheumatoid arthritis
  allergies, 103
  aspirin, 50
  Lyme disease, 72, 77
  medications and drugs, 302
  Sjogren's syndrome, 221, 222
Rift Valley fever
  Senegal-Mauritania outbreak,
  329
Right-to-die laws, 207–209, 247
Rimbaud, Arthur
  absinthe hallucinations, 164–
  165
Ringworm
  naftifine, 299
Rivalry, *see* Sibling rivalry
RJR Nabisco
  cigarette advertising, 322
Robins, A. H., Company
  Dalkon Shield, 277
Rocking
  infant colic, 185
Rocky Flats nuclear power plant
  (Boulder, Colo.)
  toxic wastes, 273
Roferon, *see* Alpha-interferon
Rogaine, *see* Minoxidil
Rolled oats, *see* Oat bran
Romania
  heart disease, 328
ROP, *see* Retinopathy of
  prematurity
Rosacea
  metronidazole, 299
Rosenbaum, Jean
  aerobic dance, 92
Roseola
  herpesvirus-6, 313
Rossini, Gioacchino
  gonorrhea, 158
Rostenkowski, Dan
  Medicare Catastrophic Coverage
  Act, 284
Rotator cuff tear
  magnetic resonance imaging,
  250–251
Roughage, *see* Fiber, dietary
Roundworms
  raw fish, 264–265
Rousseau, Jean-Jacques
  gonorrhea, 158
Rowasa, *see* Mesalamine
Rubber band ligation
  hemorrhoids, 203
Rubella
  maternal, prematurity due to,
  168
RU 486
  abortion drug, *278, 279*
Russia, *see* Union of Soviet
  Socialist Republics
Rynacrom, *see* Cromolyn sodium

S

Saatchi & Saatchi DFS Compton
  tobacco advertising, 322
Safety
  aspirin use, 47
  children's car safety seats, 314
  eye injuries, 276–277
  liquid protein diet, 308
  medicine cabinet, 218–220
  salad bar, 232–233
  seat belts, 107, 111
  sun, 4–15
Safe Drinking Water Act
  lead solder, 274
St. Catherine of Siena
  anorexia nervosa, *164,* 165
St. Vitus' dance, *see* Chorea
Salad bar, 232–233
Salicin
  pain relief, 48
Salicylate
  arthritis, 50
Salicylic acid
  aspirin, 47–48
Salieri, Antonio
  Mozart, Wolfgang Amadeus,
  162
Saliva
  AIDS, 326–327
  Sjogren's syndrome, 221–223
  see also Dry mouth
Salmonella **bacteria**
  eggs, 264
  food poisoning, 102, 233
Salofalk, *see* Mesalamine
Salt, *see* Sodium
Sandostatin, *see* Octreotide
Sashimi
  intestinal infections, 264–265
Saskatchewan
  abortion, 287
Saturated fat
  affluence-linked diseases, 329
  cholesterol levels, 36
  oils, labeling of, 307
  pork, 39
  recommended percentage in
  diet, 306, 318
  stearic acid, 306–307
Sausage
  dietary fat, 45
Savannah River nuclear plant
  (S.C.)
  toxic wastes, 273
Scars
  gelatin matrix implant, 321
Schizophrenia
  electroconvulsive therapy, 197–
  198
  genetics, 303
  imaging, 304
  manic-depression, differentiated,
  133
  speed-induced paranoia, 254–
  255
School Daze (movie), 84
Schubert, Franz
  syphilis, 162
Schulman, Lawrence E.
  osteoporosis and exercise, 89–
  90
Schumann, Robert
  manic-depression, 162
Scleroderma
  Sjogren's syndrome, 221
Sclerotherapy
  hemorrhoids, 203
Scratch test
  allergies, 98, 103
Seafood, *see* Fish
Sealants
  tooth decay prevention, 325
Searle, G. D., Company
  free medications for indigent
  patients, *300*

Seat belts
  children, 314
  employee fitness-wellness
  programs, 107, 111
Seattle
  emergency heart attack
  treatment, 291
Secondhand smoke
  Canadian government policies
  and programs, 287, 322
  U.S. government policies and
  programs, 322, 323
Seizures
  cocaine, 254
  electroconvulsive therapy, 197–
  198
  fluoxetine, 301
  manic-depression symptoms,
  141
  meningitis, 312
Seldane, *see* Terfenadine
Selegiline
  Parkinson's disease, 301–302
Self-esteem
  abusive parents, 192
  dance, 82, 91, 92, 93
  dyslexia, 215, 216, 217
  exercise, 242
  overweight children, 118, 129
  toilet training, 224
Self-help groups
  child abuse and neglect, 193
  cocaine addiction, 267
  employee fitness-wellness
  programs, 114–115
  Sjogren's syndrome, 223
  weight loss, 92
Senegal
  Rift Valley fever, 329
Senility, *see* Alzheimer's disease
Serotonin
  depression, 142
Sex crimes
  abused children, 191
  HIV transmission, 201
  rape victims' dissociation, 305
Sex differences, *see* Gender
Sexual abuse, *see* Sex crimes
Sexual dysfunction, *see* Impotence
Sexuality
  AIDS transmission, 243–244,
  265, 328
  impotence, 234–235
  see also Intercourse
Sexually transmitted diseases,
  319–321
  genital warts, 298
  historical figures, 158, 161–162
  HIV transmission, 244
  infertility, 150
  IUDs, 278
  premature infants, 170
  see also AIDS
Shapiro, Bruce, *135*
Shapiro, Sam
  cancer research award, 259,
  260
Shepherd, Cybill
  beef advertising, 39
Shingles
  chicken pox, 230
Shinsplints
  low-impact aerobics, 82
Shock
  cocaine, 254
Shock treatment, *see*
  Electroconvulsive therapy
Shoulder
  problems, diagnosing, 250–251
Sibling rivalry, 16–23
  toilet training regression, 225
Sickle-cell anemia
  bone marrow transplants, 314
  hemoglobin abnormality, 182
Side effects of therapeutic agents
  AIDS medications, 201, 244
  allergies, 96
  anemia, 182, 183
  antibiotics, 189

antidepressant drugs, 138, 141–142, 301
antihistamines, 100
artificial heart, 294
aspirin, 56–57
bronchodilators, 101
chemotherapy, 183
cyclosporine, 261
decongestants, 100
electroconvulsive therapy, 143, 198
FDA drug approval, 180
genetics as basis for, 281–282
head and neck tumor surgery, 266
hypertension drugs, 300
impotence, 234
insulin nasal sprays, 262
interferon, 299
L-dopa, 302
mood stabilizing drugs, 138, 141–142
oral contraceptives, 251–252
painkillers, 218
ParaGard IUD, 277–278
penile prostheses, 235
retinoids, 236, 237–238
Spectraprobe-PLR, 297
steroids, 141, 189, 313
yeast infection medications, 189–190
SIDS, *see* Sudden infant death syndrome
Sigmoidoscopy
hemorrhoids, 202
Silent ischemia, 291–292
Silver jewelry
malignant mesothelioma, 317
Sinequan, *see* Doxepin
Single parenthood
adolescent abortion consent, 249
child abuse and neglect, 192–193
Sitz baths
hemorrhoids, 202
64K autoantibody
diabetes, 261
Sjogren's syndrome, 221–223
Sjogren's Syndrome Foundation, 223
Skeletal trauma
treatment, 249–250
Skin, 320–321
allergic reactions, 97–102
disease and global warming, 272
eczema, 314
impetigo, 298
infection from chicken pox, 231
irritation relief, 218–219
medications and drugs, 299
retinoids, 180, 236–238, 256
Sjogren's syndrome, 221–222
sun's effects, 4–15
yeast infection, 189
Skin cancer
early detection, 228, 229
retinoids, 237, 238, 256
risk factors, 229
ultraviolet light, 6–9, 13, 15
Sleep
cocaine, 254
Sleep apnea, *see* Apnea
SleepTight
infant colic, 185
SmithKline & French Laboratories
employee fitness-wellness program, 114
Smog
pollution, 272
Smokeless tobacco
cancer, 256
Smoking, 322–325
addictive behavior, 256
Africa and Asia, 329
atherosclerosis and impotence, 234, 235
Canadian policies, 287–288, 322, 323

cancer risk, 229, *259*, 293
employee fitness-wellness programs, 106, 107, 109, 111–113
maternal, prematurity due to, 168
Nigerian advertising ban, 329
oral contraceptives, 252, 293
stroke, 251, 252
Sn-protoporphyrin
newborn infant jaundice, 170
Soap, *see* Toiletries
Socioeconomic conditions
affluence-related diseases, 328–329
child abuse and neglect, 192
children with AIDS, 200–201
delayed childbearing, 145, 155
obesity, 125
premature babies, 168
rheumatic fever, 210
Sodium
recommended intake, 306, 309, 318
Softball
base-sliding injuries, 318
Sokolof, Philip
saturated fats, *307*
Soluble fiber
cholesterol lowering, 176–177
Sonography (ultrasound)
delayed pregnancy, 152
obstetrics and gynecology, 310–311
premature infants, 170
Sorenson, Jackie
aerobic dance videos, 82
Soviet Union, *see* Union of Soviet Socialist Republics
Soy products
allergies, 103
Spectraprobe-PLR Catheter
blocked blood vessels, 297
Speech
computer aid, 31
hearing aid, perception with, 265, 266
impairment from cancer surgery, 266
stroke, 251
Speed
nervous system effects, 254
Sperm
infertility, 96, 151
Spermicides
cervical cap, 278
condoms, 319
SPF (Sun Protection Factor), 6, 10–11
Spine
back problems, 106, 111
cocaine and stroke, 254
imaging, 250–251
injury treatment, 250
osteoporosis prevention, 89–90
Spirochetes
Lyme disease, 73, 76
Spleen
anemia, removal for, 182
autoimmune diseases, removal for, 295
human tissue ownership, 247
Spontaneous abortion, *see* Miscarriage
Sports
handicapped persons, 32–33
softball base-sliding injuries, 318
see also Exercise; Physical fitness
Sprains
ice, 220
Squamous cell carcinoma, 9
Square dancing, 88, 90
Squint, *see* Strabismus
Staphylococcus aureus
food poisoning, 233
Stearic acid
cholesterol, 306–307
Steelcase, Inc.
employee fitness-wellness program, 112, 116

Steere, Allen C.
Lyme disease, 72
Steinbeck, John
alcohol abuse, 165
Steinberg, Joel
child abuse, 191, 192
Steinberg, Lisa (Elizabeth)
child abuse, 191, 192
Stelazine, *see* Trifluoperazine
Stem cells
anemia, 183
Sterility, *see* Infertility
Sterilization (birth control method)
laparoscopy, 312
Sterling Drug Inc.
aspirin, 48
Steroids
alcoholic hepatitis, 294
asthma, 313
idiopathic thrombocytopenic purpura, 295
manic-depression symptoms, 141
meningitis, 312
yeast infection, 189
StieVAA, *see* Tretinoin
Stillbirth, *see* Pregnancy
Stomach
aspirin intolerance, 56–57
infant colic, 184–185
Stomach cancer
Napoleon Bonaparte, 163
Stools
blood in, 170–171, 202, 227, 228, 256, 264
hemorrhoids, 202–203
laxatives, 219
toilet training, 225
see also Diarrhea
Strabismus
botulinum toxin, 276
Strax, Philip
cancer research award, *259*, 260
Streptase, *see* Streptokinase
Strep throat
rheumatic fever, 210–212
Streptococcus bacteria
Mozart's infections, 162
premature infants, 170
rheumatic fever, 210–211, 212
Streptokinase
aspirin and heart attack, 54, 291
Stress, emotional
allergies, 103
child abuse and neglect, 192–193
exercise, 242
hospital visitors, 186, 188
immune system, 304–305
impotence, 234
older women's infertility, 150
parental, infant colic causing, 185
parents of premature infants, 172–173, 174
posttraumatic stress disorder, 305–306
silent ischemia, 292
toilet training, 224, 225
Strokes
aspirin, 52–53
cocaine, 254
famous composers, 162
nutrition and diet, 306
prevention and treatment, 251–253
Subacute lupus erythematosus
anemia, 182
Submandibular-sublingual glands
inhibition of AIDS virus, 327
Substance abuse, *see* Alcoholism; Drug abuse
Substantia nigra
depression, 304
Parkinson's disease, 304
Sudden infant death syndrome
premature infants, 174
Suffolk County (N.Y.)
video display terminals law, 316

Sugar
childhood obesity, 127
tooth decay, 194, 223
U.S. surgeon general's recommendations, 309
see also Blood sugar; Glucose
Sugar substitutes, *see* Sweeteners, artificial
Suicide
depression, 134–135, 137, 143
Huntington's disease, 282
Sulfa drugs
rheumatic fever, 212
Sulfur dioxide
air pollution, 273
Sunburn, 13
remedies, 219
Sunette, *see* Acesulfame potassium
Sunglasses, 12, 315
Sunlight
health and safety, 4–15, 315
skin cancer, 7–9, 229
tretinoin, 237, 238
Sun Protection Factor, *see* SPF
Sunscreens, 6, 10–13
Sunstroke, 13
Suppositories
hemorrhoids, 202–203
yeast infections, 189–190
Supreme Court, Canada
abortion, 286
Supreme Court, U.S.
adolescent abortion consent, 249
random drug testing, 267
Surgeon general, U.S.
abortion, 286
nutrition, 286, 306, 309, 318
radon, 316
smoking, 322
Surgery
cancer, 256
carotid endarterectomy, 252
Cesarean deliveries, 154–155
cochlear implants, 265–266
dental, 213–214
elderly patients, 240
head and neck tumors, 266
hemorrhoids, 202, 203
impotence, 235
laparoscopy, 312
laser, 296, 297, 303
malignant melanoma, 9
orthopedic, 249–250
premature infants, 171, 172, 173, 174
spleen removal, 182
Sushi
intestinal infections, *263*, 264–265
Swallowing difficulty, *see* Dysphagia
Sweat glands
Sjogren's syndrome, 222
Sweeteners, artificial
acesulfame potassium (Sunette), 307
tooth decay prevention, 326
Syphilis
historical figures, 161–162
premature infants, 170
upswing, 320
Systemic anaphylaxis
allergies, 97–98
Systemic lupus erythematosus
Sjogren's syndrome, 221

T

Tagamet, *see* Cimetidine
Talal, Norman
Sjogren's syndrome, 222
Tamoxifen
breast cancer, 256, 257
Tanning machines
health effects, 6, 14–15, 315

Tanning products, 14–15
Tap dancing, 84–85, 89
Taylor, John
  Bach, Johann Sebastian, 162
T cells (T lymphocytes)
  AIDS drugs, 244–245
  children with AIDS, 199, 200
Tears
  infant colic, 184
  Sjogren's syndrome, 221–223
Technology
  aids for the handicapped, 24–33
  lean meat, 39–41
  see also Medical technology
Teenagers, *see* Adolescents
Teeth and gums, 325–327
  dental implants, 213–214
  fluoridation, 194–196
  Sjogren's syndrome, 222, 223
Tegison, *see* Etretinate
Tegretol, *see* Carbamazepine
Television viewing
  aerobic dance videotapes, 82, 88
  childhood obesity, 125, 128
Temperature
  food storage, 232
  global warming, 269–273
Temperature, body
  aspirin for fever, 49
  internal thermometer, 301
  pacemaker sensitivity, 296–297
  premature babies, 169
  sunstroke, 13
Tension-fatigue syndrome
  allergies, 103
Terazol, *see* Terconazole
Terazosin
  hypertension, 299–300
Terconazole
  yeast infections, 299
Terfenadine
  allergies, 100
Testicles
  varicose veins and infertility, 151
Testicular cancer
  early detection, 228
  risk factors, 229
Testosterone
  impotence, 234, 235
Tests, home, *see* Home medical tests
Test-tube babies, *see* In vitro fertilization
Tetracycline
  gonorrhea, 320
  Lyme disease, 78
  photosensitive reaction, 7
Thalassemia
  anemia, 183
Theater
  hearing aids, 265
Theophylline
  allergies and asthma, 10
Therapy, *see* Behavioral therapies; Psychotherapy
Thermometer
  internal, 301
Thigh
  bone fracture treatment, 249–250
Thioridazine
  psychosis, 138
Thompson, Francis
  opium use, 165
Throat, 265–266
  allergies, 97
  cough remedies, 219
  culture, 212
  epiglottitis, 298
  Sjogren's syndrome, 221, 222
  strep infection, 210–212
Thromboxane A$_2$
  aspirin and platelet aggregation, 54
Thymus gland
  aspirin, 50

disease symptoms and manic-depression confusion, 141
TIAs, *see* Transient ischemic attacks
Ticks
  Lyme disease, 71–79
Tissue plasminogen activator (TPA)
  heart attacks, 291
Tissues
  fetal, 246, 255, 261
  guided tissue regeneration, 326
  human, ownership issue, 247
  see also Transplantation of organs and tissues
Titanium
  dental implants, 213
T lymphocytes, *see* T cells
Tobacco, *see* Smoking
Tofranil, *see* Imipramine
Toiletries
  allergies, 99
  feminine hygiene sprays, 189
  moisturizers, 11, 13, 218, 223
  photosensitive reaction, 7
  sunscreens, 10–11, 12, 13
Toilet training, 224–225
Tooth, *see* Teeth and gums
Tooth decay
  diet to prevent, 309
  fluoride, 194–196, 325–326
  Sjogren's syndrome, 222, 223
Tooth extraction, *see* Dental surgery
Tooth fillings
  back teeth, 327
Tooth loss, *see* Dental implants
Toothpaste
  fluoride, 195, 196, 325
Toxemia
  delayed pregnancy, 153
Toxic reactions, *see* Allergies; Poisoning; Side effects of therapeutic agents
Toxic wastes
  greenhouse effect, 270–273
  nuclear plants, 273
TPA, *see* Tissue plasminogen activator
Trademarks, *see* Patents
Tranquilizers
  anxiety, 138
  photosensitive reaction, 7
  rheumatic fever, 211
Transfusions, *see* Blood transfusions
Transient ischemic attacks (TIAs)
  aspirin, 53
  stroke precursor, 252, 254
Transplantation of organs and tissues
  artificial heart, 293–294
  bioethics, 246, 247–249
  bone marrow, 183, 314
  cornea, 277
  cytomegalovirus immune globulin, 297–298
  fetal, 246, 255, 261
  genes, 257–258
  internal thermometer for heart, 301
  immune defense system, 256, 257–258
  liver, 294–295
  organ donations and brain death criteria, 207
  organ life extension, 248–249
  pancreas, 261
Tranylcypromine
  depression, 138
Trauma
  long-term effects, 305–306
  orthopedic surgical techniques, 249–250
Traveling and health
  smoking restrictions, 322, *323*
Treatment INDs (treatment investigational new drugs), *see* Experimental drugs

Trees and grasses
  allergies, 96, 99
Tretinoin
  photoaging, 237, 238, 321
  skin disorders, 236–238
  wrinkles, 321
Trichinosis
  food poisoning, 233
Trichomonas vaginalis
  itching, 189
Tricyclic antidepressants
  depression, 138
Trifluoperazine
  psychosis, 138
Trimetrexate
  AIDS-related pneumonia, 244
  FDA regulation, 180
Tubal ligation
  laparoscopy, 312
Tuberculosis
  historical figures, 159–160
Tumor-infiltrating lymphocytes
  genetic engineering, 257–258
Tumors
  eye, 259, 280
  genetic engineering, 257–258
  head and neck, 266
  manic-depression symptoms, 141
Turkey, *see* Poultry
TV, *see* Television viewing
Twelve Step programs
  cocaine addiction, 267
Twins
  delayed pregnancy incidence, 155
  manic-depression, 138–139
  obesity, 121
  prematurity, 168
  schizophrenia, 303
Tylenol, *see* Acetaminophen
Type A behavior
  heart attack survival, 289
  hypomania, 134
Type B behavior
  heart attack survival, 289
Type I diabetes, *see* Insulin-dependent diabetes mellitus
Type II diabetes, *see* Non-insulin-dependent diabetes mellitus
Typhoid fever
  vaccine, 318
Tyrosine hydroxylase
  manic-depression, 140

U

Ulcerative colitis
  mesalamine, 302
Ulcers, genital, *see* Genital ulcers
Ulcers, peptic, *see* Peptic ulcers
Ulcers, stomach
  aspirin hazards, 56
Ultrasound, *see* Sonography
Ultraviolet light
  cataracts, 315
  premature babies, 170
  safety, 4–15
Ultroid
  hemorrhoids, 203
Under the Eye of the Clock, 253
Union of Soviet Socialist Republics
  alcoholism, 329
  mysterious children's disease, 329
University of Arkansas
  eczema, 314
University of California (Berkeley)
  alcohol-cancer link, 282
  personality and heart attack survival, 289
University of California (Irvine)
  ozone pollution, 272

University of California (Los Angeles) Medical Center
  human tissue ownership issue, 247
University of California (San Diego)
  anti-oncogenes, 281
University of Michigan
  breakaway bases (softball), 318
University of Minnesota
  familial personality traits, 303
University of Ontario
  carotid surgery study, 252
University of Utah Medical Center
  genetics and colorectal cancer study, 260, 281
University of Western Ontario
  sex-linked differences study, 281
University of Wisconsin
  liver transplant, 295
Unstable angina, *see* Angina pectoris
Upjohn Company
  hormone contraceptive, 279
Urethra
  ejaculation, 234
  stricture, historical figures, 158
  yeast infections, 190
Urinary system
  circumcision and infections, 315
  gonorrhea and infections, 158
  maternal infection, prematurity due to, 168
  toilet training, 224–225
  yeast infections, 189, 190
  see also Bladder; Kidneys
Urine tests
  diabetes and kidney failure, 261
  drug abuse, 267
Ursodiol
  gallstones, 302
USDA, *see* Agriculture, U.S. Department of
USSR, *see* Union of Soviet Socialist Republics
Utah
  genetics and colorectal cancer study, 260, 281
  smoking policies, 325
Uterine cancer
  early detection, 226–228
  infertility, 150
  risk factors, 229
Uterus
  abnormalities, prematurity due to, 168
  blood supply and preeclampsia, 54, 153
  childbirth contractions, 49
  infertility, 150

V

Vaccination, *see* Immunization; Vaccines
Vaccines
  chicken pox, 230, 231
  children with AIDS, 200
  Hib bacteria, 298, 317
  measles, *313*, 315
  meningitis, 298, 317–318
  typhoid fever, 318
  whooping cough, 317
Vagina
  contraceptives, 278–279
  Sjogren's syndrome, 221, 222, 223
  sonography, 310–311
  tumors and diethylstibestrol, 180
  yeast infections, 189–190, 299
Valvuloplasty, balloon, *see* Balloon valvuloplasty
Vander Zalm, Bill
  abortion, 286

Vane, Sir John
  aspirin-prostaglandin link, 49, 51
Van Gogh, Vincent
  absinthe hallucinations, *162,* 163–164
Varicella-zoster virus
  chicken pox, 230–231
Varicose veins
  testicular and infertility, 151
VDTs, *see* Video display terminals
Veal, 37, 38, 42
Vegetables
  beta-carotene, 256
  cholesterol lowering, 176, 177
  recommended intake, 306
  salad bar, 233
Venereal diseases, *see* AIDS; Sexually transmitted diseases
Video display terminals
  occupational hazards, 315–316
Videotapes, *see* Television viewing
Virginia
  no-fault obstetrical insurance, 206
Viruses
  AIDS-related, 199–201, 242–246, 265–266, 327–328
  Alzheimer's disease, 241
  chicken pox, 230–231
  condoms, 319
  fifth disease, 317
  infection distinguished from strep infection, 212
  medications and drugs, 297–298, 321
  non-A, non-B hepatitis, 294
  Rift Valley fever, 329
  roseola, 313
Vision
  ultraviolet light, 7, 14–15, 315
Visual impairment
  AIDS-related, 245, 297–298
  children, 275–277
  dyslexia, 215–216
  eye injuries, 276–277
  glaucoma, 276, 303
  "living lens," 277
  reading aids, 30
  retinopathy of prematurity, 171, 275–276
  Sjogren's syndrome, 221–222
  stroke, 251, 252
  tanning products, 14, 15
Vitamin A
  cancer prevention, 256
  retinoids, 180, 236–238
  retinopathy of prematurity, 276
Vitamin A Acid, *see* Tretinoin

Vitamin B complex
  pernicious anemia, 183
  recommended requirement, 37
Vitamin D
  psoriasis, 320–321
  sunlight producing, 9
Vitamin E
  retinopathy of prematurity, 276
Vitamins
  childhood weight-loss dietary supplement, 129
  see also specific vitamin
Voltaren, *see* Diclofenac
Vulva, *see* Vagina
V-Z virus, *see* Varicella-zoster virus

W

Walking
  cardiovascular benefits, 290
  osteoporosis prevention, 242
Walleye
  botulinum toxin, 276
Warts
  genital, 298, 321
  skin cancer, 6, 9, 228
Wassenaar, Admiral de, 158
Waste Isolation Pilot Plant (Nev.)
  toxic wastes, 273
Waste materials
  greenhouse effect, 270–272
  nuclear plants, 273
Water
  fluoridation, 194–196
  greenhouse effect, 271–272
  lead content, 274, 316–317
  nuclear wastes, 273
  pollution, 271–273, 329
  sunlight effects, 11
Water fountains
  lead, 316–317
Watkins, James D.
  AIDS antidiscrimination law, 285
Waxman, Henry
  aspirin, 55
Weather
  heat wave and drought, 269–273
  sunstroke, 13
Weight
  children's diet, 129
  dancing, 82, 90–91
  diet pills, 254

  employee fitness-wellness programs, 111
  fat cells, 120–121
  liquid protein diet, 307–308
  U.S. surgeon general's recommendations, 309
  yo-yo syndrome, 309
  see also Obesity
Weight Watchers
  aerobic dance, 92
Wheelchairs, 26, 27, 29, 33
Wheezing
  asthma, 97, 313
  food allergies, 102
WHO, *see* World Health Organization
Whooping cough
  vaccine, 317
Will
  living, *208,* 209
Wilms' tumor
  genetics, 259
Winfrey, Oprah
  liquid protein diet, 307, *308*
Wisconsin Clinical Cancer Center
  breast cancer study, 256
Women
  AIDS, 200, 201, 244
  calcium and iron, 309
  cancer risk factors, 229
  cancer tests, 226–228, 229, 260, 284
  delayed childbearing, 144–155
  dental visit anxiety, 327
  depression, 133, 139
  heart attack factors, 292, 293
  recommended nutrients, 36–37
  Sjogren's syndrome, 222
  skills linked to hormone levels, 281
  syphilis, 320
  yeast infections, 189–190
  see also Abortion; Gender; Miscarriage; Mothers; Obstetrics and gynecology; Pregnancy
Workplace, *see* Employment
World health news, 327–329
  Stockholm meeting on AIDS, 243
World Health Organization
  AIDS, 327
Worldwatch Institute
  livestock report, 37
Worms
  raw fish, 264–265
Wound
  home care, 218, 220

Wrinkles
  gelatin matrix implant, 321
  photoaging, 6
  retinoids, 236, 237, 238, 321
Wrist
  trauma treatment, 250

X

Xanax, *see* Alprazolam
X chromosome
  manic-depression, 139
Xeroderma pigmentosum
  retinoids, 256
X rays
  mammography, 227, 229, 260, 284
  musculoskeletal dye tests, 250
  penile, 235
Xylitol
  tooth decay, 326

Y

Yale University
  Alzheimer's disease, 241
Yeast
  food contamination, 232
Yeast infections, 189–190
  antifungal agents, 299
Yogurt
  yeast infections, 190
Yo-yo syndrome
  weight loss/gain back, 309

Z

Zadai, Cynthia
  dance, 88
Zantac, *see* Ranitidine
Zebu, 40
Zestril, *see* Lisinopril
Zidovudine, *see* Azidothymidine
Zinc oxide
  sunscreens, 10, 12
Zovirax, *see* Acyclovir
Zyderm, *see* Bovine collagen
Zyplast, *see* Bovine collagen

Photo/Art Credits